Contemporary Management of Civilian Trauma

Editors

OSCAR D. GUILLAMONDEGUI
BRADLEY M. DENNIS

SURGICAL CLINICS
OF NORTH AMERICA

www.surgical.theclinics.com

Consulting Editor
RONALD F. MARTIN

October 2017 • Volume 97 • Number 5

ELSEVIER

1600 John F. Kennedy Boulevard • Suite 1800 • Philadelphia, Pennsylvania, 19103-2899

http://www.surgical.theclinics.com

SURGICAL CLINICS OF NORTH AMERICA Volume 97, Number 5
October 2017 ISSN 0039–6109, ISBN-13: 978-0-323-54690-4

Editor: John Vassallo, j.vassallo@elsevier.com

Developmental Editor: Colleen Dietzler

Surgical Clinics of North America (ISSN 0039–6109) is published bimonthly by Elsevier Inc., 360 Park Avenue South, New York, NY 10010-1710. Months of publication are February, April, June, August, October, and December. Business and Editorial Offices: 1600 John F. Kennedy Blvd., Suite 1800, Philadelphia, PA 19103-2899. Periodicals postage paid at New York, NY and additional mailing offices. Subscription prices are $386.00 per year for US individuals, $756.00 per year for US institutions, $100.00 per year for US students and residents, $469.00 per year for Canadian individuals, $958.00 per year for Canadian institutions, $525.00 for international individuals, $958.00 per year for international institutions and $250.00 per year for Canadian and foreign students/residents. To receive student/resident rate, orders must be accompanied by name of affiliated institution, date of term, and the *signature* of program/residency coordinator on institution letterhead. Orders will be billed at individual rate until proof of status is received. Foreign air speed delivery is included in all *Clinics* subscription prices. All prices are subject to change without notice. POSTMASTER: Send address changes to *Surgical Clinics*, Elsevier Health Sciences Division, Subscription Customer Service, 3251 Riverport Lane, Maryland Heights, MO 63043. **Customer Service (orders, claims, online, change of address): Telephone: 1-800-654-2452 (U.S. and Canada); 314-447-8871 (outside U.S. and Canada). Fax: 314-447-8029. E-mail: journalscustomerservice-usa@elsevier.com (for print support); journalsonline support-usa@elsevier.com (for online support).**

Reprints. For copies of 100 or more, of articles in this publication, please contact the Commercial Reprints Department, Elsevier Inc., 360 Park Avenue South, New York, New York 10010-1710. Tel. 212-633-3874, Fax: 212-633-3820, E-mail: reprints@elsevier.com.

The Surgical Clinics of North America is also published in Spanish by McGraw-Hill Interamericana Editores S.A., P.O. Box 5-237 06500 Mexico D.F. Mexico; and in Portuguese by Interlivros Edicoes Ltda., Rua Comandante Coelho 1085, CEP 21250, Rio de Janeiro, Brazil; and in Greek by Paschalidis Medical Publications, Athens Greece.

The Surgical Clinics of North America is covered in *MEDLINE/PubMed (Index Medicus), EMBASE/Excerpta Medica, Current Contents/Clinical Medicine, Current Contents/Life Sciences, Science Citation Index,* and *ISI/BIOMED.*

Contributors

CONSULTING EDITOR

RONALD F. MARTIN, MD, FACS
Colonel (ret.), United States Army Reserve, Department of Surgery, York Hospital, York, Maine, USA

EDITORS

OSCAR D. GUILLAMONDEGUI, MD, MPH, FACS
Professor of Surgery, Trauma Medical Director, Division of Trauma, Surgical Critical Care, Emergency General Surgery, Professor, Department of Surgery, Vanderbilt University Medical Center, Nashville, Tennessee, USA

BRADLEY M. DENNIS, MD, FACS
Assistant Professor of Surgery, Division of Trauma, Surgical Critical Care, Emergency General Surgery, Department of Surgery, Vanderbilt University Medical Center, Nashville, Tennessee, USA

AUTHORS

BRIAN BELDOWICZ, MD
Surgical Critical Care Fellow, UC Davis Health, Sacramento, California, USA; Uniformed Services University of Health Sciences, Bethesda, Maryland, USA

SETH A. BELLISTER, MD
Fellow, Division of Trauma, Surgical Critical Care, Emergency General Surgery, Department of Surgery, Vanderbilt University Medical Center, Nashville, Tennessee, USA

RICHARD D. BETZOLD, MD
Fellow, Division of Trauma, Surgical Critical Care, Emergency General Surgery, Department of Surgery, Vanderbilt University Medical Center, Nashville, Tennessee, USA

INDERMEET BHULLAR, MD, FACS
Director of Acute Care Surgery Fellowship, Director of Scholarly Activity, Orlando Regional Medical Center, Orlando, Florida, USA

STEVEN E. BROOKS, MD, FACS
Assistant Professor of Surgery, Trauma Medical Director, Medical Director, Geriatric Trauma Unit, Surgical Director, Pediatric Intensive Care Unit, Division of Trauma, Surgical Critical Care, Acute Care Surgery, Department of Surgery, John A. Griswold Trauma Center, Texas Tech University Health Sciences Center, Lubbock, Texas, USA

JOSHUA BROWN, MD, MSc
General Surgery Resident, UPMC Department of Surgery, University of Pittsburgh Medical Center, Pittsburgh, Pennsylvania, USA

PAUL M. CANTLE, MD, MBT, FRCSC
Trauma Fellow, McGovern Medical School, The University of Texas Health Science Center at Houston, Red Duke Trauma Institute, Memorial Hermann, Houston, Texas, USA

JEFFREY A. CLARIDGE, MD, MS, FACS
Professor of Surgery, Division of General Surgery, Trauma, Surgical Critical Care, Department of Surgery, MetroHealth Medical Center, Case Western Reserve University School of Medicine, Cleveland, Ohio, USA

JAMIE J. COLEMAN, MD
Assistant Professor, Department of Surgery, Indiana University School of Medicine, Indianapolis, Indiana, USA

BRYAN A. COTTON, MD, MPH, FACS
Professor of Surgery, McGovern Medical School, University of Texas Health Science Center at Houston, Red Duke Trauma Institute, Memorial Hermann, Houston, Texas, USA

MARIE L. CRANDALL, MD, MPH, FACS
Professor of Surgery, Division of Acute Care Surgery, Department of Surgery, Health Science Center Jacksonville, University of Florida, Jacksonville, Florida, USA

BRADLEY M. DENNIS, MD, FACS
Assistant Professor of Surgery, Division of Trauma, Surgical Critical Care, Emergency General Surgery, Department of Surgery, Vanderbilt University Medical Center, Nashville, Tennessee, USA

JOE DuBOSE, MD, FACS
Associate Professor of Surgery, Uniformed Services University of the Health Sciences, Bethesda, Maryland, USA; Associate Professor of Surgery–Volunteer, David Grant USAF Medical Center, Travis Air Force Base, Fairfield, California, USA; Divisions of Vascular Surgery and Trauma, Acute Care Surgery, and Surgical Critical Care, University of California, Davis, Davis, California, USA

MATTHEW J. ECKERT, MD, FACS
Department of Surgery, General Surgery, Madigan Army Medical Center, Tacoma, Washington, USA

DAFYDD EDWARDS, FRCS (Tr&Orth)
Centre for Blast Injury Studies, Imperial College London, London, United Kingdom; Royal Centre for Defence Medicine, Birmingham, United Kingdom

STEPHEN GONDEK, MD, MPH
Assistant Professor of Surgery, The Center for Trauma and Critical Care, The George Washington University, Washington, DC, USA

OSCAR D. GUILLAMONDEGUI, MD, MPH, FACS
Professor of Surgery, Trauma Medical Director, Division of Trauma, Surgical Critical Care, Emergency General Surgery, Professor, Department of Surgery, Vanderbilt University Medical Center, Nashville, Tennessee, USA

JOSEPH A. IBRAHIM, MD, FACS
Director of Acute Care Surgery Fellowship, Director of Scholarly Activity, Trauma Medical Director, Associate General Surgery Program Director, Orlando Health Physicians Surgical Group, Orlando Regional Medical Center, Orlando, Florida, USA

NIELS V. JOHNSEN, MD
Resident, Urological Surgery, Department of Urological Surgery, Vanderbilt University Medical Center, Nashville, Tennessee, USA

GREGORY J. JURKOVICH, MD
Vice Chair of Surgery, UC Davis Health, University of California, Davis, Sacramento, California, USA

PATRICK K. KIM, MD
Associate Professor of Clinical Surgery, Division of Traumatology, Surgical Critical Care, and Emergency Surgery, Department of Surgery, Perelman School of Medicine at the University of Pennsylvania, Penn Presbyterian Medical Center, Philadelphia, Pennsylvania, USA

MATTHEW J. MARTIN, MD, FACS
Department of Surgery, General Surgery, Madigan Army Medical Center, Tacoma, Washington, USA; Trauma and Emergency Surgery Service, Legacy Emanuel Medical Center, Portland, Oregon, USA

MAHER M. MATAR, MD, MHA, FRCSC
Assistant Professor of Surgery, The University of Ottawa Trauma and Acute Care Surgery, The Ottawa Hospital, Ottawa, ON, Canada

MAYUR B. PATEL, MD, MPH, FACS
Assistant Professor of Surgery, Neurosurgery, Hearing and Speech Sciences, Division of Trauma, Surgical Critical Care, and Emergency General Surgery, Department of Surgery, Section of Surgical Sciences, Center for Health Services Research, Vanderbilt Brain Institute, Vanderbilt University Medical Center, Surgical Services, Nashville Veterans Affairs Medical Center, Tennessee Valley Healthcare System, Nashville, Tennessee, USA

ALLAN B. PEETZ, MD
Assistant Professor of Surgery, Division of Trauma, Surgical Critical Care, Emergency General Surgery, Vanderbilt University Medical Center, Nashville, Tennessee, USA

DANIELLE A. PIGNERI, MD
Surgical Critical Care Fellow, UC Davis Health, University of California, Davis, Sacramento, California, USA

NITIN SAJANKILA, BS
Medical Student, Department of Surgery, MetroHealth Medical Center, Case Western Reserve University School of Medicine, Cleveland, Ohio, USA

JOSEPH V. SAKRAN, MD, MPH, MPA, FACS
Assistant Professor of Surgery Associate Chief, Division of Acute Care Surgery Director, Emergency General Surgery, Adult Trauma Services, Baltimore, MD, USA

BABAK SARANI, MD
Associate Professor of Surgery, The Center for Trauma and Critical Care, The George Washington University Hospital, Washington, DC, USA

MARY E. SCHROEDER, MD
Assistant Professor of Surgery, The Center for Trauma and Critical Care, The George Washington University Hospital, Washington, DC, USA

RICHARD SIDWELL, MD, FACS
Trauma Surgeon, The Iowa Clinic / Iowa Methodist Medical Center, Clinical Adjunct
Professor, Department of Surgery, University of Iowa Carver College of Medicine,
Iowa City, IA, USA

NICOLE A. STASSEN, MD, FACS, FCCM
Director, Surgical Critical Care Fellowship and Surgical Sub-Internship, Professor of
Surgery, University of Rochester, Director, Kessler Burn & Trauma Center, Intensive Care
Unit, University of Rochester Medical Center, Rochester, New York, USA

DANIEL J. STINNER, MD
Centre for Blast Injury Studies, Imperial College London, London, United Kingdom;
US Army Institute of Surgical Research, San Antonio, Texas, USA; Associate Professor,
Department of Surgery, Uniformed Services University of the Health Sciences, Bethesda,
Maryland, USA

PEDRO G.R. TEIXEIRA, MD
Associate Professor of Surgery, Department of Surgery and Perioperative Care,
Associate Trauma Director, University Medical Center Brackenridge, Dell Seton Medical
Center at the University of Texas, Austin, Texas, USA

MICHAEL A. VELLA, MD, MBA
Fellow, Divisions of Traumatology, Surgical Critical Care, Emergency General Surgery,
Department of Surgery, University of Pennsylvania, Philadelphia, Pennsylvania, USA;
Department of Surgery, Section of Surgical Sciences, Vanderbilt University Medical
Center, Nashville, Tennessee, USA

BEN L. ZARZAUR, MD, MPH
Associate Professor, Department of Surgery, Indiana University School of Medicine,
Indianapolis, Indiana, USA

Contents

Trauma is the leading cause of death among patients 46 years or younger, and having a system in place for the care of the injured is of paramount importance to the health of a community. The growth and development of civilian trauma systems has not been an easy process. The concept of regionalized health care that the trauma system models has been emulated by other specialized and time-sensitive areas of medicine, notably stroke and acute cardiac events. Continued process improvement, public education, support and involvement, a sound infrastructure, and integrated technology should remain the focus.

The organization of prehospital care for trauma patients began in the military arena. At the urging of multiple stakeholders and providers, these lessons were applied to the civilian setting and emergency medical services were created across the nation. Advances have taken place in the triage, transport, and management of severely injured patients. Many issues remain in the care of trauma patients in the prehospital environment. Collaboration between stakeholders and providers, regionalization of trauma care, and protocol-driven care may be solutions to some of these issues. Further research is necessary to dictate standard of care in this early phase after injury.

The golden hour of trauma represents a crucial period in the management of acute injury. In an efficient trauma resuscitation, the primary survey is viewed as more than simple ABCs with multiple processes running in parallel. Resuscitation efforts should be goal oriented with defined endpoints for airway management, access, and hemodynamic parameters. In tandem with resuscitation, early identification of life-threatening injuries is critical for determining the disposition of patients when they leave the trauma bay. Salvage strategies for profoundly hypotensive or pulseless patients include retrograde balloon occlusion of the aorta and resuscitative thoracotomy, with differing populations benefiting from each.

Over the past decade substantial knowledge has been gained in understanding both the coagulopathy of trauma and the complications associated with aggressive crystalloid-based resuscitation. Balanced resuscitation, which includes permissive hypotension, limiting crystalloid use, and the transfusion of blood products in ratios similar to whole blood, has changed the previous standard of care. Prompt initiation of massive transfusion and the protocolled use of 1:1:1 product ratios have improved the morbidity and mortality of patients with trauma in hemorrhagic shock. Balanced resuscitation minimizes the impact of trauma-induced coagulopathy, limits blood product waste, and reduces the complications that occur with aggressive crystalloid resuscitation.

Traumatic brain injury (TBI) is a leading cause of death and disability in patients with trauma. Management strategies must focus on preventing secondary injury by avoiding hypotension and hypoxia and maintaining appropriate cerebral perfusion pressure (CPP), which is a surrogate for cerebral blood flow. CPP can be maintained by increasing mean arterial pressure, decreasing intracranial pressure, or both. The goal should be euvolemia and avoidance of hypotension. Other factors that deserve important consideration in the acute management of patients with TBI are venous thromboembolism, stress ulcer, and seizure prophylaxis, as well as nutritional and metabolic optimization.

Injuries to the spinal column and spinal cord frequently occur after high-energy mechanisms of injury, or with lower-energy mechanisms, in select patient populations like the elderly. A focused yet complete neurologic examination during the initial evaluation will guide subsequent diagnostic procedures and early supportive measures to help prevent further injury. For patients with injury to bone and/or ligaments, the initial focus should be spinal immobilization and prevention of inducing injury to the spinal cord. Spinal cord injury is associated with numerous life-threatening complications during the acute and long-term phases of care that all acute care surgeons must recognize.

Management of chest trauma is integral to patient outcomes owing to the vital structures held within the thoracic cavity. Understanding traumatic chest injuries and appropriate management plays a pivotal role in the overall well-being of both blunt and penetrating trauma patients. Whether the injury includes rib fractures, associated pulmonary injuries, or tracheobronchial tree injuries, every facet of management may impact the short- and long-term outcomes, including mortality. This article elucidates the workup and management of the thoracic cage, pulmonary, and tracheo-bronchial injuries.

Seth A. Bellister, Bradley M. Dennis, and Oscar D. Guillamondegui

Patients with traumatic cardiac injuries can present with wide variability in their severity of illness. The most severe will present in cardiac arrest, whereas the most benign may be altogether asymptomatic; most will fall somewhere in between. Management of cardiac injuries largely depends on mechanism of injury and patient physiology. Understanding the spectrum of injuries and their associated manifestations can help providers react more quickly and initiate potentially life-saving therapies more efficiently when time is critical. This article discusses the workup and management of both blunt and penetrating cardiac injuries.

Niels V. Johnsen, Richard D. Betzold, Oscar D. Guillamondegui,
Bradley M. Dennis, Nicole A. Stassen, Indermeet Bhullar, and
Joseph A. Ibrahim

Surgery used to be the treatment of choice in patients with solid organ injuries. This has changed over the past 2 decades secondary to advances in noninvasive diagnostic techniques, increased availability of less invasive procedures, and a better understanding of the natural history of solid organ injuries. Now, nonoperative management (NOM) has become the initial management strategy used for most solid organ injuries. Even though NOM has become the standard of care in patients with solid organ injuries in most trauma centers, surgeons should not hesitate to operate on a patient to control life-threatening hemorrhage.

Jamie J. Coleman and Ben L. Zarzaur

Hollow viscus injury is common with penetrating trauma to the torso and infrequent with a blunt traumatic mechanism of injury. The diagnosis in hemodynamically unstable patients is often made in the operating room. In hemodynamically stable patients, the diagnosis can be difficult due to additional injuries. Although computed tomography remains the diagnostic tool of choice in hemodynamically stable patients, it has lower reported sensitivity and specificity with hollow viscus injury. However, even short delays in diagnosis increase morbidity and mortality significantly. Operative management of stomach, duodenal, small bowel, and colon injuries is reviewed.

Daniel J. Stinner and Dafydd Edwards

Musculoskeletal injuries cause a significant burden to society and can have a considerable impact on patient morbidity and mortality. It was initially thought that these patients were too sick to undergo surgery and later believed that they were too sick not to undergo surgery. The pendulum has subsequently swung back and forth between damage control orthopedics and early total care for polytrauma patients with extremity injuries and has settled on providing early appropriate care (EAC). The decision-making process in providing EAC is reviewed in an effort to optimize patient outcomes following severe extremity trauma.

Vascular injuries remain among the most challenging entities encountered in trauma care. Improvements in diagnostic capabilities, resuscitation approaches, vascular techniques, and prosthetic device options have afforded considerable advancement in the care of these patients. This evolution in care capabilities continues. Despite advances, uncontrolled hemorrhage due to major vascular injury remains one of the most common causes of death after trauma. Successful management of vascular injury requires the timely diagnosis and control of bleeding sources. To facilitate this task, trauma providers must appreciate the capabilities and limitations of diagnostic imaging modalities and understand when and how to effectively apply these strategies.

The doubling of the geriatric population over the next 20 years will challenge the existing health care system. Optimal care of geriatric trauma patients will be of paramount importance to the health care discussion in America. These patients warrant special consideration because of altered anatomy, physiology, and the resultant decreased ability to tolerate the stresses imposed by traumatic insult. Despite increased risk for worsened outcomes, nearly half of all geriatric trauma patients will be cared for at nondesignated trauma centers. Effective communication is crucial in determining goals of care and arriving at what patients would consider a meaningful outcome.

Conventional radiography (plain film), ultrasonography, and computed tomography (CT) are important modalities for the evaluation of patients with trauma. In meta-stable or unstable patients, the combination of chest radiograph, pelvis radiograph, and focused assessment for sonography in trauma (FAST) or extended FAST rapidly triages the torso. CT has become a standard for definitive imaging in blunt trauma. CT angiography is the modality of choice for suspected vascular injuries of the neck and extremities. The impact of ionizing radiation (effective dose) from CT scans may be significant at the population level. Imaging strategies in trauma should be evaluated continuously.

Trauma education and injury prevention are essential components of a robust trauma program. Educational programs address specific knowledge gaps and provide focused and structured learning. Advanced Trauma Life Support is the most well known. Each offering seems to be valid, although it has been difficult to prove improved patient care outcomes owing specifically to any of them. Injury prevention offers the best opportunity to limit death and disability owing to trauma. Injury prevention initiatives have paid tremendous dividends in reducing the mortalities for motor vehicle crashes. Modern injury prevention efforts focus on reducing distracted driver rates and increasing helmet use.

SURGICAL CLINICS
OF NORTH AMERICA

ISSUE OF RELATED INTEREST

Clinics in Plastic Surgery, July 2017 (Vol. 44, Issue 3)
Burn Care: Rescue, Resuscitation, and Resurfacing
Charles Scott Hultman and Michael W. Neumeister, *Editors*
Available at: www.plasticsurgery.theclinics.com

THE CLINICS ARE AVAILABLE ONLINE!
Access your subscription at:
www.theclinics.com

Foreword

Trauma 2017

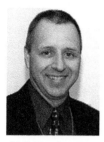

Ronald F. Martin, MD, FACS
Consulting Editor

As we choose the topics for the *Surgical Clinics of North America* series, we follow a general plan of coming to back to most topics, at least in the broad context, about every five to seven years, roughly the length of a postgraduate training program in surgery. At first look, it appears to be a somewhat cyclical approach, but in reality, it is far more like a spiral than a circle since the axis of time is always moving as we trace out our path forward or back to certain topics. We don't keep an absolutely rigid schedule for lots of reasons: some topics evolve faster than others, sometimes a completely new topic emerges, sometimes we change the lens through which we a view a topic (laparoscopy leaps to mind), and sometimes an overarching changing event comes up that we need to insert (such as the training hours regulations and the impact they had). Yet, as we take the distanced look, the patterns continue to replicate and the broad view frequently yields a clearer understanding than the narrowly focused view.

One of the observations that has always struck me is how good ideas for one topic filter into other disciplines and branches of medicine; or even more so, how they do not get there. The discipline of trauma surgery is a wonderful example of the good aspect of this. One view of the study of trauma could be that it is the study of the dissipation of energy (kinetic, thermal, electrical, chemical, or otherwise) through a human. And on at least one level, that is accurate. If the study of trauma stopped there, it would still have a truly fascinating history, but it doesn't stop there. One can add on the advances in critical care support, some of the advances in sepsis, coagulation, and much more on an individual patient basis. Even more important perhaps is the concept of systems and coordination.

As pretty much every treatise on trauma care will state, the history of trauma is largely the history of war. So it should come as no surprise that war is usually waged by states and that states usually keep records. Our recent notable exception of large-scale violence being perpetrated by non–state actors is a fairly substantial outlier on that history but still an outlier. Furthermore, most of the advances in trauma care that have been developed and propagated during these unusual times were still achieved by state

Surg Clin N Am 97 (2017) xiii–xiv
http://dx.doi.org/10.1016/j.suc.2017.08.004
0039-6109/17/© 2017 Published by Elsevier Inc.

surgical.theclinics.com

actors in their responses to the advent of sustained asymmetric warfare. Governments and their militaries in particular are notoriously meticulous record keepers and systems fanatics. This of course is borne of the truism that those with better tactics and operations win battles, while those with better logistics win wars. As always it seems, better large-scale systems trump superior small-scale or individual efforts. The rest of society generally benefits in some measure from the lesson learned from war being tested and where applicable being applied to the civilian population.

Long before there was a "medical home," long before there was an emphasis on stents and statins over bypass grafting, the trauma systems of the United States were reaching well beyond the venue of hospital-based care. Regional trauma centers, standardized teaching of advanced trauma life support (especially to nonsurgeons), improved training of prehospital personnel and first responders through prehospital trauma life support, and the inclusion of prehospital personnel in performance evaluation have all contributed significantly to the success of trauma programs the country over.

Beyond the effort of improving treatment of the trauma patient, our regional and national organizations, including the various trauma societies and the efforts of the American College of Surgeons through its Committee on Trauma, have markedly contributed to the prevention of traumatic injuries through their collaboration with industry to make safer products and improved social awareness of injury prevention. It is perhaps all the more remarkable when one stops to consider that we are collectively trying to create conditions that will curtail or eliminate our livelihood as those who care for trauma patients. That is in fact putting one's money where one's mouth is! There are very few examples of other disciplines in medicine being as effective at widespread prevention and reduction of undesired medical outcomes, with the possible exceptions of immunization programs and contraception. (Editor's note: this last sentence is an observation, not necessarily advocacy. Also, it is the sole observation of the Consulting Editor, R.F. Martin, and does necessarily represent the views of the Guest Editors of this issue, the contributors, or the publishers.)

Drs Guillamondegui and Dennis have provided us with an excellent collection of articles that summarize the global arc of trauma care with expertise and skill. These articles will be of great benefit to anyone who wants to become familiar for the first time with trauma care or become more expert than he/she already is. We are deeply indebted to them for their time and efforts in providing us with this insight.

We will undoubtedly return to trauma care some number of years in the future, as we do with all topics. In the meantime, I look forward to seeing how much of what these experts have taught us filters into other realms of patient care. I encourage you to do what you can to learn from others and teach others the special skills you have. It makes us all better at what we do and it makes for a more capable system. Who knows—you or your loved ones may be the recipients of this improved care.

Ronald F. Martin, MD, FACS
Colonel (ret.), United States Army Reserve
Department of Surgery
York Hospital
16 Hospital Drive, Suite A
York, ME 03909, USA

E-mail address:
rmartin@yorkhospital.com

Preface

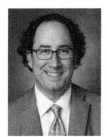
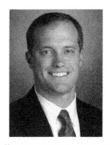

Oscar D. Guillamondegui, MD, MPH, FACS   Bradley M. Dennis, MD, FACS

Editors

We love trauma. We love caring for trauma patients, thinking about trauma care, challenging current dogma, and applying new treatment and approaches to improve outcomes. However, we also recognize that our patients have no love for trauma. For many, the day of their injury is the worst day of their life—a day that shatters all they knew and marks the beginning of a new normal. As a result, we constantly push ourselves and our colleagues to advance care in order to save more lives and restore health to more patients.

Trauma is an organic specialty. Dynamic changes come from dynamic individuals pushing the bounds of care. Over the years since the last Trauma issue of *Surgical Clinics of North America*, there have been some major advances in the management of trauma patients. Innovations, such as resuscitative balloon occlusion of the aorta, and adaptations, such as thromboelastogram-based resuscitation and tranexamic acid treatment of hyperfibrinolysis-mediated hemorrhage, have changed the way trauma is practiced. In this ever-changing field, one thing remains the same: improving the health and well-being of our population, day in and day out.

We have amassed a compendium of trauma care and methods that should provide a concerted strategy utilizing current recommendations for every major area in the management of the trauma patient. The experts we have gathered from both the military and the civilian trauma worlds all share the same passion for improving the outcomes of those we treat, every day. We chose each author for the considerable amount of time they spend in the clinical arena actually managing these injuries. We are truly indebted to their service and their expertise.

We hope this issue of *Surgical Clinics of North America* meets the educational and informational needs of all who manage the complex trauma patient. We start with the historical perspective of how we got here and attempt to work through every aspect of current trauma care. From prehospital issues through current trauma educational opportunities, we believe the knowledge held in these pages grows from the previous works of civilian and military prowess and holds true to progression of the craft of

Surg Clin N Am 97 (2017) xv–xvi
http://dx.doi.org/10.1016/j.suc.2017.08.003
0039-6109/17/© 2017 Published by Elsevier Inc.   **surgical.theclinics.com**

traumatology. It is truly an honor and a privilege to be given the opportunity to put this issue together, and we are proud to be members of the trauma community.

Oscar D. Guillamondegui, MD, MPH, FACS
Vanderbilt University Medical Center
Division of Trauma and Critical Care
1211 21st Avenue South
404 Medical Arts Building
Nashville, TN 37212, USA

Bradley M. Dennis, MD, FACS
Vanderbilt University Medical Center
Division of Trauma and Critical Care
1211 21st Avenue South
404 Medical Arts Building
Nashville, TN 37212, USA

E-mail addresses:
oscar.guillamondegui@vanderbilt.edu (O.D. Guillamondegui)
bradley.m.dennis@vanderbilt.edu (B.M. Dennis)

Trauma Systems
Origins, Evolution, and Current Challenges

Danielle A. Pigneri, MD[a], Brian Beldowicz, MD[a,b],
Gregory J. Jurkovich, MD[c,*]

KEYWORDS

- Trauma systems • Regionalized care • Governmental oversight
- Trauma as major cause of death

KEY POINTS

- Trauma is a major cause of death and major cause of life-years lost.
- Outcomes within trauma systems are markedly improved compared with areas without trauma systems.
- The growth and development of trauma systems is reliant on governmental oversight, financial support, and public interest.

Trauma is the leading cause of death in the United States for people younger than 45, and more children die of injuries than all other causes combined. Trauma is the fifth leading cause of death overall, and accounts for 25% of all life-years lost, more than cancer and heart disease combined. More than 130,000 Americans die every year in our communities from injury, and the combination of health care expenditure and loss of productivity due to injury is estimated to be $675 billion per year.[1] Trauma systems are an effort to address a real and pressing need, and the trauma system effectiveness is a key determinant of the health of a community. Not only does injury happen at unpredictable moments, but the elapsed time from injury to definitive care dramatically affects outcomes. For these reasons, a system that is organized, prepared, and has dedicated providers is of paramount importance. The ideal trauma system design is often referenced to a document published by the Health Services Research Administration in 1992.[2,3] Hallmarks of that report were the recognition that a well-functioning trauma system must integrate all phases of care to allow for

[a] Division of Trauma, Acute Care, and General Surgery, Department of Surgery, UC Davis Health, 2315 Stockton Boulevard, Room OP 512, Sacramento, CA 95817, USA; [b] Division of Trauma, Acute Care, and General Surgery, Department of Surgery, Uniformed Services University of Health Sciences, 4301 Jones Bridge Road, Bethesda, MD 20814, USA; [c] Division of Trauma, Acute Care, and General Surgery, Department of Surgery, UC Davis Health, 2221 Stockton Boulevard, Cypress #3111, Sacramento, CA 95817, USA
* Corresponding author.
E-mail address: gjjurkovich@ucdavis.edu

Surg Clin N Am 97 (2017) 947–959
http://dx.doi.org/10.1016/j.suc.2017.06.011
0039-6109/17/© 2017 Elsevier Inc. All rights reserved.

smooth management of and transitions between recognition, stabilization, transport, treatment, and rehabilitation of the injured. There must be appropriate availability of specialists without overcrowding the system. A wide breadth of specialists should be concentrated in the centers that deal with the most gravely injured patients, and a network of lower severity hospitals should expediently transfer severely injured patients, once stabilized, to these centers. The location of these centers with various capabilities should be based on need, meaning it is to some extent an exclusionary system. Standards of care must be defined, adhered to, and constantly reexamined for opportunities for improvement. Injury prevention outreach should be instituted to decrease the total burden of injury within a community. The ideal trauma system would enable data sharing to effectively analyze care, identify shortcomings, and provide a mechanism for continued improvement in quality.

Although organized civilian trauma systems and the designation of a trauma center are fairly new, the concept of triaged trauma care is as old as war. Many of the lessons learned regarding treatment of traumatic injury were first learned on the battlefield. The Civil War is attributed with being the first time that resources, including anesthetics, were organized to support the surgeon at the scene. The first and second World Wars are credited with the first use of blood transfusions and the first recognition of the effect of time to treatment on outcomes.[4,5] With further scientific advancement in pharmacology, antisepsis and surgical technique available in each successive war of the nineteenth, twentieth, and now twenty-first century, the systematic application of triage, evacuation, and resource allocation exerted as much influence on mortality as the weapons of war themselves. A 1961 study of Army personnel highlighted the prevalence of delayed diagnosis and inappropriate treatment in soldier deaths, calling for improved organization of military medical care for the injured. The high concentration of complex injuries observed in war demanded time-sensitive transportation of injured soldiers to strategically distributed medical assets with specialized capability. Inadequate supply or inefficient use of such assets could be detected by a measurable, and preventable, loss of lives.

As advances were made on the battlefield, the value of applying these principles to the care of injured civilians was recognized. The first formalized civilian trauma center is commonly recognized as the Birmingham Accident Hospital and Rehabilitation Center located in Birmingham, United Kingdom, which opened its doors to the injured in 1941. This hospital was the first to separate injured patients from medically ill patients and structured treatment plans to include all phases of care, from initial resuscitation to rehabilitation.[6]

The first organized civilian US committee dedicated to the care of the injured was the Committee on Fractures, founded in 1922 and chaired by Charles L. Scudder. This was later merged with the American College of Surgeons (ACS) Committee on Industrial Medicine and Traumatic Surgery in 1939 to create the Committee on Fractures and Other Trauma. Over time, the focus of this committee expanded to include visceral injuries in addition to the continued attention to skeletal injuries. Reflecting this change, in 1950 the committee was given its current name, the ACS Committee on Trauma (COT).[7] The ACS COT has defined national standards for the care of the injured. The Optimal Hospital Resources for Care of the Seriously Injured was first published by the ACS COT in 1976 and defined the hospital-based resources for the care of the injured.[8] A seemingly subtle name change to this document occurred in 1990, renaming the iteration as *Resources for Optimal Care of the Injured Patient* in an effort to account for more than just the hospital resources needed.[9] This "bible" of trauma center resources is now in its eighth edition (2014). The first trauma unit in the United States was opened at the University of Maryland by Dr R. Adams Cowley in

1961.[10] Shortly thereafter, additional hospitals followed suit by opening their own trauma centers. Dr Robert Freeark and Dr Robert Baker organized the opening of a trauma unit at Cook County in Chicago in 1966.[11] Under the guidance of Dr George Sheldon, the University of California San Francisco General Hospital received both a trauma center designation and a large multidisciplinary research grant in 1972.[12]

The development of academic departments of surgery with a strong interest in caring for the injured patients and its related research was stimulated by the growing recognition of a need, but also by the return to civilian life of surgeons from the Korean War and the Vietnam War. A critical motivation was also a landmark report by the National Academy of Sciences' National Research Council entitled, "Accidental Death and Disability: The Neglected Disease of Modern Society."[13] This was published in 1966 and examined the prevalence and need for organized trauma care. The investigators highlighted the urgent need for improved organization, resource allocation, data collection, research, and education in the comprehensive management of injured patients.[13] Congress responded to this report by passing the National Highway Safety Act of 1966, which identified and funded changes to improve the communication, coordination, and transportation of injured patients after motor vehicle accidents.[5]

Maryland, Florida, and Illinois used this opportunity to create some of the first organized trauma systems, which more formally integrated prehospital transport within an interconnected system of trauma centers. In Maryland, this took the form of a cooperative organization between the University of Maryland, the Shock-Trauma Center in Baltimore, the state police, helicopter crews, and prehospital providers. Implementation of this cooperative resulted in a marked reduction in mortality.[14] Jacksonville, Florida, instituted similar systems to improve prehospital care and coordination between prehospital providers and hospitals, with a demonstrated 38% reduction in vehicular deaths.[15]

Illinois is credited with creating the first statewide trauma system in the early 1970s, which included governmental support and leadership from the governor himself. The Illinois system identified 5 key components for a trauma system: designated trauma centers, special trauma training for providers, ambulance design for safe transport of injured patients, technology to allow immediate communication between providers, and constant reevaluation of care via trauma registries.[11] In 1971, Illinois became the first state to legislate the designation of trauma centers. Review of the Illinois outcomes in 2 studies demonstrated improved mortality among patients treated in trauma centers after the implementation of legislated trauma systems, whereas mortality rates among injured patients treated at undesignated centers remained constant.[16,17] When these data were examined by region, a much more dramatic improvement in mortality was noted among patients injured in a rural setting, demonstrating the importance of access to prompt and high-quality trauma center care.[17]

The demonstrated mortality benefit of trauma systems in Maryland, Florida, and Illinois prompted additional legislation that fueled further development. The Emergency Medical Services Systems Act of 1973 granted approximately $300 million for the development and operation of statewide emergency medical services (EMS) systems with a focus on ensuring improved rural access to specialized emergency care.[5,18] These EMS geographic boarders defined following this act are still used as the current EMS regions and agencies in all states, and typically are the beneficiaries of money directed at emergency medical care and devices. This act remains a large reason why EMS agencies exist and have modern equipment, even in rural settings.

As EMS services improved and expanded, the need for more formalized hospital designations became apparent. The idea of rating or categorizing emergency departments was first discussed by the National Academy of Sciences at their 1966 National

Research Council meeting. It was not until 1971 that the American Medical Association Commission on EMS formulated a system of designation based on emergency department capabilities.[19] Five years later, the COT published the first iteration of Optimal Hospital Resources for Care of the Injured Patient, which defines the key components of a trauma center and stressed the importance of a trauma center's function within a trauma system. These fundamental elements of a trauma system remain the accepted standard today and include injury prevention outreach; access to trauma care; prehospital triage, care, and transportation; acute hospital care at capable centers; rehabilitation services; and ongoing research (Resources for optimal care of the injured patient 2014).

In the 1980s, a series of articles was published that fueled the public's demand for the growth of trauma systems. As noted previously, the efficacy of trauma centers had been demonstrated in Maryland; Jacksonville, Florida; and Illinois systems. Conversely, as the efficacy of trauma systems was coming to light, the inadequacy of medical care in areas without trauma systems was sorely noted. In the late 1970s to mid-1980s, 3 areas specifically noted and studied this disparity in health care as related to preventable death rates. West and colleagues[20] published a landmark article in 1979 demonstrating dramatically worse outcomes in Orange County, California, when compared with San Francisco, California. At the time, no formalized trauma system existed in Orange County, and all injured patients were taken to the closest available hospital. In contrast, severely injured patients in San Francisco were directed to a single, central Level I trauma center. Despite the Orange County patients having been younger and less injured, outcomes were markedly worse. In the cases reviewed during the study period, 1.1% of trauma deaths were deemed potentially preventable in San Francisco, whereas 28% of the central nervous system (CNS) injury deaths and 73% of the non-CNS deaths were deemed potentially preventable in Orange County. The study cited lack of organized trauma care, lack of structured resuscitation, and lack of aggressive surgical intervention for injured patients as the cause of this disparity in outcomes.[20] With assistance of local government, a trauma system was implemented with subsequent improvement in trauma outcomes.[21]

In 1983, poor outcomes were reported in Portland, Oregon, and implementation of a trauma system was suggested. Oregon's government responded by instituting a statewide trauma system, with a strategic designation of trauma centers. Two elements of Oregon's approach to trauma system creation were novel at the time. First, they declined several of the centers that applied for trauma center status. Second, they expanded their network to include rural centers, which were designated as Level IV centers. Through this, they were able to widen their catchment area while concentrating high-level trauma care into fewer, more specialized centers.[5]

The success of the Oregon trauma system encouraged its neighbor, Washington State, to examine the health care of its injured patients, which identified enough problems to motivate the legislature of Washington State to fund an analysis of trauma care system design and implementation, which was completed in 1987. This, in turn, led to the creation of the Washington State trauma system under the direction of the State Department of Health, which remarkably was passed unanimously into law in 1990.[22,23]

Following similar reports of unacceptable trauma outcomes, San Diego County also developed a regionalized trauma center (1 Level I center, 4 Level II centers, 1 pediatric trauma center, and an EMS network) in 1984. A follow-up study conducted by Shackford and colleagues[24] reviewed the trauma outcomes data for the 12-month period following implementation of this new regionalized system. The investigators demonstrated a marked increase in survival among the most critically injured trauma patients when treated within their trauma system. Specifically, survival among severely injured blunt trauma patients increased from 18% to 29% and survival for severe penetrating injuries increased from 8% to 20%.

Simultaneous to the development of these trauma systems was a call from Congress for a follow-up evaluation of trauma outcomes nationwide. The resulting report, *Injury in America: A Continuing Public Health Problem*,[25] was published in 1985 and demonstrated that despite the improvements that had been seen within individual trauma systems, traumatic injury remained a significant threat to public health on the national scale. In addition to benchmarking trauma outcomes, the report advocated for increased efforts related to traumatic epidemiologic studies, injury prevention outreach, and research focused on rehabilitation.[25] Following publication of this report, the Center for Injury Control was founded and established as a branch within the Centers for Disease Control and Prevention (CDC).[5] This followed considerable discussion and debate on the appropriate federal funding home for trauma research, with many advocates disappointed that the National Institute of Trauma Research within the National Institutes of Health was not funded. This proved to be prophetic, as in 1996 (Public Law 104–208) the CDC was barred by Congress from funding gun-violence research programs, and shortly after drifted entirely away from funding clinically relevant trauma-related research.

In 1987, West and colleagues[26] conducted a national survey to determine the level of ubiquity of trauma systems in the United States. EMS directors, health department authorities, and state chairpersons on the COT from each state were contacted. All 50 states and the District of Columbia responded. Eight criteria were used to assess adequacy of the trauma systems. These included (1) the presence of a governing agency with legal authority to designate trauma centers; (2) the use of a structured process for designation of trauma centers; (3) the use of the ACS COT standards for trauma centers; (4) the use of a geographically remote survey team in trauma center designation; (5) restricting the number of trauma centers in an area based on community need; (6) written triage criteria that guide transport of injured patients to designated trauma centers; (7) ongoing assessment of trauma centers; and (8) statewide trauma center coverage. Only 2 states, Virginia and Maryland, were found to have complete trauma systems with statewide coverage.

In 1990, the *Trauma Care Systems and Development Act* (Public Law 101–590) allocated development grants to a total of 35 states for initiation of a new trauma system or revision of an existing system.[18] This federal legislation was in response to the statements from some states and EMS regions that they could not afford to develop the infrastructure of a trauma system. At the same time, it was also evident there was considerable pressure from individual hospitals, agencies, and physician groups to forgo trauma system development due to concerns regarding loss of autonomy, excess governmental oversight of clinical practice, and the cost of meeting the requirements of a trauma centers. The progress of trauma system development was also thwarted by declining health care reimbursements and a change to diagnosis-related group (DRG) payment system. This resulted in equivalent reimbursement for acute care hospitals compared with trauma centers, despite patients with higher severity of a given diagnosis being cared for at Level I centers. Referring hospitals could now cherry-pick the most profitable cases, passing along those patients who would require greater resource consumption without a compensatory adjustment in reimbursement. The result was increased cost of care provided at Level I centers with unadjusted reimbursement.[5]

An analysis of cost in New York State demonstrated that trauma patients in the same DRG cost $27.5 million more when compared with nontrauma patients.[27] A total of 61 regional trauma centers shut down between 1988 and 1991, with an additional center closing later that decade.[28] Inadequate reimbursement was cited as a major cause of trauma center closure.[29] Centers that downgraded from trauma center status could continue to care for patients with lower severity of injury, while transporting the higher-severity patients within a given DRG to Level I centers, thereby compounding the problem. Additionally, Level I centers were caring for a disproportionate number of self-pay and Medicare/Medicaid patients when compared with community hospitals, leading to even further reimbursement disparity.[27]

Being involved in the care of the injured as non-Level 1 centers would allow lower-level centers to "transfer up" those patients who cost the most to care for, and often (usually) had inadequate insurance/reimbursement resources. Hence, there was, and remains, a financial incentive to be a lower-level trauma center within a community that generally has a higher income and better insurance penetration as long as a Level I center is nearby. These centers are able to care for mildly injured patients and are not required to accept the severely injured in the same way that Level I centers are. This may continue to contribute to the proliferation of Level II and III centers in states without the governmental ability or will to regulate trauma centers, one of the tenets of the original Health Resources and Services Administration (HRSA) trauma system design document. As demonstrated in Florida, increasing the number of trauma centers alone does not improve the quality of care provided to injured patients within a community. Rather, improving care relies on providing access to seasoned trauma centers with adequate volume of trauma experience to continually adjust and improve treatment paradigms.[30]

As the landscape of trauma care changed in the 1990s, the need for an increased focus on systems of trauma centers became apparent. Despite guidance from the ACS COT regarding optimal resources within each individual hospital designated as a trauma center, there was little national guidance regarding the creation and organization of the larger trauma systems themselves. This decision making was left to individual states and EMS systems. To address this need, HRSA released their *Model Trauma Care Systems Plan* in 1992, which hoped to serve as a template for each individual state during the process of trauma system development or adjustment. This document stressed the importance of consistent legislative and financial support, and cited the lack of these elements as key to the failure and closure of many trauma systems and centers. A follow-up study was conducted by Bazzoli and colleagues[18] to evaluate the progress of trauma development in the early 1990s. A 23-page questionnaire was sent to existing trauma systems. The questions included in the questionnaire were designed to address the 8 components of a trauma system addressed in the 1987 study by West and colleagues.[26] Only 5 states (Maryland, Florida, Nevada, New York, and Oregon) were found to have complete statewide trauma systems. This demonstrated only a modest improvement since the 1987 study by West and colleagues.[26] Notably, the most common deficiency was the failure to regulate the number of trauma centers within the statewide system, likely secondary to the financial incentives for Level II and III centers. This specific deficiency was responsible for Virginia being removed from the list of complete trauma systems.

Despite the advancements made in civilian trauma system organization over a quarter-century, medical support for America's first armed conflict since the Vietnam War fell short of expectations in 1992 with Operations Desert Shield and Desert Storm. A report published by the Government Accountability Office that same year indicated how the military had fallen behind its civilian counterparts in developing a mature system of regionalized trauma care (GAO/NSIAD-92–175, 1992).[31]

In 1996, Michael DeBakey delivered a lecture at the 50th Anniversary Meeting of the Society of Medical Consultants to the Armed Forces in which he challenged civilian and military medical experts to remain vigilant and focused on the requirements of military readiness. "I expect that you will be called upon should our nation ever face another national emergency," DeBakey said, himself a retired US Army Colonel. "I know that you will be ready to accept that call, and I am confident that you will execute your task at the highest level of excellence."[32]

The military-civilian shared ideology that had been paramount in the early development of trauma centers and systems would come full circle. In 2004, the ACS COT would prove instrumental in the US military's development of the largest trauma system in the world to support the wars in Iraq and Afghanistan. Spanning more than 9000 miles, the Joint Theater Trauma System was the culmination of trauma system development in the early twenty-first century. Based on the ACS COT's *Resources for Optimal Care of the Injured Patient*,[9] the system incorporated data-driven resource distribution intended to efficiently sustain multiple high-intensity, open-ended conflicts. The plan also required the Joint Theater Trauma Registry to collect, organize, analyze, and distribute casualty information from the point of injury through evacuation to definitive care stateside for the purposes of research, performance improvement, and quality assurance. A library of clinical practice guidelines was also developed and distributed in an effort to standardize evidence-based best practices throughout various levels of casualty care. The system collectively reduced the mortality rate of combat casualties to less than 9%, roughly half that observed in the Vietnam War when trauma systems were in their infancy.

The benefits of well-orchestrated trauma systems extend beyond mortality statistics. In combat, they exert confidence in the fighting soldier. For civilians, they impart a similar perception of safety that influences the way communities thrive. HRSA published a report in 2002 citing public support, and the resultant state and federal support, as a mandatory element for the success of civilian trauma system growth and development (**Fig. 1**). A follow-up report by Champion and colleagues[33] published

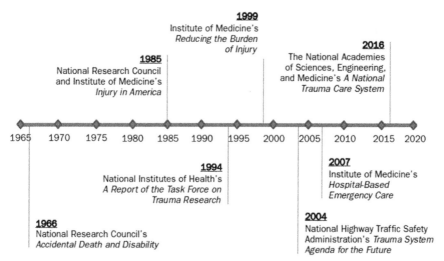

Fig. 1. Timeline of assessments relevant to civilian trauma research. (*From* National Academies of Sciences, Engineering, and Medicine. A national trauma care system: integrating military and civilian trauma systems to achieve zero preventable deaths after injury. Washington, DC: The National Academies Press; 2016; with permission.)

in 2006 demonstrated several prominent public misconceptions regarding the state of trauma systems of care. First, nearly 90% of Americans polled felt that an organized and coordinated system for the delivery of trauma care should exist and be a priority. Nearly two-thirds of Americans were confident that such a system existed near them, such that they would receive this care if they were injured. Additional findings included more than 60% of Americans being unaware of the prevalence of death from serious injury and the prevalent misconception that a formalized trauma system existed in every state. However, at the time, only 8 states were deemed to have complete state-wide systems for trauma care. This knowledge gap by the general public is likely responsible for the lack of consistent state and federal prioritization of the development and constant improvement of trauma systems.

In 2006, HSRA released *Model Trauma System Planning and Evaluation*, their updated version of the 1992 *Model Trauma Care System Plan*[2] and one that presented trauma as a public health problem. This document specified the discrete element of a trauma system, to which the ACS COT references during their discussion of trauma system dynamics. The 3 key functions of a trauma system defined within the *Model Trauma Systems Planning and Evaluation* report are ongoing assessment of injury epidemiology, policy development focused on protecting the public from injury, and ensuring high-quality care through regulation. The 10 services essential to achieving these 3 functions are (1) constant monitoring of the community health status and needs; (2) diagnosis and investigation of public health issues and hazards; (3) public engagement through education and empowerment; (4) community partnerships aimed at diagnosing and treating local health problems; (5) development of policies that support identified health care needs; (6) enforcement of laws and regulations designed to ensure health and safety; (7) a network for linking patients to their needed health resources with a route for access to care that may be locally unavailable; (8) quality assurance of the health care work force; (9) ongoing assessment of the effectiveness, accessibility, and quality of health services rendered; and (10) research initiatives to seek new solutions to current health problems.

A ubiquitous, effective, and efficient EMS service is inherent to the ability of any trauma system to meet the previously listed criteria. Like police departments, fire departments, and EMS services, trauma systems can arguably be considered a community need, funded and regulated like these other public health entities. EMS not only provides the initial assessment and stabilization of injured patients, but they also decide to which hospitals patients will be taken. Triage to the level of care appropriate for the definitive management of a patient's injuries may conflict with the immediate need for stabilization and geographic. For this reason, field triage criteria were developed in tandem with trauma system growth.[34] These algorithms also require frequent reassessment and amendment to ensure appropriate attention to the needs of the community served.

Although room for improvement of trauma systems remains, the national improvement in trauma care through the development of regionalized trauma systems has been clearly demonstrated.[35] Additionally, this improvement has not been without notice from outside sectors of the medical community. Perhaps the most notable endorsement of this success comes from the trend toward regionalization of other aspects of medical care. Over the past few decades, there has been a national push for regionalization of cardiac care, acute stroke treatments, cancer diagnosis and treatment, and bariatric surgery care. These fields have aimed to create regionalized systems not unlike the regionalized trauma systems platform. In a similar manner to trauma, these sectors aim to concentrate specialists in the field into centers of excellence. These centers are often chosen in areas with the best access to epidemiologic data, most current systems of care, and a high degree of ongoing research aimed at finding innovative treatments for their specific health challenges. The American Heart Association (AHA) has taken this 1 step further and in 2010 called for a regionalized system more extensive that a system of centers of concentrated care providers. The AHA called for a regionalized system to include EMS in the stabilization and triage of patients who suffer cardiac arrest outside of the hospital. In this call-to-action address, improved outcomes with coordinated trauma systems was used as evidence that regionalized systems improve care.[36,37]

What is next for trauma systems? Can they be improved, or are the economic forces too powerful to allow regionalization of health care? The care of patients injured in a rural setting has long presented a unique challenge. Population concentration in these regions does not support the development or sustainment of Level I centers in these regions. Yet time from injury to definitive treatment remains an undeniable factor in trauma outcomes. The historic approach to this unique problem has been to expand the catchment net for urban-based trauma systems. However, this approach has led to a large volume of mildly or moderately injured patients being transferred to urban Level I or II centers. When patients are over triaged to these urban centers, a reasonable amount of emotional and financial distress can be created for the patient and family. The message is relayed to the family that their loved one is so gravely injured that he or she requires triage to a high level of trauma care. Additionally, emergency travel to urban centers may be inconvenient, expensive, or dangerous for elderly or emotionally distraught loved ones. Historically and currently, rural centers are trained to provide initial stabilization and rapid transfer for injured patients who present at their door. This should remain true and mandatory for severely injured patients or patients whose needs exceed the care available at the receiving hospital. However, most injured patients are mildly injured and do not require such transfer. Improved communication between EMS providers and receiving hospitals may allow us to spare a large number of patients from unnecessary transfer.[38]

Another challenge facing the success of trauma system design and implementation is the unregulated opening of trauma centers, most notably Level II trauma centers. In states and regions that fail to control the number and distribution of trauma centers, there has been a proliferation of trauma centers near populations that generally have a higher socioeconomic status, are more insured, and have a low volume of penetrating trauma. This has led to the decrease in patient volume in the Level I center, along with decreasing reimbursement that jeopardizes the existence of the Level I center. Unlike the trauma center crisis 1989 to 1991, this is the result of high reimbursement for Level II trauma centers, that then want to keep patients, with the resultant loss of volume for training and experience with uncommon injuries, as well as income, for the Level I centers.[39] Notable examples are Florida, Colorado, and Texas.[40,41]

In August 2015, the ACS COT convened a consensus conference to develop the Needs-Based Assessment of Trauma Systems (NBATS) tool to assist in determining the number of trauma centers required for a region[42] (**Table 1**). Although legislative authority to determine the number and need of trauma centers has been an essential component of trauma system design since 1992, it has, until the most recent decade, been largely unnecessary, as most hospitals did not want to participate in trauma care. This is changing and bringing new challenges to trauma system survival.[2]

The background for this changing approach to trauma care and the view of the ACS COT are nicely outlined in a discussion (by Mike Rotondo) of the article by Uribe-Leitz and colleagues,[43] the only peer-reviewed publication to date on the use of this tool and the source of **Table 1**. The NBATS tool is available on the ACS Web site

Table 1
NBATS criteria and assumptions used for NBATS model for missing data source

		Assumptions		
	Range of Possible Points	Base Case	Lower Range	Higher Range
1. Population size	2–10	N/A	N/A	N/A
2. Median transport times	0–4	0	0	4
3. Community support	0–5	0	0	5
4. Number of patients with ISS >15 at nontrauma centers (non-Level I/II or III centers)	0–4	0	0	4
5. Number of Level I, II, or III trauma centers	0 to negative number based on multiplier	N/A	N/A	N/A
6. Estimated number of patients with ISS >15 based on number of trauma centers vs actual number seen at Level I/II centers	−2 to 2	0	−2	2

Abbreviations: ISS, injury severity score; N/A, not applicable (no missing data); NBATS, Needs-Based Assessment of Trauma Systems.

From Uribe-Leitz T, Esquivel MM, Knowlton LM, et al. The American College of Surgeons needs-based assessment of trauma systems: estimates for the State of California. J Trauma Acute Care Surg 2017;82(5):861–6; with permission.

(https://www.facs.org/quality-programs/trauma/tscp/nbats; accessed June 13, 2017) as well as documents that include the list of participants and some introductory notes.[44] The tool assesses 6 specific factors, assigning positive or negative points to each factor. These factors are as follows:

1. Population size
2. Median transport times
3. Lead agency/community support presence
4. Severely injured not cared for at any trauma center
5. Number of current Level I centers
6. Number of severely injured seen at a Level I and II trauma center already in the system

Criticisms of this tool are that by including both Level I and II in the final point, the tool fails to make the distinction of care (or costs, or margin) between these 2 types of trauma centers, and that it does not reward volume performance, nor the importance of training and teaching. The more points on this tool scale, the more trauma centers a region should have, again, not differentiating between Level I or II centers.

This tool was largely developed from discussions that had been occurring in Florida, and as a result, this tool lacks any legislative authority to implement the suggestions based on its results. The ACS COT has deferred any authority to deciding which hospitals should be trauma centers based on need, allowing that the local regulatory agencies of the EMS services should have that authority, and if they are unwilling, the ACS COT lacks the authority. In many regions, it would appear that the current state of trauma system design and hospital designation is based on political pressures, economic factors, and last, on patient need.

In the age of technology, there is certainly room for technological advancements aimed at improving communication among EMS, receiving hospitals, rehabilitation centers, and long-term providers. An integrated electronic medical system (EMR) could allow trauma specialists at Level I centers to review imaging and prepare for a patient before the patient's arrival, expediting the delivery of time-sensitive care. The same system could allow trauma surgeons to follow patients or opine on critical events that occur after patients have moved to rehabilitation facilities. EMS crews enabled with video-conferencing technology would allow physicians to drive decision making regarding triage and field care when needed. A nationally integrated EMR system based on permanent patient identifiers, such as fingerprints, could allow immediate access to patient history in the trauma bay, which would likely prove most useful for our elderly and comorbid patients. In rural and geographically difficult to access regions, video-enabled drones could allow for early assessment and triage planning before EMS crew arrival at the scene. The degree to which these changes will influence patient outcomes remains to be seen. However, the previously documented outcomes improvement when patients are managed by trauma specialists at Level I centers would argue that these specialists driving other areas of decision making during other vulnerable phases of care would likely lead to similar improvements. The primary obstacle to a technology-rich fully integrated national trauma system will likely be the need for layered mechanisms for protection of personal health information. Additional issues may be encountered at the interface between existing EMR systems. As we push forward, overcoming these obstacles may prove worthwhile if we are better able to use the golden hour, improve communication between providers, and ensure patient safety through their period of rehabilitation.

The evolution of trauma care in America is far from over. As new weapons reach the streets and we step into a time of political uncertainty, the specific challenges that lie ahead remain unknown. We must ask ourselves how our past experiences impact our vision for the care of injured patients now and in the future? An ideal state would be formulated through a network of highly functioning and interconnected trauma systems that provide complete coverage to the entire United States without significant redundancy or overlap. Such a system would require a consistent source of financial support for both ongoing operations as well as research and development. Innovative technologies would focus on improved communication between phases of care to create a truly integrated experience at the level of each individual patient. Such a system would require governmental oversight and regulation, specifically related to restricting the number of trauma centers to those truly needed within each individual trauma system to meet the community need. Continued data collection within each trauma center, within each trauma system, and within larger cohorts, such as the Joint Theater Trauma System and national Trauma Quality Improvement Program, will be necessary to continue improving the routes through which care is provided. Finally, improved public awareness and support would serve as the backbone on which our efforts rest.

REFERENCES

1. Berwick DM, Downey AS, Cornett EA. A national trauma care system to achieve zero preventable deaths after injury recommendations from a National Academies of Sciences, Engineering, and Medicine report. JAMA 2016;316(9): 927–8.

2. Administration, H.R.a.S. Model trauma system planning and evaluation. U.S. Department of Health and Human Services; 1992.

3. Jurkovich GJ. Regionalized health care and the trauma system model. J Am Coll Surg 2012;215(1):1–11.
4. Trunkey DD. History and development of trauma care in the United States. Clin Orthop Relat Res 2000;(374):36–46.
5. Mullins RJ. A historical perspective of trauma system development in the United States. J Trauma 1999;47(3 Suppl):S8–14.
6. Great Britain. Inter-departmental committee on rehabilitation of persons injured by accidents. [from old catalog], et al. Final report of the Inter-departmental committee on the rehabilitation of persons injured by accidents. 1939, London: H. M. Stationery off. vi, 194 p. incl. illus. (plans) tables, diagrs.
7. Surgeons, C.o.T.o.t.A.C.o. Blue book: a guide to organization, objectives, and activities. 2007.
8. Optimal hospital resources for care of the seriously injured. Bull Am Coll Surg 1976;61(9):15–22.
9. American College of Surgeons. Committee on Trauma. Resources for optimal care of the injured patient. Chicago: American College of Surgeons, Committee on Trauma; 1990. p. iii, 79.
10. Edlich RF, Wish JR. An organized approach to trauma care: legacy of R Adams Cowley. J Long Term Eff Med Implants 2004;14(6):481–511.
11. Boyd DR. How Illinois' trauma and EMS system of care helped shape the industry. J Emerg Med Serv 2015.
12. Surgery, D.o.O. Our history. University of California, San Francisco OrthoWeb; 2011.
13. Accidental death and disability: the neglected disease of modern society. Washington, DC: 1966.
14. Cowley RA, Hudson F, Scanlan E, et al. An economical and proved helicopter program for transporting the emergency critically ill and injured patient in Maryland. J Trauma 1973;13(12):1029–38.
15. Waters JM Jr, Wells CH. The effects of a modern emergency medical care system in reducing automobile crash deaths. J Trauma 1973;13(7):645–7.
16. Mullner R, Goldberg J. The Illinois Trauma System: changes in patient survival patterns following vehicular injuries. JACEP 1977;6(9):393–6.
17. Mullner R, Goldberg J. An evaluation of the Illinois trauma system. Med Care 1978;16(2):140–51.
18. Bazzoli GJ, Madura KJ, Cooper GF, et al. Progress in the development of trauma systems in the United States. Results of a national survey. JAMA 1995;273(5):395–401.
19. Mehrotra A, Sklar DP, Tayal VS, et al. Important historical efforts at emergency department categorization in the United States and implications for regionalization. Acad Emerg Med 2010;17(12):e154–60.
20. West JG, Trunkey DD, Lim RC. Systems of trauma care. A study of two counties. Arch Surg 1979;114(4):455–60.
21. Cales RH. Trauma mortality in Orange County: the effect of implementation of a regional trauma system. Ann Emerg Med 1984;13(1):1–10.
22. Mullins RJ, Mann NC, Hedges JR, et al. Preferential benefit of implementation of a statewide trauma system in one of two adjacent states. J Trauma 1998;44(4):609–16 [discussion: 617].
23. Bulger K, Maier. Journal of Trauma Acute Care Surgery Open. in press.
24. Shackford SR, Mackersie RC, Hoyt DB, et al. Impact of a trauma system on outcome of severely injured patients. Arch Surg 1987;122(5):523–7.
25. Injury in America: a continuing public health problem. Washington, DC: 1985.

26. West JG, Williams MJ, Trunkey DD, et al. Trauma systems. Current status–future challenges. JAMA 1988;259(24):3597–600.

27. Joy SA, Lichtig LK, Knauf RA, et al. Identification and categorization of and cost for care of trauma patients: a study of 12 trauma centers and 43,219 statewide patients. J Trauma 1994;37(2):303–8 [discussion: 308–13].

28. U.S. trauma center crisis: lost in the scramble for terror resources. National Foundation for Trauma Care; 2004. p. 1–13.

29. Dailey JT, Teter H, Cowley RA. Trauma center closures: a national assessment. J Trauma 1992;33(4):539–46 [discussion: 546–7].

30. Pracht EE, Langland-Orban B, Tepas JJ, et al. Analysis of trends in the Florida Trauma Systems (1991-2003) changes in mortality after establishment of new centers. Surgery 2006;140(1):34–43.

31. Affairs, O.o.P. Operation Desert Storm: full army medical capability not achieved. NSAID 1992;92(175).

32. Mil Med 1996;161(12):711–6.

33. Champion HR, Mabee MS, Meredith JW. The state of US trauma systems: public perceptions versus reality–implications for US response to terrorism and mass casualty events. J Am Coll Surg 2006;203(6):951–61.

34. Sasser SM, Hunt RC, Sullivent EE, et al. Guidelines for field triage of injured patients. Recommendations of the National Expert Panel on Field Triage. MMWR Recomm Rep 2009;58(RR-1):1–35.

35. Mann NC, Mullins RJ, MacKenzie EJ, et al. Systematic review of published evidence regarding trauma system effectiveness. J Trauma 1999;47(3 Suppl): S25–33.

36. Nichol G, Soar J. Regional cardiac resuscitation systems of care. Curr Opin Crit Care 2010;16(3):223–30.

37. Nichol G, Aufderheide TP, Eigel B, et al. Regional systems of care for out-of-hospital cardiac arrest: a policy statement from the American Heart Association. Circulation 2010;121(5):709–29.

38. McSwain N, Rotondo M, Meade P, et al. A model for rural trauma care. Br J Surg 2012;99(3):309–14.

39. Simon R, Stone M, Cucuzzo J. The impact of a new trauma center on an existing nearby trauma center. J Trauma 2009;67(3):645–50.

40. Tepas JJ 3rd, Kerwin AJ, Ra JH. Unregulated proliferation of trauma centers undermines cost efficiency of population-based injury control. J Trauma Acute Care Surg 2014;76(3):576–9 [discussion: 579–81].

41. Ciesla DJ, Pracht EE, Leitz PT, et al. The trauma ecosystem: the impact and economics of new trauma centers on a mature statewide trauma system. J Trauma Acute Care Surg 2017;82(6):1014–22.

42. American College of Surgeons Committee on Trauma. Statement on trauma center designation based upon system need. Bull Am Coll Surg 2015;100(1):51–2.

43. Uribe-Leitz T, Esquivel MM, Knowlton LM, et al. The American College of Surgeons needs-based assessment of trauma systems: estimates for the State of California. J Trauma Acute Care Surg 2017;82(5):861–6.

44. Available at: https://www.facs.org/quality-programs/trauma/tscp/nbats. Accessed July 28,2017.

Prehospital Assessment of Trauma

Joshua Brown, MD, MSc[a], Nitin Sajankila, BS[b], Jeffrey A. Claridge, MD, MS[c],*

KEYWORDS

- Prehospital • Emergency medical services • Trauma • Triage • Air medical
- Transport

KEY POINTS

- A significant amount of variability exists between the various prehospital trauma systems that provide early postinjury care in the United States.
- This variability includes differences in emergency medical services provided, types of transport available, protocols guiding care, and cooperation between hospitals and providers involved.
- Although advances have been made to prehospital care, more research is necessary to see how uniformly these advances are implemented.
- Further research on determining the best care practices and the development of uniform protocols is also necessary.

INTRODUCTION AND HISTORY OF PREHOSPITAL TRAUMA CARE

As with many of the advancements in trauma care, prehospital trauma care has evolved significantly with periods of military conflict. Most credit Baron Dominique Jean Larrey, Napoleon's surgeon, with the concept of the ambulance in 1792.[1] The genesis of an organized ambulance corps in the military, however, was not until the United States Civil War. This experience was furthered in World War II, when medical personnel were assigned to combat companies to provide care at the point of wounding, becoming the first combat medics. It was then during the Korean War and Vietnam conflict that en route care by medics for the wounded solider became the standard, alongside the rapid transport of patients to higher levels of care through air evacuation.[2]

Disclosure Statement: The authors have nothing to disclose.
[a] Department of Surgery, University of Pittsburgh Medical Center, 200 Lothrop Street, Pittsburgh, PA 15213, USA; [b] Department of Surgery, MetroHealth Medical Center, Case Western Reserve University School of Medicine, 2500 MetroHealth Drive, Cleveland, OH 44109, USA; [c] Division of General Surgery, Trauma, and Surgical Critical Care, Department of Surgery, MetroHealth Medical Center, Case Western Reserve University School of Medicine, 2500 Metrohealth Drive, Cleveland, OH 44109, USA
* Corresponding author.
E-mail address: jclaridge@metrohealth.org

http://dx.doi.org/10.1016/j.suc.2017.06.007
0039-6109/17/© 2017 Elsevier Inc. All rights reserved.
surgical.theclinics.com

In the United States, the National Academy of Sciences' 1966 white paper *Accidental Death and Disability: The Neglected Disease of Modern Society* is considered the birth of modern civilian emergency medical services (EMS) and prehospital trauma care. This landmark paper called for standardized training, funding, and organization of ambulance services.[3] Dr J.D. Farrington brought these issues to surgeons' attention when he published "Death in a Ditch" in the June 1967 *American College of Surgeons Bulletin*; in this piece, he outlines simple first aid techniques that he taught to local rescue volunteers.[4] The EMS Systems Act of 1973 identified key elements of an EMS service and provided funding and authorization for the Department of Health, Education, and Welfare to establish EMS systems throughout the United States. As trauma care and systems developed through the 1960s and 1970s, EMS systems continued to grow.

The advent of the Advanced Trauma Life Support course in 1978 was followed shortly by the first Prehospital Trauma Life Support course in 1984, aimed at training prehospital providers in the systematic approach to the injured patient.

PREHOSPITAL TRAUMA SYSTEMS

Since the early days of EMS and trauma systems, significant advancements in technology and medical practice have matured these services. In the United States, tremendous variation exists in prehospital trauma systems owing to differences in resource availability and varying levels of regional need. Regulatory authority for EMS systems, including treatment protocols and licensure of individual providers, is at the state level. Many states designate regional EMS councils to provider further local oversight. A recent survey demonstrated 38 states had either mandatory or model treatment protocols for EMS agencies, and the remainder allowed the development of protocols at the local level.[5]

Prehospital trauma care is provided by a variety of agencies. Some areas provide prehospital care and transport through the local fire department. EMS providers may comprise a separate division within the fire department or may be fully cross-trained as firefighters. Other areas may have separate standalone EMS agencies. These agencies exclusively provide prehospital medical care and often work with local fire departments, which then provide first response before the arrival of dedicated EMS personnel.

Another distinction is the EMS agency ownership. Many areas use municipal EMS agencies that fall under the jurisdiction of the city or town. In more rural areas, a county itself may provide EMS services. Municipal services are usually subsidized by taxes of the municipality residents. Other areas use private EMS agencies. Several large private EMS corporations exist throughout the United States that contract with municipalities directly to provide emergency prehospital care or supplement the local municipal EMS agency's response capacity.

Depending on the demand for service, EMS agencies may be composed of paid or volunteer providers. Larger services with a higher volume generally hire paid EMS personnel. More rural or less active services often employ volunteer members. These members may take block volunteer shifts or provide service on an on-call basis when the EMS agency is activated for a response. Finally, a number of agencies employ a core of paid providers with coverage supplemented by volunteers.

EMERGENCY MEDICAL SERVICES LEVEL OF CARE

Perhaps the greatest distinction of prehospital trauma care is the scope of practice. At the provider level, this ranges from the emergency medical technician (EMT) providing basic life support (BLS) care to the paramedic who provides advanced life support (ALS) care. BLS trauma care generally allows for vital sign measurement and patient assessment, noninvasive airway and ventilation techniques, oxygen administration, basic hemorrhage control, and splinting. ALS trauma care generally allows for more invasive airway methods including endotracheal intubation (ETI), chest decompression, intravenous (IV) access and fluid administration, as well as administration of cardiac and vasoactive medications.

Most states license providers for several levels of care between the EMT and paramedic. In 1996, the National Highway Traffic Safety Administration identified 44 different levels of EMS provider certification and 39 different state licensure levels between EMT and paramedic.[6] This has led to a national push by the National Highway Traffic Safety Administration and the National Registry of Emergency Medical Technicians to adopt a standardized scope of practice for a defined set of provider certification levels, including EMT, advanced EMT, and paramedic. The advanced EMT level is able to establish supraglottic airways as well as IV access with fluid administration. This standardization is intended to reduce variation in the scope of practice for EMS providers nationally.

Unlike many European and Asian countries, there is little direct physician participation in prehospital trauma care in the United States. Most physicians involved in prehospital systems are emergency medicine trained, serving as medical directors to provide administrative and educational support, develop protocols, and provide quality assurance. Some physicians, with various levels of training, staff aeromedical units as well.

PREHOSPITAL TRAUMA EDUCATION

Provider courses vary with state licensure requirements; however, a typical EMT course is composed of 120 to 150 hours of instruction including didactic and psychomotor skills. The advanced EMT course may require up to 300 hours to complete. Paramedic courses are typically conducted as a 2-year associate program.

Most initial and recertification courses contain a modular trauma education course. There are 2 main courses in the United States that focus on prehospital trauma care (**Table 1**). The first is the Prehospital Trauma Life Support course developed by the American College of Surgeons Committee on Trauma and the National Association of Emergency Medical Technicians. The course is framed around Advanced Trauma Life Support principles and approach. The second course is International Trauma Life Support. This course emphasizes a flexible, team-centered algorithmic approach and is endorsed by the American College of Emergency Physicians.

CHALLENGES OF THE PREHOSPITAL ENVIRONMENT

The prehospital environment presents several challenges that may be unfamiliar to the hospital-based provider. The most important issue EMS providers must constantly keep in mind is their own safety. The primary foundation taught to all prehospital providers is to first ensure scene safety before proceeding with any assessment or treatment. Threats to the EMS provider can come in many forms, including hostile patients or bystanders, unstable structures or vehicles, exposure to hazardous chemicals, or inattentive road traffic. Furthermore, prehospital providers are at a significantly increased risk of injury and death from ambulance crashes.[7,8]

The prehospital setting also poses environmental hazards and access to injured patients may be challenging owing to difficult terrain and patient entrapment. Depending on geography, providers must endure temperature extremes, as well as be prepared

Table 1
Similarities and differences in prehospital trauma care education

	Prehospital Trauma Life Support[a]	International Trauma Life Support[b]
Society endorsement	American College of Surgeons Committee on Trauma	American College of Emergency Physicians
Global reach	59 countries	35 countries
Types of courses offered	Provider, refresher, instructor	Provider, refresher, instructor
Special courses offered	First Responders, for care before EMS arrival	Military, Pediatric, Motor Vehicle Collision Access
Duration of provider course	16 h (instruction and skills training)	16 h (instruction and skills training)
Basic content	Scene assessment, patient assessment/management, organ system or region of injury, mechanism of injury, special populations: pediatric, geriatric, burns	
Additional content	Disaster management, mass casualties, wilderness medicine, role of civilians	Trauma in pregnancy, trauma arrest

[a] *Data from* National Association of Emergency Medical Technicians. Available at: http://www.naemt.org/education/PHTLS/phtls.aspx.
[b] *Data from* International Trauma Life Support. Available at: https://www.itrauma.org/education/itls-provider/.

to treat their patients for these issues. EMS agencies are integral in the first response to natural disasters and providers are subject to the attendant hazards.

Finally, the prehospital environment is limited in the availability of resources. Prehospital providers must quickly assess and treat patients on presumptive findings, because there are few diagnostic modalities available to them. Supplies are limited to what can be carried to the patient initially and subsequently what can be stored in the ambulance. Environmental and temperature issues may further limit the supplies that can be stocked.

TRIAGE

Field triage is one of the most important aspects of prehospital trauma care, because EMS providers using limited data must decide whether an injured patient requires transport to a trauma center for specialized care. The ASCOT and the Centers for Disease Control and Prevention jointly developed the National Field Triage Guidelines, which are based on the stepwise identification of 4 aspects of clinical presentation that are readily identifiable to prehospital providers at the scene of injury (**Fig. 1**).[9] These include physiologic criteria, anatomic criteria, mechanism of injury criteria, and special considerations criteria that are evaluated in a sequential fashion to identify patients who should be transported to a trauma center. Physiologic and anatomic criteria should prompt providers to transport patients to the highest level of trauma care in the system, whereas patients with only mechanism or special consideration criteria may be taken to lower levels of care.

Performance of the field triage guidelines has demonstrated high specificity, particularly for physiologic and anatomic criteria, although the sensitivity is variable.[10–14] Some have shown that all sequential steps are necessary to prevent unacceptable rates of undertriage.[15,16] There is also increasing evidence that geriatric patients are often undertriaged,[17–20] leading to some to develop geriatric-specific criteria.[13,21–23] The most recent revision of the guidelines notes that a normal systolic blood pressure may represent hypotension in the geriatric population.[24] More objective criteria have shown promise, such as prehospital lactate and automatic crash notification data, and are subject to ongoing study.[25–29]

An increasingly relevant aspect of field triage is mass casualty triage. When the demand of patients overwhelms existing resources, a shift in focus is required. The philosophy of mass casualty triage is to do the greatest good for the greatest number of patients. This includes rapid identification of salvageable patients and prioritization for evacuation and transport. Resources are not expended on patients who have a low likelihood of survival. Several mass casualty triage systems exist. Multiple emergency medicine and trauma association endorse the SALT algorithm (Sort, Assess, Life-saving interventions, Treatment/Transport).[30] This algorithm (**Fig. 2**) begins with global assessment of patients who can walk, have purposeful movement, and those who are not moving or have obvious life-threatening injuries. This is followed by individual assessment and provision of simple life-saving maneuvers, such as basic hemorrhage control and opening the airway. This allows the on-scene triage of patients into 4 categories of minimal, delayed, immediate, and dead/expectant to prioritize patients for treatment and transport. Commercially available triage tags are often used to designate patients during the triage process with color-coded tags: black for dead or expectant, red for immediate, yellow for delayed, and green for minimal.

PREHOSPITAL PROVIDER ASSESSMENT AND CARE

Even in the prehospital environment, a systematic approach to the injured patient is required. Most prehospital providers follow a familiar approach of the ABCDs. Prehospital providers perform their assessment with attention to cervical spine precautions and immobilization first. This is applied liberally; however, some states have introduced more selective cervical spine protocols for the injured patient.[31] Some have also moved away from use of long backboards and focus on cervical spine motion restriction only. A good example of patients who do not need to be immobilized are patients with penetrating trauma. In fact, in these patients, it could be detrimental.

Airway

Prehospital providers begin with an immediate assessment of the airway, often by attempting to communicate with the patient. In patients with airway concerns, the first step is to attempt simple maneuvers to open the airway. This is usually a jaw thrust in the trauma patient, owing to cervical spine precautions. Additional adjuncts include placement of an oral pharyngeal or nasal pharyngeal airway and can be performed by BLS providers.

ALS providers can perform ETI. Indications most commonly include failure to protect the airway followed by inadequate ventilation or oxygenation. Depending on state and local protocols, paramedics may be able to perform rapid sequence intubation using pharmacologic sedation and paralysis. Controversy exists as to the benefit of prehospital ETI in trauma patients. Several groups have demonstrated worse outcomes in trauma patients undergoing ETI,[32–38] whereas others have shown improved outcomes.[39–41] Episodes of hypoxia, bradycardia, and inadvertent hyperventilation, as well as procedural complications and errors have been postulated to contribute to worse outcomes,[34,36,38] suggesting the need for rigorous performance improvement and continual training to maintain skill levels.[42] An option with increasing popularity is the use of supraglottic airways in the trauma patient. These airways require

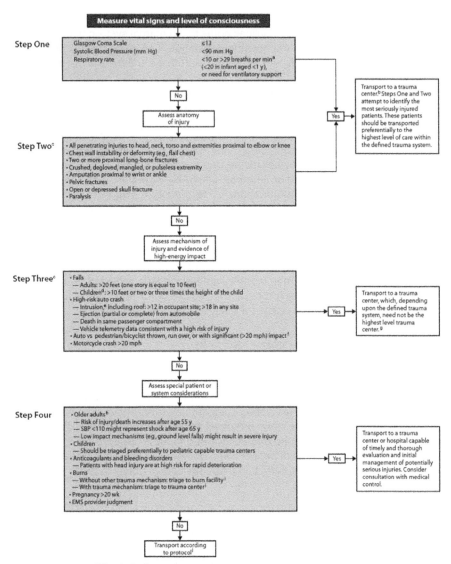

Fig. 1. American College of Surgeons Committee of Trauma and Centers for Disease Control National Trauma Triage Protocol, 2011. EMS, emergency medical services. [a] The upper limit of respiratory rate in infants is greater than 29 breaths per minute to maintain a higher level of overtriage for infants. [b] Trauma centers are designated levels I to IV. A level I center has the greatest amount of resources and personnel for care of the injured patient and provides regional leadership in education, research, and prevention programs. A level II facility offers similar resources to a level I facility, possibly differing only in continuous availability of certain subspecialties or sufficient prevention, education, and research activities for a level I designation; level II facilities are not required to be resident or fellow education centers. A level III center is capable of assessment, resuscitation, and emergency surgery, with severely injured patients being transferred to a level I or II facility. A level IV trauma center is capable of providing 24-hour physician coverage, resuscitation, and stabilization to injured patients before transfer to a facility that provides a higher level of trauma care. [c] Any injury noted in

less skill maintenance and may take less time in the field to place.[43,44] These are not, however, definitive airways and thus trauma personnel must be familiar with these devices and be prepared to replace it with a definitive airway when receiving a patient with this type of airway placed by EMS.

Many EMS systems also include protocols for surgical airway placement. This may take the form of needle cricothyrotomy or surgical cricothyrotomy. This skill is rarely used in the prehospital environment, but may be the only option to secure an airway in patients with severe maxillofacial or laryngeal trauma.[45]

Breathing

After confirming a patent airway or securing one, attention is turned to breathing. Most trauma patients are placed on supplemental oxygen. Options include nasal cannula or a nonrebreather mask for patients maintaining their own airway. Prehospital providers will also provide ventilations using a bag–valve mask for patients not adequately ventilating. BLS providers are trained to provide bag–valve mask respirations in conjunction with the oral or nasal airway adjuncts noted. For patients with an advanced airway placed in the field, respirations are provided using a bag–valve mask. Some agencies have access to transport ventilators that can be quite sophisticated, allowing for different volume or pressure control modes of ventilation and provide user-defined levels of positive end-expiratory pressure.

EMS providers are also trained to assess respirations with auscultation. In the trauma patient, they assess for signs of pneumothorax and signs of tension; however, subtle examination findings are difficult to appreciate in the prehospital environment. ALS providers are able to perform chest decompression for suspected tension pneumothorax. Patients with diminished breath sounds or signs of respiratory distress such as increased work of breathing, poor oxygen saturation, or signs of shock may be candidates for decompression.

Standard technique includes insertion of a 14-gauge angiocatheter in the second intercostal space in the midclavicular line. Several studies have shown that standard angiocatheters are not long enough to adequately decompress the pleural space.[46–48] This concern has led many agencies to use longer and stiffer commercial products designed specifically for chest decompression. Further, placement of the catheter or even finger thoracostomy in the fourth or fifth intercostal space anterior axillary line has become an acceptable alternative based on studies that the chest wall may be thinner in this location.[49,50]

---

step 2 or mechanism identified in step 3 triggers a "yes" response. [d] Age less than 15 years. [e] Intrusion refers to interior compartment intrusion, as opposed to deformation, which refers to exterior damage. [f] Includes pedestrians or bicyclists thrown or run over by a motor vehicle or those with estimated impact of greater than 20 mph with a motor vehicle. [g] Local or regional protocols should be used to determine the most appropriate level of trauma center within the defined trauma system; need not be the highest-level trauma center. [h] Age greater than 55 years. [i] Patients with both burns and concomitant trauma for whom the burn injury poses the greatest risk for morbidity and mortality should be transferred to a burn center. If the nonburn trauma presents a greater immediate risk, the patient may be stabilized in a trauma center and then transferred to a burn center. [j] Patients who do not meet any of the triage criteria in steps 1 through 4 should be transported to the most appropriate medical facility as outlined in local EMS protocols. (*From* Sasser SM, Hunt RC, Faul M, et al. Guidelines for field triage of injured patients: recommendations of the National Expert Panel on Field Triage, 2011. MMWR Recomm Rep 2012;61:1–20.)

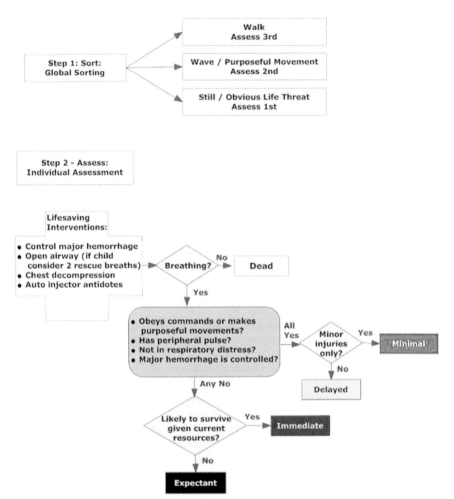

Fig. 2. Sort, Assess, Lifesaving interventions, Treatment/Transport (SALT) algorithm. (*From* SALT mass casualty triage: concept endorsed by the American College of Emergency Physicians, American College of Surgeons Committee on Trauma, American Trauma Society, National Association of EMS Physicians, National Disaster Life Support Education Consortium, and State and Territorial Injury Prevention Directors Association. Disaster Med Public Health Prep 2008;2(4):245; with permission.)

Circulation

Once the airway is secure and the patient is adequately ventilating, attention is turned to the patient's circulatory needs. Because it remains a major cause of morbidity and mortality, significant attention is given to active hemorrhage. A patient can bleed to death internally in the chest, abdomen, pelvis, or thigh. Furthermore, a patient can exsanguinate externally from many sites especially extremities and scalp. For life-threatening external hemorrhage, care can involve providing adequate fluid or blood products, if necessary and possible, and applying external hemorrhage control techniques.

Many of the current recommendations stem from the US military's recent experience in Iraq and Afghanistan, where there were increased rates of external hemorrhage.[51–56]

An increased focus on preparedness for active shooter scenarios[57,58] and awareness of the importance of early hemorrhage control in all trauma patients[54] has inspired specific guidelines for civilian settings as well. Several methods for external hemorrhage control exist today, including packing or pressure dressing, with or without hemostatic agents, as well as commercially available tourniquets. However, the most traditional method of curbing an active bleed and also the initial step in first aid is to apply direct manual pressure with or without gauze or cloth dressing to sites of hemorrhage until hemostasis is achieved.[59,60]

When direct pressure is not possible (eg, owing to limited staff or resources, unsafe scene of injury, or the need for complicated transportation of the patient) or when direct pressure alone is futile (eg, significant arterial bleed), tourniquets should be used for controlling external hemorrhage, especially at amenable extremity sites.[54,56,59,60] Commercially tested tourniquets are regarded as superior to improvised ones and should always be used first,[54,61–63] although improvised tourniquets may be beneficial in limited civilian settings when no commercial one is available.[64–66] Several types of commercial tourniquets exist, with windlass, pneumatic, or ratcheting types preferred by the American College of Surgeons Committee on Trauma, although this recommendation is based on limited data. Use of a narrow, elastic, or bungee-type device may worsen hemorrhage owing to venous occlusion without adequate arterial occlusion.[54]

Regardless of which tourniquet is selected, it is likely best to keep effective tourniquets in place until definitive treatment can be provided; however, exceptions may exist such as long transport times.[54] When placed properly, tourniquets have been shown to adequately control bleeding.[53,63–69] However, it is important to understand that this method of hemorrhage control is not without a risk of complications, for example, compartment syndrome, nerve damage, vascular damage, and amputation.[60] The rate of these complications, however, remains very low.[53,63–69] Despite well-documented evidence backing the early use of tourniquets, average prehospital care provider knowledge of this hemorrhage control technique may still be poor and highlights the need for further education and protocols.[70] Nonextremity tourniquets such as junctional tourniquets, designed for hemorrhage from the axilla or groin, have also shown some promise and there are multiple devices that have been approved by the US Food and Drug Administration,[59,71] although efficacy data are too sparse to make any recommendations on their use and this remains an open area for investigation.[54]

For anatomic regions that are not amenable to tourniquet use, such as neck, trunk, axillae, or groin wounds, and when direct pressure is simply not enough, topical hemostatic agents with packing or dressing may be useful.[54,56,60,72] Several agents have shown promise, including chitosan-based HemCon[73] and zeolite-based QuikClot.[74] Currently, the military uses kaolin-infused QuikClot Combat Gauze, which has some evidence backing its use,[75] as well as chitosan-based gauze products.[62] The ACS has recommended that regardless of which hemostatic agent is used, based on military experience, it should be used with gauze as the applicator; however, little evidence exists to make clear guidelines on the subject at this time.[54]

After assessing the patient for external bleeding and applying the appropriate hemorrhage control techniques, ALS providers will attempt to establish IV access when feasible; however, this should not delay transport, which can significantly increase prehospital time.[76,77] Attempts to establish peripheral IV access should be limited to 2 in the field, after which alternative routes should be attempted if necessary.[78] Intraosseous access has gained popularity among prehospital providers, owing to its technical ease and speed to obtain access for fluid and medication delivery.[79]

Crystalloid remains the de facto resuscitation fluid for prehospital care. It is inexpensive, widely available, and durable in the prehospital environment. Current practice has moved away from large crystalloid volumes in the prehospital setting as it has in hospital, starting with the landmark trial by Bickell and colleagues,[80] which demonstrated increased mortality in penetrating torso injury patients receiving prehospital crystalloid. Although several others have reported increased mortality with greater volumes of crystalloid, particularly in patients with normal blood pressure,[76,81,82] this has not been a universal finding and some report benefits in select populations, such as traumatic brain injury (TBI) and hypotensive patients.[78,81,83–89] Thus, a goal-directed protocol of judicious crystalloid use based on mental status and avoiding hypotension may be the best approach.[78]

The potential deleterious effects of crystalloid have led to an investigation of the use of prehospital blood products. United States and United Kingdom military have implemented prehospital transfusion of packed red blood cells for casualties at the point of wounding,[51,90] with promising results.[91–93] This practice has heightened interest in the civilian prehospital community, although generally limited to well-developed air medical transport programs.[94,95] However, initial evidence suggests that the use of packed red blood cells and plasma improves early outcomes in severely injured patients, including reductions in early mortality, indices of shock and coagulopathy, and need for in-hospital transfusion.[96–98]

Disability

Disability is, in essence, a neurologic evaluation. For EMS providers, assessing the patient's level of consciousness is of particular importance in evaluating TBI. Several scales exist to stratify deficits in consciousness; a classic scale for assessing consciousness is the AVPU or Alert, Responds to Voice, Responds to Pain, Unresponsive scale, which was initially a component of the primary survey by Advanced Trauma Life Support.[99] However, this scale has largely been replaced by the Glasgow Coma Scale (GCS) score. First devised in 1974, the GCS consists of 3 components based on the patient's arousal, awareness, and activity: eye opening (scored out of 4), verbal response (scored out of 5), and best motor response (scored out of 6). Patients receive a score out of 15, with a score of 3 being the lowest score possible and indicating significant deficits.[100]

Multiple studies have shown that the GCS collected in the field by prehospital providers is similar to that collected by the accepting emergency department with good interrater reliability[101,102]; however, as the GCS worsens, there may be more significant differences.[103,104] Also, it is important to note that for shorter response times, the GCS recorded in the field may be inaccurate if recorded during a "concussive" period after injury. Regardless, prehospital GCS[105,106] and delta, or change in GCS from field to arrival,[107] have both been shown to be predictive of outcome. More recently, the GCSm, or the motor subscale of the GCS, which can be measured even in intubated patients, has been shown to be a suitable replacement for predicting outcomes.[108,109] In the prehospital setting, a GCSm of 5 or less has been shown to be more specific and less sensitive compared to a GCS of 13 or less and may better predict trauma center need.[110]

In the context of TBI, serial GCS scores can be helpful in evaluating suspected increased intracranial pressure (ICP). If a patient begins to show signs of cerebral herniation (eg, asymmetric pupil sizes >1 mm, dilated and fixed pupils, extensor posturing, or a decline in GCS by 2 points from an initial score of ≤8), it is important that measures are taken in the field to lower ICP.[111,112] These may include hyperventilating the patient or providing pharmacologic or hyperosmolar agents; however, these interventions should not slow down transfer to definitive neurosurgical care.[111]

Although hyperventilation, with resultant hypocarbia, is a classic measure for reducing ICP in the setting of acute brainstem herniation in TBI, excessive hyperventilation may result in further damage owing to reduced cerebral blood flow.[111,113] The latest Brain Trauma Foundation guidelines on prehospital management recommend that hyperventilation, ETCO$_2$ of less than 35 mm Hg, only be used when there are clear signs of herniation; otherwise, the goal ETCO$_2$ of 35 to 40 mm Hg should be used to guide ventilation.[114] Failure to achieve these targets is an indicator of severe injury and has been shown to predict poor outcome.[115] Despite guidelines limiting the use of hyperventilation to those with clear signs of herniation, there seems to be a disparity between the guidelines and actual prehospital practice.[111] To avoid excessive use or even prophylactic use of hyperventilation, some have suggested either uniform normoventilation in the prehospital setting or stricter adherence of the Brain Trauma Foundation guidelines.[113] We strongly suggest that normoventilation should be the standard default practice in the field for the vast majority of cases.

With regard to hyperosmolar therapy, mannitol and hypertonic saline are both well-known methods of lowering ICP; however, there are very few efficacy data on their use in the prehospital setting.[114] The management of an increased ICP in the prehospital setting is still an emerging field and there is no clear consensus between the various guidelines that exist on which prehospital interventions to recommend.[116] In general, guidelines for managing TBI patients in the prehospital setting are sparse. However, the appropriate transfer and triage of these patients has been shown to have a positive effect on outcome.[117] In fact, some areas of the country have been able to demonstrate both improved short- and long-term outcomes in patients with TBI after the creation of a regional trauma system.[118,119]

TRANSPORT TO THE TRAUMA CENTER

A key function of the EMS system is to deliver the patient to the trauma center for further assessment and care. For trauma patients, controversy exists in the philosophical approach to this, often characterized as the "scoop and run" approach compared with the "stay and play" approach. Scoop and run postulates that time is the most important factor and EMS providers should transport the patient as rapidly as safely possible, providing minimal or no interventions in the prehospital setting. Several groups have reported no benefit to the use of ALS interventions among trauma patients.[77,120–122] Conversely, the stay and play approach advocates providing critical interventions to the injured patients in the field, proponents of which argue will occur much more quickly than if delayed to be performed in the hospital. Some investigators have demonstrated improved outcomes with prehospital interventions in select populations.[41]

Likely a balance between these approaches is necessary to provide optimal prehospital trauma care, avoiding a "one size fits all" approach. There is evidence that existing field triage criteria, including hypotension, penetrating injury, and flail chest can identify patients with truly time-sensitive injuries that may benefit from limited prehospital time.[123] For example, the Northern Ohio Trauma System developed and implemented both scene and interhospital transfer criteria with the philosophy of getting the "right patient to the right place at the right time." This policy was demonstrated to be an independent predictor of improved survival.[124] Regionalization and the appropriate transport of patients to an experienced level 1 center, has also been shown to reduce mortality in those requiring an exploratory trauma laparotomy[125] (**Fig. 3**).

Another issue prehospital providers must consider is the mode of transport to the trauma center. In general, this is a decision between ground and air transport. At

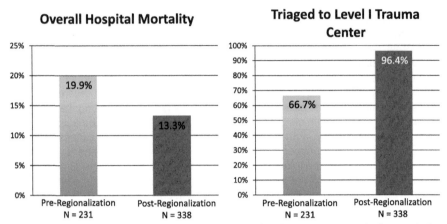

Fig. 3. Overall hospital mortality and triage rate to a level 1 trauma center before and after regionalization of a trauma network.

the individual patient level, this becomes a highly complex decision, because providers must consider physiologic and anatomic injury severity of the patient, distance to the trauma center, traffic and weather conditions, and the availability of EMS resources in the local area.

Patients may benefit from air medical transport for several reasons. First, it is widely accepted that air is faster than ground transport. Prehospital trauma care from air medical crews may also benefit patients, either owing to advanced capabilities or "regionalized" prehospital trauma care, because these providers are more familiar with caring for severely injured patients.[97,126] For example, several studies suggest airway management in the hands of air medical providers have better outcomes when compared with ground EMS providers.[36,37,40,42,123] Finally, air transport may expand access to trauma care for patients who otherwise would be taken to a nontrauma center.[127]

Again, there is conflicting evidence regarding the potential benefits of air medical transport. Several studies have found no survival benefit for patients undergoing transport,[128–132] whereas others report significant improvements in mortality among patients transported by air.[126,133–137] Additionally, some only report a benefit from air medical transport in selected groups of patients.[128,130,138,139] However, overtriage of patients to air medical transport is common, even among studies reporting benefits.[123,133,136] Given the costs of this trauma system resource and aviation risk, patient selection becomes paramount.[7,8,140,141] Few studies have examined the issue of air medical transport triage until recently.[142,143] The development of the Air Medical Prehospital Triage score (criteria for air transport displayed in **Table 2**) has been the first attempt at an evidence based approach to air medical triage; preliminary data have shown it to be successful in discriminating between patients who have a survival benefit from air medical transport and those who do not, based on a subset of field triage criteria.[144,145]

INTERFACILITY TRANSPORT

Although transport time from the scene of injury to an accepting facility is one component of prehospital care, another equally important aspect is the transport of patients to their appropriate final destination based on their needs. In an ideal world, EMS will

Table 2	
Air AMPT criteria	
Criterion	**Points**
Glasgow Coma Scale <14	1
Respiratory rate <10 or >29 breaths/min	1
Unstable chest wall fractures	1
Suspected hemothorax or pneumothorax	1
Paralysis	1
Multisystem trauma	1
Any 1 physiologic criterion[a] plus any 1 anatomic criterion[b] from the ACSCOT national field triage guidelines	2
Consider Helicopter Transport if AMPT Score ≥2 points	

Abbreviations: AMPT, Air medical prehospital transport; ACSCOT, American College of Surgeons Committee on Trauma.

[a] ACSCOT Physiologic Criterion: GCS of 13 or greater, systolic blood pressure of less than 90 mm Hg, respiratory rate of less than 10 or greater than 29 breaths per minute (<20 in infants aged <1 y), or need for ventilator support.

[b] ACSCOT anatomic criterion: All penetrating injuries to head, neck, torso, and extremities proximal to elbow or knee; chest wall instability or deformity (eg, flail chest); amputation proximal to wrist or ankle; 2 or more proximal long bone fractures (ie, femur and humerus); crushed, degloved, mangled, or pulseless extremity; pelvic fractures; open or depressed skull fracture; paralysis.

From Brown JB, Gestring ML, Guyette FX, et al. Development and validation of the air medical prehospital triage score for helicopter transport of trauma patients. Ann Surg 2016;264(2):382; with permission.

triage and directly transport the most severely injured patients to level 1 trauma centers. However, several situations may exist where interfacility transfers, from lower level centers or community hospitals to level 1 centers, are inevitable. In rural regions, as a consequence of the scarcity of trauma centers, patients may need to be stabilized at local community hospitals first. Studies have shown that, in such regions, this pattern of transport versus direct transport to a trauma center does not worsen mortality,[146] although in the rural setting this pattern may result in more transfers of minimally injured patients owing to inexperience or overtriage by the transferring hospital.[147]

In urban regions with more mature trauma systems, initial undertriage of patients, to ease the burden on level 1 trauma centers, may later result in increased interfacility transports. Although this pattern of transport uses significant resources at lower level centers and is overall more expensive, it has minimal impact on mortality.[148] The cost burden from inefficient triage and subsequent interfacility transfers may be due to repeat procedures and imaging at the final destination,[149] as well as an increased emergency department duration of stay.[150] Similar to the debate on air versus ground scene of injury transport, more research is needed on interfacility transport to find specific populations that may benefit from particular transportation modes. Although more severely injured patients, an Injury Severity Score of greater than 15, may benefit from helicopter transport in interfacility transfers,[139] when crew experience and ALS capabilities are controlled for there may also be no difference in outcomes.[151] However, distance between facilities may also play a role in this decision.

REGIONALIZATION OF SYSTEMS AND UNIFORM PROTOCOLS

The goal of our prehospital trauma systems is to essentially "get the right patient to the right place at the right time."[152] However, the question of what is the right place for each patient may vary depending on the needs of the patient, the severity of injury, distance to each potential caregiving facility, and the capabilities of these accepting facilities to provide appropriate care. This question of what is the right place will vary region to region, because some urban corridors may have an abundance of trauma centers per capita, whereas other more rural areas may have almost none. In regions covered by multiple separate trauma systems and EMS or in regions that cross local or state borders, competition and differences in care pathways may further complicate this issue.

"Regionalization" and Regional Trauma Networks have evolved as 1 approach to standardizing and streamlining the prehospital care of the severely injured patient. By coordinating the effort and resources between all local EMS, hospitals, and hospital networks, the balance between optimal care, resource limitations and competition may be better addressed.[153,154] This may require Regional Trauma Networks to be inclusive, containing all trauma centers within a region regardless of affiliation or ownership, and also comprehensive, containing multiple lower level centers (level 2 or 3) in addition to level 1 trauma centers.[155] Many international studies on Regional Trauma Networks have shown that regionalization can reduce mortality, while improving functional outcomes.[156–161] Although data in the United States are scarcer, implementation of an inclusive and collaborative Regional Trauma Networks, with a uniform triage and transfer protocol and a single call center, has been shown to significantly improve mortality and outcomes.[118,119,125,152] These benefits may result from an increased use of lower level trauma centers for less severe injuries, less competition between centers allowing for adequate patient volume, and proper coordination between EMS and all trauma centers involved.[152,162–164]

SUMMARY

The prehospital period is an important phase in the care of all trauma patients. Because the effectiveness of early triage, interventions, and transport may be the only chance some patients have to survive, trauma providers and their networks must increasingly assess and improve this period of care. When the prehospital phase of care is implemented appropriately, it may have substantial impacts on the definitive management and long-term morbidity and mortality of trauma patients.

One particularly interesting development in prehospital care is the role of the public in providing early interventions. After the Sandy Hook Elementary School shooting that shocked the nation, a working group, later known as the Hartford Consensus, was convened to suggest national policy for enhancing survivability after intentional mass casualty and active shooter events.[58] Because uncontrolled hemorrhage remains a preventable prehospital cause of death and morbidity, a movement known as "Stop The Bleed" was created to make tourniquets more accessible to the public and to empower bystanders to act as first responders for such injuries.[165]

Although there has been much accomplished in the field of prehospital care since its genesis, there remain many open avenues for improvement and investigation. For instance, there is an incredible amount of variability in EMS prehospital provider training. Further, even more variability exists in how EMS prehospital systems are organized and function within a geographic area. Without clear, data-driven protocols guiding the appropriate triage and transfer of patients across a region, the use of local resources and facilities to care for the severely injured will be far from optimal. Achieving these goals will require more open cooperation from all stakeholders, local government, EMS providers, and hospital networks, as well as further research into best practices.

REFERENCES

1. Goniewicz M. Effect of military conflicts on the formation of emergency medical services systems worldwide. Bogucki S, ed. Acad Emerg Med 2013;20(5): 507–13.
2. Mullins RJ. A historical perspective of trauma system development in the United States. J Trauma 1999;47(3 Suppl):S8–14.
3. National Research Council. Accidental death and disability: the neglected disease of modern society. Washington, DC: National Academy of Sciences; 1966.
4. Farrington JD. Death in a ditch. Bull Am Coll Surg 1967;52(3):121–30.
5. Kupas DF, Schenk E, Sholl JM, et al. Characteristics of statewide protocols for emergency medical services in the United States. Prehosp Emerg Care 2015; 19(2):292–301.
6. National Highway Traffic Safety Administration. National EMS scope of practice model. 2007. Available at: https://www.ems.gov/education/EMSScope.pdf. Accessed January 10, 2017.
7. Blumen IJ, Lees D. Air medical safety: your first priority. In: Blumen IJ, Lemkin DL, editors. Principles and direction of air medical transport. Salt Lake City (UT): Air Medical Physician Association; 2006. p. 519–32.
8. National Highway Traffic Safety Administration. NHTSA and ground ambulance crashes. 2014. Available at: http://www.ems.gov/pdf/GroundAmbulanceCrashes Presentation.pdf. Accessed April 4, 2015.
9. Sasser SM, Hunt RC, Faul M, et al. Guidelines for field triage of injured patients: recommendations of the National Expert Panel on Field Triage, 2011. MMWR Recomm Rep 2012;61(RR-1):1–20.
10. Faul M, Wald MM, Sullivent EE, et al. Large cost savings realized from the 2006 Field Triage Guideline: reduction in overtriage in U.S. trauma centers. Prehosp Emerg Care 2012;16(2):222–9.
11. Newgard CD, Fu R, Zive D, et al. Prospective validation of the national field triage guidelines for identifying seriously injured persons. J Am Coll Surg 2016;222(2):146–58.e2.
12. Newgard CD, Hsia RY, Mann NC, et al. The trade-offs in field trauma triage: a multiregion assessment of accuracy metrics and volume shifts associated with different triage strategies. J Trauma Acute Care Surg 2013;74(5): 1298–306 [discussion: 1306].
13. Newgard CD, Richardson D, Holmes JF, et al. Physiologic field triage criteria for identifying seriously injured older adults. Prehosp Emerg Care 2014;18(4): 461–70.
14. Newgard CD, Zive D, Holmes JF, et al. A multisite assessment of the American College of Surgeons Committee on Trauma field triage decision scheme for identifying seriously injured children and adults. J Am Coll Surg 2011;213(6): 709–21.
15. Brown JB, Stassen NA, Bankey PE, et al. Mechanism of injury and special consideration criteria still matter: an evaluation of the National Trauma Triage Protocol. J Trauma 2011;70(1):38–44 [discussion: 44–5].
16. Haider AH, Chang DC, Haut ER, et al. Mechanism of injury predicts patient mortality and impairment after blunt trauma. J Surg Res 2009;153(1):138–42.
17. Chang DC, Bass RR, Cornwell EE, et al. Undertriage of elderly trauma patients to state-designated trauma centers. Arch Surg 2008;143(8):776–81 [discussion: 782].

18. Lehmann R, Beekley A, Casey L, et al. The impact of advanced age on trauma triage decisions and outcomes: a statewide analysis. Am J Surg 2009;197(5): 571–4 [discussion: 574–5].

19. Nakamura Y, Daya M, Bulger EM, et al. Evaluating age in the field triage of injured persons. Ann Emerg Med 2012;60(3):335–45.

20. Rogers A, Rogers F, Bradburn E, et al. Old and undertriaged: a lethal combination. Am Surg 2012;78(6):711–5.

21. Caterino JM, Raubenolt A, Cudnik MT. Modification of Glasgow Coma Scale criteria for injured elders. Acad Emerg Med 2011;18(10):1014–21.

22. Werman HA, Erskine T, Caterino J, et al, Members of the Trauma Committee of the State of Ohio EMSB. Development of statewide geriatric patients trauma triage criteria. Prehosp Disaster Med 2011;26(3):170–9.

23. Brown JB, Gestring ML, Forsythe RM, et al. Systolic blood pressure criteria in the National Trauma Triage Protocol for geriatric trauma: 110 is the new 90. J Trauma Acute Care Surg 2015;78(2):352–9.

24. Oyetunji TA, Chang DC, Crompton JG, et al. Redefining hypotension in the elderly: normotension is not reassuring. Arch Surg 2011;146(7):865–9.

25. Guyette F, Suffoletto B, Castillo JL, et al. Prehospital serum lactate as a predictor of outcomes in trauma patients: a retrospective observational study. J Trauma 2011;70(4):782–6.

26. Guyette FX, Meier E, Kerby J, et al. Prehospital lactate for identification of the need for resuscitative care in trauma patients transported by air. Chicago: American Heart Association; 2014.

27. Guyette FX, Meier EN, Newgard C, et al. A comparison of prehospital lactate and systolic blood pressure for predicting the need for resuscitative care in trauma transported by ground. J Trauma Acute Care Surg 2015;78(3):600–6.

28. Ayoung-Chee P, Mack CD, Kaufman R, et al. Predicting severe injury using vehicle telemetry data. J Trauma Acute Care Surg 2013;74(1):190–4 [discussion: 194–5].

29. Davidson GH, Rivara FP, Mack CD, et al. Validation of prehospital trauma triage criteria for motor vehicle collisions. J Trauma Acute Care Surg 2014;76(3): 755–61.

30. SALT mass casualty triage: concept endorsed by the American College of Emergency Physicians, American College of Surgeons Committee on Trauma, American Trauma Society, National Association of EMS Physicians, National Disaster Life Support Education Consortium, and State and Territorial Injury Prevention Directors Association. Disaster Med Public Health Prep 2008;2(4): 245–6.

31. White CCT, Domeier RM, Millin MG, Standards and Clinical Practice Committee, National Association of EMS Physicians. EMS spinal precautions and the use of the long backboard - resource document to the position statement of the National Association of EMS Physicians and the American College of Surgeons Committee on Trauma. Prehosp Emerg Care 2014;18(2):306–14.

32. Bukur M, Kurtovic S, Berry C, et al. Pre-hospital intubation is associated with increased mortality after traumatic brain injury. J Surg Res 2011;170(1): e117–21.

33. Chou D, Harada MY, Barmparas G, et al. Field intubation in civilian patients with hemorrhagic shock is associated with higher mortality. J Trauma Acute Care Surg 2016;80(2):278–82.

34. Davis DP, Peay J, Sise MJ, et al. The impact of prehospital endotracheal intubation on outcome in moderate to severe traumatic brain injury. J Trauma 2005; 58(5):933–9.
35. Irvin CB, Szpunar S, Cindrich LA, et al. Should trauma patients with a Glasgow Coma Scale score of 3 be intubated prior to hospital arrival? Prehosp Disaster Med 2010;25:541–6.
36. Wang HE, Peitzman AB, Cassidy LD, et al. Out-of-hospital endotracheal intubation and outcome after traumatic brain injury. Ann Emerg Med 2004;44(5): 439–50.
37. Cudnik MT, Newgard CD, Wang H, et al. Distance impacts mortality in trauma patients with an intubation attempt. Prehosp Emerg Care 2008;12(4):459–66.
38. Davis DP, Hoyt DB, Ochs M, et al. The effect of paramedic rapid sequence intubation on outcome in patients with severe traumatic brain injury. J Trauma 2003; 54(3):444–53.
39. Bernard SA, Nguyen V, Cameron P, et al. Prehospital rapid sequence intubation improves functional outcome for patients with severe traumatic brain injury: a randomized controlled trial. Ann Surg 2010;252(6):959–65.
40. Davis DP, Peay J, Sise MJ, et al. Prehospital airway and ventilation management: a trauma score and injury severity score-based analysis. J Trauma 2010;69(2):294–301.
41. Meizoso JP, Valle EJ, Allen CJ, et al. Decreased mortality after prehospital interventions in severely injured trauma patients. J Trauma Acute Care Surg 2015; 79(2):227–31.
42. Fakhry SM, Scanlon JM, Robinson L, et al. Prehospital rapid sequence intubation for head trauma: conditions for a successful program. J Trauma 2006;60(5): 997–1001.
43. Burns JBJ, Branson R, Barnes SL, et al. Emergency airway placement by EMS providers: comparison between the King LT supralaryngeal airway and endotracheal intubation. Prehosp Disaster Med 2010;25(1):92–5.
44. Kajino K, Iwami T, Kitamura T, et al. Comparison of supraglottic airway versus endotracheal intubation for the pre-hospital treatment of out-of-hospital cardiac arrest. Crit Care 2011;15(5):R236.
45. Fortune JB, Judkins DG, Scanzaroli D, et al. Efficacy of prehospital surgical cricothyrotomy in trauma patients. J Trauma Acute Care Surg 1997;42(5):832–8.
46. Ball CG, Wyrzykowski AD, Kirkpatrick AW, et al. Thoracic needle decompression for tension pneumothorax: clinical correlation with catheter length. Can J Surg 2010;53(3):184–8.
47. Carter TE, Mortensen CD, Kaistha S, et al. Needle decompression in Appalachia: do obese patients need longer needles? West J Emerg Med 2013;14(6): 650–2.
48. Stevens RL, Rochester AA, Busko J, et al. Needle thoracostomy for tension pneumothorax: failure predicted by chest computed tomography. Prehosp Emerg Care 2009;13(1):14–7.
49. Chang SJ, Ross SW, Kiefer DJ, et al. Evaluation of 8.0-cm needle at the fourth anterior axillary line for needle chest decompression of tension pneumothorax. J Trauma Acute Care Surg 2014;76(4):1029–34.
50. Deakin CD, Davies G, Wilson A. Simple thoracostomy avoids chest drain insertion in prehospital trauma. J Trauma 1995;39(2):373–4.
51. Eastridge BJ, Mabry RL, Seguin P, et al. Death on the battlefield (2001–2011). J Trauma Acute Care Surg 2012;73:S431–7.

52. Kelly JF, Ritenour AE, McLaughlin DF, et al. Injury severity and causes of death from Operation Iraqi Freedom and Operation Enduring Freedom: 2003-2004 versus 2006. J Trauma 2008;64(2 Suppl):S21–6 [discussion: S26–7].
53. Beekley AC, Sebesta JA, Blackbourne LH, et al. Prehospital tourniquet use in Operation Iraqi Freedom: effect on hemorrhage control and outcomes. J Trauma 2008;64(Supplement):S28–37.
54. Bulger EM, Snyder D, Schoelles K, et al. An evidence-based prehospital guideline for external hemorrhage control: American College of Surgeons Committee on Trauma. Prehosp Emerg Care 2014;18(2):163–73.
55. Kragh JF, Swan KG, Smith DC, et al. Historical review of emergency tourniquet use to stop bleeding. Am J Surg 2012;203(2):242–52.
56. Butler FK, Blackbourne LH. Battlefield trauma care then and now: a decade of tactical combat casualty care. J Trauma Acute Care Surg 2012;73(6 Suppl 5): S395–402.
57. Walls RM, Zinner MJ. The Boston Marathon Response. JAMA 2013;309(23): 2441.
58. Pons PT, Jerome J, McMullen J, et al. The Hartford Consensus on active shooters: implementing the continuum of prehospital trauma response. J Emerg Med 2015;49(6):878–85.
59. Drew B, Bennett BL, Littlejohn L. Application of current hemorrhage control techniques for backcountry care: part one, tourniquets and hemorrhage control adjuncts. Wilderness Environ Med 2015;26(2):236–45.
60. Singletary EM, Charlton NP, Epstein JL, et al. Part 15: first aid. Circulation 2015; 132(18 suppl 2):S574–89.
61. Kragh JF, Walters TJ, Baer DG, et al. Practical use of emergency tourniquets to stop bleeding in major limb trauma. J Trauma 2008;64(2 Suppl):S38–49 [discussion: S49–50].
62. Callaway DW, Smith ER, Cain J, et al. Tactical emergency casualty care (TECC): guidelines for the provision of prehospital trauma care in high threat environments. J Spec Oper Med 2011;11(3):104–22.
63. Kragh JF. Use of tourniquets and their effects on limb function in the modern combat environment. Foot Ankle Clin 2010;15(1):23–40.
64. Inaba K, Siboni S, Resnick S, et al. Tourniquet use for civilian extremity trauma. J Trauma Acute Care Surg 2015;79(2):232–7 [quiz: 332–3].
65. Schroll R, Smith A, McSwain NE, et al. A multi-institutional analysis of prehospital tourniquet use. J Trauma Acute Care Surg 2015;79(1):10–4 [discussion: 14].
66. Kue RC, Temin ES, Weiner SG, et al. Tourniquet use in a civilian emergency medical services setting: a descriptive analysis of the Boston EMS Experience. Prehosp Emerg Care 2015;19(3):399–404.
67. Lakstein D, Blumenfeld A, Sokolov T, et al. Tourniquets for hemorrhage control on the battlefield: a 4-year accumulated experience. J Trauma 2003;54(5 Suppl):S221–5.
68. Ode G, Studnek J, Seymour R, et al. Emergency tourniquets for civilians. J Trauma Acute Care Surg 2015;79(4):586–91.
69. Kragh JF Jr, Walters TJ, Baer DG, et al. Survival with emergency tourniquet use to stop bleeding in major limb trauma. Ann Surg 2009;249(1):1–7.
70. Wall PL, Welander JD, Smith HL, et al. What do the people who transport trauma patients know about tourniquets? J Trauma Acute Care Surg 2014;77(5):734–42.
71. Kragh JF, Kotwal RS, Cap AP, et al. Performance of junctional tourniquets in normal human volunteers. Prehosp Emerg Care 2015;19(3):391–8.

72. Littlejohn L, Bennett BL, Drew B. Application of current hemorrhage control techniques for backcountry care: part two, hemostatic dressings and other adjuncts. Wilderness Environ Med 2015;26(2):246–54.
73. Wedmore I, McManus JG, Pusateri AE, et al. A special report on the chitosan-based hemostatic dressing: experience in current combat operations. J Trauma 2006;60(3):655–8.
74. Rhee P, Brown C, Martin M, et al. QuikClot use in trauma for hemorrhage control: case series of 103 documented uses. J Trauma 2008;64(4):1093–9.
75. Shina A, Lipsky AM, Nadler R, et al. Prehospital use of hemostatic dressings by the Israel Defense Forces Medical Corps. J Trauma Acute Care Surg 2015;79: S204–9.
76. Sampalis JS, Tamim H, Denis R, et al. Ineffectiveness of on-site intravenous lines: is prehospital time the culprit? J Trauma Acute Care Surg 1997;43(4): 608–17.
77. Smith JP, Bodai BI, Hill AS, et al. Prehospital stabilization of critically injured patients: a failed concept. J Trauma Acute Care Surg 1985;25(1):65–70.
78. Cotton BA, Jerome R, Collier BR, et al. Guidelines for prehospital fluid resuscitation in the injured patient. J Trauma Acute Care Surg 2009;67(2):389–402.
79. Frascone RJ, Jensen JP, Kaye K, et al. Consecutive field trials using two different intraosseous devices. Prehosp Emerg Care 2007;11(2):164–71.
80. Bickell WH, Wall MJJ, Pepe PE, et al. Immediate versus delayed fluid resuscitation for hypotensive patients with penetrating torso injuries. N Engl J Med 1994; 331(17):1105–9.
81. Brown JB, Cohen MJ, Minei JP, et al. Goal-directed resuscitation in the prehospital setting: a propensity-adjusted analysis. J Trauma Acute Care Surg 2013; 74(5):1207–12 [discussion: 1212–4].
82. Haut ER, Kalish BT, Cotton BA, et al. Prehospital intravenous fluid administration is associated with higher mortality in trauma patients: a National Trauma Data Bank analysis. Ann Surg 2011;253(2):371–7.
83. Dula DJ, Wood GC, Rejmer AR, et al. Use of prehospital fluids in hypotensive blunt trauma patients. Prehosp Emerg Care 2002;6(4):417–20.
84. Dutton RP, Mackenzie CF, Scalea TM. Hypotensive resuscitation during active hemorrhage: impact on in-hospital mortality. J Trauma 2002;52(6):1141–6.
85. Eckstein M, Chan L, Schneir A, et al. Effect of prehospital advanced life support on outcomes of major trauma patients. J Trauma Acute Care Surg 2000;48: 643–8.
86. Shackford SR. Prehospital fluid resuscitation of known or suspected traumatic brain injury. J Trauma 2011;70(5 Suppl):S32–3.
87. Turner J, Nicholl J, Webber L, et al. A randomised controlled trial of prehospital intravenous fluid replacement therapy in serious trauma. Health Technol Assess 2000;4(31):1–57.
88. Wald SL, Shackford SR, Fenwick J. The effect of secondary insults on mortality and long-term disability after severe head injury in a rural region without a trauma system. J Trauma 1993;34(3):377–81 [discussion: 381–2].
89. Hampton DA, Fabricant LJ, Differding J, et al. Pre-hospital intravenous fluid is associated with increased survival in trauma patients. J Trauma Acute Care Surg 2013;75(1):S9–15.
90. Malsby RF, Quesada J, Powell-Dunford N, et al. Prehospital blood product transfusion by U.S. army MEDEVAC during combat operations in Afghanistan: a process improvement initiative. Mil Med 2013;178(7):785–91.

91. Apodaca A, Olson CM, Bailey J, et al. Performance improvement evaluation of forward aeromedical evacuation platforms in Operation Enduring Freedom. J Trauma Acute Care Surg 2013;75(2 Suppl 2):S157–63.

92. Morrison JJ, Oh J, DuBose JJ, et al. En-route care capability from point of injury impacts mortality after severe wartime injury. Ann Surg 2013;257(2):330–4.

93. O'Reilly DJ, Morrison JJ, Jansen JO, et al. Prehospital blood transfusion in the en route management of severe combat trauma: a matched cohort study. J Trauma Acute Care Surg 2014;77(3 Suppl 2):S114–20.

94. Berns KS, Zietlow SP. Blood usage in rotor-wing transport. Air Med J 1998;17(3): 105–8.

95. Higgins GL, Baumann MR, Kendall KM, et al. Red blood cell transfusion: experience in a rural aeromedical transport service. Prehosp Disaster Med 2012; 27(3):231–4.

96. Brown JB, Cohen MJ, Minei JP, et al. Pretrauma center red blood cell transfusion is associated with reduced mortality and coagulopathy in severely injured patients with blunt trauma. Ann Surg 2014;261:997–1005.

97. Brown JB, Sperry JL, Fombona A, et al. Pre-trauma center red blood cell transfusion is associated with improved early outcomes in air medical trauma patients. J Am Coll Surg 2015;220(5):797–808.

98. Holcomb JB, Donathan DP, Cotton BA, et al. Prehospital transfusion of plasma and red blood cells in trauma patients. Prehosp Emerg Care 2014;19(1):1–9.

99. Zadravecz FJ, Tien L, Robertson-Dick BJ, et al. Comparison of mental-status scales for predicting mortality on the general wards. J Hosp Med 2015; 10(10):658–63.

100. Barlow P. A practical review of the Glasgow Coma Scale and Score. Surgeon 2012;10(2):114–9.

101. Arbabi S, Jurkovich GJ, Wahl WL, et al. A comparison of prehospital and hospital data in trauma patients. J Trauma 2004;56(5):1029–32.

102. Menegazzi JJ, Davis EA, Sucov AN, et al. Reliability of the Glasgow Coma Scale when used by emergency physicians and paramedics. J Trauma 1993;34(1): 46–8.

103. Kerby JD, MacLennan PA, Burton JN, et al. Agreement between prehospital and emergency department Glasgow Coma Scores. J Trauma 2007;63(5):1026–31.

104. Winkler JV, Rosen P, Alfry EJ. Prehospital use of the Glasgow Coma Scale in severe head injury. J Emerg Med 1984;2(1):1–6.

105. Cudnik MT, Werman HA, White LJ, et al. Prehospital factors associated with mortality in injured air medical patients. Prehosp Emerg Care 2012;16(1):121–7.

106. Durant E, Sporer KA. Characteristics of patients with an abnormal Glasgow Coma Scale score in the prehospital setting. West J Emerg Med 2011;12(1): 30–6.

107. Davis DP, Serrano JA, Vilke GM, et al. The predictive value of field versus arrival Glasgow Coma Scale score and TRISS calculations in moderate-to-severe traumatic brain injury. J Trauma 2006;60(5):985–90.

108. Healey C, Osler TM, Rogers FB, et al. Improving the Glasgow Coma Scale score: motor score alone is a better predictor. J Trauma 2003;54(4):671–8 [discussion: 678–80].

109. Haukoos JS, Gill MR, Rabon RE, et al. Validation of the simplified motor score for the prediction of brain injury outcomes after trauma. Ann Emerg Med 2007; 50(1):18–24.

110. Brown JB, Forsythe RM, Stassen NA, et al. Evidence-based improvement of the National Trauma Triage Protocol. J Trauma Acute Care Surg 2014;77(1):95–102.

111. Stiver SI, Manley GT. Prehospital management of traumatic brain injury. Neurosurg Focus 2008;25(4):E5.
112. Goldberg SA, Rojanasarntikul D, Jagoda A. The prehospital management of traumatic brain injury. In: Jordan Grafman, Andres Salazar, editors. Traumatic brain injury, Part I. Handbook of clinical neurology, vol. 127. Amsterdam, Netherlands: Elsevier; 2015. p. 367–78.
113. Dumont TM, Visioni AJ, Rughani AI, et al. Inappropriate prehospital ventilation in severe traumatic brain injury increases in-hospital mortality. J Neurotrauma 2010;27(7):1233–41.
114. Badjatia N, Carney N, Crocco TJ, et al. Guidelines for prehospital management of traumatic brain injury 2nd edition. Prehosp Emerg Care 2008;12(Suppl 1): S1–52.
115. Caulfield EV, Dutton RP, Floccare DJ, et al. Prehospital hypocapnia and poor outcome after severe traumatic brain injury. J Trauma 2009;66(6):1577–83.
116. Hoogmartens O, Heselmans A, Van de Velde S, et al. Evidence-based prehospital management of severe traumatic brain injury: a comparative analysis of current clinical practice guidelines. Prehosp Emerg Care 2014;18(2):265–73.
117. Sugerman DE, Xu L, Pearson WS, et al. Patients with severe traumatic brain injury transferred to a level I or II trauma center: United States, 2007 to 2009. J Trauma Acute Care Surg 2012;73(6):1491–9.
118. Kelly ML, Banerjee A, Nowak M, et al. Decreased mortality in traumatic brain injury following regionalization across hospital systems. J Trauma Acute Care Surg 2015;78(4):715–20.
119. Kelly ML, Roach MJ, Banerjee A, et al. Functional and long-term outcomes in severe traumatic brain injury following regionalization of a trauma system. J Trauma Acute Care Surg 2015;79(3):372–7.
120. Sampalis JS, Lavoie A, Williams JI, et al. Impact of on-site care, prehospital time, and level of in-hospital care on survival in severely injured patients. J Trauma 1993;34(2):252–61.
121. Seamon MJ, Fisher CA, Gaughan J, et al. Prehospital procedures before emergency department thoracotomy: "scoop and run" saves lives. J Trauma 2007; 63(1):113–20.
122. Stiell IG, Nesbitt LP, Pickett W, et al. The OPALS Major Trauma Study: impact of advanced life-support on survival and morbidity. CMAJ 2008;178(9):1141–52.
123. Brown JB, Rosengart MR, Forsythe RM, et al. Not all prehospital time is equal: influence of scene time on mortality. J Trauma Acute Care Surg 2016;81(1): 93–100.
124. Claridge JA, Allen D, Patterson B, et al. Regional collaboration across hospital systems to develop and implement trauma protocols saves lives within 2 years. Surgery 2013;154(4):875–84.
125. Schechtman D, He JC, Zosa BM, et al. Trauma system regionalization improves mortality in patients requiring trauma laparotomy. J Trauma Acute Care Surg 2017;82(1):58–64.
126. Brown JB, Gestring ML, Guyette FX, et al. Helicopter transport improves survival following injury in the absence of a time-saving advantage. Surgery 2016; 159(3):947–59.
127. Branas CC, MacKenzie EJ, Williams JC, et al. Access to trauma centers in the United States. JAMA 2005;293(21):2626–33.
128. Brathwaite CE, Rosko M, McDowell R, et al. A critical analysis of on-scene helicopter transport on survival in a statewide trauma system. J Trauma 1998; 45(1):140–4 [discussion: 144–6].

129. Bulger EM, Guffey D, Guyette FX, et al. Impact of prehospital mode of transport after severe injury: a multicenter evaluation from the Resuscitation Outcomes Consortium. J Trauma Acute Care Surg 2012;72(3):567–73 [discussion: 573–5]; [quiz: 803].

130. Cunningham P, Rutledge R, Baker CC, et al. A comparison of the association of helicopter and ground ambulance transport with the outcome of injury in trauma patients transported from the scene. J Trauma 1997;43(6):940–6.

131. Schiller WR, Knox R, Zinnecker H, et al. Effect of helicopter transport of trauma victims on survival in an urban trauma center. J Trauma 1988;28(8):1127–34.

132. Shatney CH, Homan SJ, Sherck JP, et al. The utility of helicopter transport of trauma patients from the injury scene in an urban trauma system. J Trauma 2002;53(5):817–22.

133. Brown JB, Stassen NA, Bankey PE, et al. Helicopters and the civilian trauma system: national utilization patterns demonstrate improved outcomes after traumatic injury. J Trauma 2010;69(5):1030–4 [discussion: 1034–6].

134. Galvagno SMJ, Haut ER, Zafar SN, et al. Association between helicopter vs ground emergency medical services and survival for adults with major trauma. JAMA 2012;307(15):1602–10.

135. Ryb GE, Dischinger P, Cooper C, et al. Does helicopter transport improve outcomes independently of emergency medical system time? J Trauma Acute Care Surg 2013;74(1):149–54 [discussion: 154–6].

136. Stewart KE, Cowan LD, Thompson DM, et al. Association of direct helicopter versus ground transport and in-hospital mortality in trauma patients: a propensity score analysis. Acad Emerg Med 2011;18(11):1208–16.

137. Sullivent EE, Faul M, Wald MM. Reduced mortality in injured adults transported by helicopter emergency medical services. Prehosp Emerg Care 2011;15(3):295–302.

138. Bekelis K, Missios S, Mackenzie TA. Prehospital helicopter transport and survival of patients with traumatic brain injury. Ann Surg 2015;261(3):579–85.

139. Brown JB, Stassen NA, Bankey PE, et al. Helicopters improve survival in seriously injured patients requiring interfacility transfer for definitive care. J Trauma 2011;70(2):310–4.

140. Delgado MK, Staudenmayer KL, Wang NE, et al. Cost-effectiveness of helicopter versus ground emergency medical services for trauma scene transport in the United States. Ann Emerg Med 2013;62(4):351–64.e19.

141. Bledsoe BE, Smith MG. Medical helicopter accidents in the United States: a 10-year review. J Trauma 2004;56(6):1325–8 [discussion: 1328–9].

142. Ringburg AN, de Ronde G, Thomas SH, et al. Validity of helicopter emergency medical services dispatch criteria for traumatic injuries: a systematic review. Prehosp Emerg Care 2009;13(1):28–36.

143. Brown JB, Forsythe RM, Stassen NA, et al. The National Trauma Triage Protocol: can this tool predict which patients with trauma will benefit from helicopter transport? J Trauma Acute Care Surg 2012;73(2):319–25.

144. Brown JB, Gestring ML, Guyette FX, et al. Development and validation of the air medical prehospital triage score for helicopter transport of trauma patients. Ann Surg 2016;264:378–85.

145. Brown JB, Gestring ML, Guyette FX, et al. External validation of the Air Medical Prehospital Triage score for identifying trauma patients likely to benefit from scene helicopter transport. J Trauma Acute Care Surg 2017;82(2):270–9.

146. Rogers FB, Osler TM, Shackford SR, et al. Study of the outcome of patients transferred to a level I hospital after stabilization at an outlying hospital in a rural setting. J Trauma 1999;46(2):328–33.
147. Sorensen MJ, von Recklinghausen FM, Fulton G, et al. Secondary overtriage: the burden of unnecessary interfacility transfers in a rural trauma system. JAMA Surg 2013;148(8):763–8.
148. Nathens AB, Maier RV, Brundage SI, et al. The effect of interfacility transfer on outcome in an urban trauma system. J Trauma 2003;55(3):444–9.
149. Gupta R, Greer SE, Martin ED. Inefficiencies in a rural trauma system: the burden of repeat imaging in interfacility transfers. J Trauma 2010;69(2):253–5.
150. Gomez D, Haas B, de Mestral C, et al. Institutional and provider factors impeding access to trauma center care: an analysis of transfer practices in a regional trauma system. J Trauma Acute Care Surg 2012;73(5):1288–93.
151. Borst GM, Davies SW, Waibel BH, et al. When birds can't fly. J Trauma Acute Care Surg 2014;77(2):331–7.
152. He JC, Kreiner LA, Sajankila N, et al. Performance of a regional trauma network. J Trauma Acute Care Surg 2016;81(1):190–5.
153. Hoyt DB, Coimbra R. Trauma systems. Surg Clin North Am 2007;87(1):21–35.
154. Eastman AB, MacKenzie EJ, Nathens AB. Sustaining a coordinated, regional approach to trauma and emergency care is critical to patient health care needs. Health Aff 2013;32(12):2091–8.
155. Bailey J, Trexler S, Murdock A, et al. Verification and regionalization of trauma systems: the impact of these efforts on trauma care in the United States. Surg Clin North Am 2012;92(4):1009–24, ix–x.
156. Cameron PA, Gabbe BJ, Cooper DJ, et al. A statewide system of trauma care in Victoria: effect on patient survival. Med J Aust 2008;189(10):546–50.
157. Gabbe BJ, Biostat GD, Lecky FE, et al. The effect of an organized trauma system on mortality in major trauma involving serious head injury: a comparison of the United Kingdom and Victoria, Australia. Ann Surg 2011;253(1):138–43.
158. Nathens AB, Brunet FP, Maier RV. Development of trauma systems and effect on outcomes after injury. Lancet 2004;363(9423):1794–801.
159. Gabbe BJ, Biostat GD, Simpson PM, et al. Improved functional outcomes for major trauma patients in a regionalized, inclusive trauma system. Ann Surg 2012;255(6):1009–15.
160. Cole E, Lecky F, West A, et al. The impact of a pan-regional inclusive trauma system on quality of care. Ann Surg 2016;264(1):188–94.
161. Janssens L, Holtslag HR, van Beeck EF, et al. The effects of regionalization of pediatric trauma care in the Netherlands. J Trauma Acute Care Surg 2012; 73(5):1284–7.
162. Haas B, Gomez D, Neal M, et al. Good neighbors? The effect of a level 1 trauma center on the performance of nearby level 2 trauma centers. Ann Surg 2011; 253(5):992–5.
163. Gagliardi AR, Nathens AB. Exploring the characteristics of high-performing hospitals that influence trauma triage and transfer. J Trauma Acute Care Surg 2015; 78(2):300–5.
164. Nathens AB, Jurkovich GJ, Maier RV, et al. Relationship between trauma center volume and outcomes. JAMA 2001;285(9):1164–71.
165. Stop the bleed: save a life. Bleeding control. Available at: http://www. bleedingcontrol.org/. Accessed March 10, 2017.

Assessment and Resuscitation in Trauma Management

Stephen Gondek, MD, MPH*, Mary E. Schroeder, MD,
Babak Sarani, MD

KEYWORDS

- Trauma assessment • Resuscitation • Primary survey • Venous access
- Emergency airway • Cavitary triage

KEY POINTS

- Initial resuscitation should focus on rapid assessment and stabilization of life-threatening injuries with management of non–life-threatening injuries deferred until the patient is stabilized.
- Damage control resuscitation includes efficient intravenous access, avoidance of hypothermia, and a preference for colloid resuscitation rather than crystalloid.
- Providers should understand indications for both emergency intubation and discretionary intubation in the trauma setting as well as options when endotracheal intubation is not possible.
- Combining plain films, physical examination, and ultrasound allows for a complete cavitary triage to be performed and will identify nearly all hemodynamically significant sites of bleeding.
- Retrograde balloon occlusion of the aorta is likely beneficial in the profoundly hypotensive patient, but is not synonymous with resuscitative thoracotomy.

INTRODUCTION

The Golden Hour was first coined by R. Adams Cowley to emphasize the importance of prompt and efficient management of the acutely injured patient. Advances in both resuscitation and diagnosis have given providers a host of new procedural and imaging options and have resulted in improved trauma care at centers of all levels.

The authors have nothing to disclose.
Center for Trauma and Critical Care, George Washington University Hospital, 2150 Pennsylvania Avenue Northwest, Washington, DC 20037, USA
* Corresponding author.
E-mail address: gondeks@gmail.com

BEYOND ADVANCED TRAUMA LIFE SUPPORT: INITIAL RESUSCITATION IN THE EMERGENCY DEPARTMENT

The Airway, Breathing, Circulation, Disability, Exposure management taught by Advanced Trauma Life Support (ATLS)[1] is an effective framework for initial evaluation and management of the injured patient and has been demonstrated to increase efficiency and quality of care.[2] As any experienced provider knows, in a well-staffed trauma center, these processes can be run in parallel and their order modified for certain exceptional cases. When performed in full, they represent a complete initial evaluation of the injured patient in an orderly and efficient manner (**Box 1**).

Airway/Access

Intravenous access

Although typically straightforward, intravenous (IV) access can be a frustrating problem in the care of the trauma patient. Standard resuscitation calls for the placement of 2 large-bore IVs, typically in the antecubital position, with ultrasound (US) assistance if necessary. Alternatives to peripheral cannulation should be performed if peripheral access is not completed quickly. There are several options for access that can be used in the trauma bay, with variability in the rate of fluid administration[3] (**Box 2**). Multiple other solutions to access have been described, including venous cutdown,[3] corpus cavernosum,[4] catheterization, direct right atrial catheterization, and umbilical vein catheterization in infants, but these are not of common utility in the trauma bay.

Central venous catheterization

Central venous catheterization (CVC) is an efficient mode of vascular access. Subclavian or femoral access is often preferred because of the ease of placement without US guidance. Caution should be maintained when using femoral access in the setting of severe trauma to the chest or abdomen, particularly penetrating injuries, because disruption or injury of the vena cava or iliac veins will prevent adequate delivery. In addition, in the case of accidental arterial access, these lines can be used in an emergency, but should be converted to venous access promptly.

Interosseous catheter

Interosseous (IO) catheter use has become widely accepted in trauma resuscitation and provides a fast alternative to CVCs. In the adult trauma patient, humeral and tibial access is preferred with success rates as high as 97%, although multiple other sites including the sternum, iliac crest, and femur have been described. Humeral IO

Box 1
The standard trauma

1. Patient arrival
2. Pulse check
   a. IV access established
   b. Manual blood pressure measurement
3. Primary survey
4. Report from Emergency Medical Services
5. Adjunctive imaging
6. Secondary survey
7. Disposition

Box 2	
Maximal infusion rate of common catheters	
Humeral IO	80 mL/min
Tibial IO	15 mL/min
32-mm 14 g IV	325 mL/min
30-mm 16 g IV	215 mL/min
30-mm 18 g IV	110 mL/min
30-mm 20 g IV	63 mL/min
9-Fr Mac distal port	508 mL/min
Proximal	200 mL/min
8.5-F Cordis	125 mL/min
7-F triple lumen distal port	38 mL/min
Medial	17 mL/min
Proximal	18 mL/min

Data from Young J, Gondek S, Kahn S, et al. Challenging IV access in the patient with septic shock. In: Diaz JJ, Efron DT, editors. Complications in acute care surgery: the management of difficult clinical scenarios. Cham (Switzerland): Springer International Publishing; 2017. p. 1–13.

catheters are preferred to tibial catheters because they provide greater flow rates but are inferior to both large-bore CVCs and IV catheters in this regard (see **Box 2**). In addition, resuscitation through a humeral IO drains into the subclavian vein, resulting in venous distention that facilities placement of a subclavian CVC when appropriate.

Airway
Indications for intubation During the initial assessment of the injured patient, a rapid decision must be made regarding control of the airway. To facilitate this, the Eastern Association for the Surgery of Trauma has produced revised guidelines for indications for emergency intubation[5] (**Box 3**).

Box 3
Indications for emergency intubation
Emergency intubation
Airway obstruction
Hypoventilation
Hypoxemia $\leq 90\%$
Severe cognitive impairment (GCS $\leq$ 8)
Severe hemorrhagic shock
Cardiac arrest
Major burn ($\leq$40%) or inhalational injury
Discretionary intubation
Facial or neck trauma
Moderate cognitive impairment (GCS 9–12)
Persistent combativeness refractory to pharmacologic intervention
Respiratory distress
Expected operative course
Cervical spinal cord injury

Although patients with a Glasgow Coma Score (GCS) of 8 or less clearly require intubation, GCS of 9 to 12 has been associated with a 33% rate of traumatic brain injury (TBI), and combativeness has been associated with a 12.7% rate of TBI.[6] Reasonable attempts should be made to support noninvasive ventilation in suspected TBI patients, and reasonable pharmacologic attempts should be made to control agitation in these settings to avoid hemodynamic compromise as well as the risk of hypoxia associated with intubation. If these measures are unsuccessful, intubation may be required to expedite computed tomography (CT) scan and subsequent TBI management. Similarly, patients with cervical spine injury that are expected to progress to respiratory insufficiency appear to benefit from early intubation, and this should be considered in the trauma bay.[7–9]

Induction agents for emergency intubation Rapid sequence intubation should be used for nearly all emergency intubations in the trauma bay. No clear data have emerged to support a preference for one pharmacologic regimen over another. Succinylcholine is the preferred paralytic agent, although high-dose rocuronium may be used when succinylcholine is contraindicated due to significant burn, crush injury, prolonged down time, or renal failure. One suggested protocol is reviewed in **Box 4**. Practitioners should be familiar with both IV and intramuscular dosing regimens, or they should be displayed in clear view in the trauma bay. In this protocol, ketamine is the preferred induction medication for its favorable hemodynamic profile and ease of dosing. Although TBI was once considered a contraindication to the use of ketamine, these concerns have since been refuted.[10] All induction medications, including ketamine, may cause hemodynamic compromise because of offloading of the sympathetic response to trauma. Propofol, however, is the most commonly cited, and its use is generally avoided. In the setting of profound hypotension, patients may benefit from noninvasive ventilation until massive transfusion protocols are initiated to avoid complete hemodynamic collapse on induction.

Alternatives to direct laryngoscopy for difficult intubation Although direct laryngoscopy (DL) is the preferred mechanism of intubation, multiple alternatives have been developed and should be considered based on familiarity and experience. All resuscitation protocols must include alternatives to DL in the trauma bay because of multiple factors increasing the difficulty of emergency intubation, including limited view due

---

Box 4
Rapid sequence intubation medication options

Preferred induction agent
  Ketamine 1 to 3 mg/kg IV

Second-line agent
  Propofol 60 to 200 mg (6–20 cc)

Third-line agent
  Etomidate 10 to 20 mg IV (5–10 cc)

AND
  Succinylcholine 80 to 100 mg (4–5 cc)

If unable to obtain IV/IO access:
  Ketamine 5 mg/kg IM
  AND
  Succinylcholine 5 mg/kg IM

to maxillofacial or neck trauma, aspirated blood or vomitus, alterations in anatomy, difficulty in patient positioning, and other factors.

Video laryngoscopy
Video laryngoscopy (VL) offers several potential benefits over DL and should be considered an option for initial attempts at intubation. The clearest benefit is the ease of supervising inexperienced providers, although VL may be superior to DL in anatomically altered or obese patients and in patients with known or suspected cervical spine injury. VL may have improved first-attempt intubation rates when compared with DL, theoretically reducing the likelihood of hypoxic episodes in emergency intubation.[5] This may be theoretically beneficial to the spinal cord injury or TBI patient, but this has not been demonstrated clinically. Practitioners should, at a minimum, be familiar with the VL options at their centers.

Supraglottic devices
Supraglottic devices, including laryngeal mask airway, Combitube (Medtronic, Minneapolis MN, USA), and King (Ambu, Ballerup, Denmark) Airways (also known as esophageal/tracheal airways), are commonly used as rescue devices by both in-hospital and prehospital providers. No one device has been demonstrated to be superior to the others, and choice of device should be determined by availability and familiarity. These devices have limited utility in the trauma bay because critically injured patients should be assumed to have a high risk of emesis, and supraglottic devices do not offer any protection against aspiration. In addition, when endotracheal intubation is not possible because of airway or vocal cord edema, supraglottic devices will also fail. Supraglottic devices should not be considered a durable airway and should be converted to an endotracheal tube or surgical airway as early as is feasible. Patients receiving supraglottic devices in the field should be evaluated and converted in the trauma bay where possible, and although a reasonable option in the prehospital setting, their use should be avoided in the trauma bay.

Surgical airway
All patients in whom emergency endotracheal intubation fails should be prepared for a surgical airway with cricothyroidotomy as the preferred option for hypoxic patients or patients who cannot be ventilated with bag valve mask or a supraglottic device. Emergency tracheostomy should be reserved for patients who are well ventilated without intubation. Both cricothyroidotomy and tracheostomy may be performed, and both may be performed open or percutaneously depending on the experience of the proceduralist. Although some data have demonstrated that emergency cricothyroidotomy does not mandate conversion to tracheostomy for short-term management, patient characteristics must be accounted for. Anecdotally, cricothyroidotomy is more likely to be accidentally dislodged in patients who require multiple transfers for imaging, patients who require multiple procedures, or those who may be agitated and difficult to sedate. In these patients, tracheostomy may be a preferred, safer option if their hemodynamics allows conversion.

BREATHING
Ventilation

Few data exist to support initial ventilation strategies specific to the trauma population, although intubation in this group should follow accepted protocols for emergency intubation. Initiation of ventilator support with a lung protective strategy is probably superior where possible. A meta-analysis found that initiation of ventilation with tidal volumes of 6 to 8 cc/kg versus higher-volume ventilation in emergency room patients has been shown to reduce rates of acute lung injury, pulmonary infection, and mortality.[11] The transition of this data to the trauma population is limited, and it should be noted that protective ventilation is associated with increases in $Paco_2$ as well as need for higher positive end-expiratory pressure, both of which may be harmful to specific subgroups of the trauma population,[11] and may require additional sedation in order to facilitate a low-volume protective strategy.[12] Ongoing trials of ventilation strategies are currently accruing patients,[13] although no specific efforts have been made in the trauma population. Clinicians should exercise clinical judgment in determining a ventilator strategy for the intubated trauma patient.

Injuries to the Chest

Hemothorax

Although significant chest injury is reviewed separately in this issue, hemothorax becomes relevant to the primary survey in the setting of hypotensive patients. Chest tube drainage should be provided in the trauma bay to aid in cavitary triage. Hemothorax is often a harbinger of other significant injuries to the chest, and these patients should be evaluated for injuries to the great vessels, lungs, or heart. Because of the negative pressure in the chest, pericardial effusion is an insufficiently sensitive indicator of cardiac injuries in patients with hemothorax, and significant injuries to the heart may be missed on US, CT, or echocardiography.

Pneumothorax

Pneumothorax in itself does not mandate emergent management, but in the presence of tension physiology, intervention during the primary survey becomes mandatory. Three methods of emergency decompression are available to the proceduralist. Needle decompression is an acceptable option in the emergent setting, although more durable options are preferred if time allows. Needle decompression can be ineffective in many patients because of inappropriate positioning, occlusion, or displacement. Cadaver models have demonstrated that a midaxillary position may be superior to anterior placement because of differences in chest well thickness in an American population.[14] More durable options include finger thoracostomy and formal chest tube placement. Finger thoracostomy does mandate later conversion to chest tube, but is efficient in a time-sensitive situation. Choice of chest tube size has not been shown to be significant,[15] and percutaneous tube thoracotomy placement may be an acceptable treatment option, but neither have come into favor for the unstable patient because of concerns regarding occlusion of the tube and provider familiarity with traditional chest tubes.

CIRCULATION
Avoidance of Hypothermia

Hypothermia has long been recognized to have a negative impact on outcomes in traumatic injury, with actively rewarmed patients having significantly better outcomes from resuscitation.[16,17] Significant alterations in coagulation have been demonstrated to begin at temperatures of 35°C.[18] Multiple mechanisms for hypothermia-related coagulopathy have been identified, including direct inhibition of the coagulation cascade, morphologic changes to platelets, reduced platelet aggregation, and diffuse microvascular thrombosis.[18] In moderately hypothermic patients (>33°C), platelet effects are the dominant cause of coagulopathy, with effects in the severely hypothermic (<33°C) driven to a larger degree by delays in the coagulation cascade.[18] Heat loss in trauma patients has been shown to increase from a baseline 60 kcal/h to as much as 400 kcal/h after acute trauma.[19] The belief that hypothermia may be protective of certain complications in trauma has been disproven, and effort should be made throughout resuscitation to avoid or correct hypothermia. Recent review of the National Trauma Data Bank has clearly demonstrated worse infectious, thromboembolic, and coagulopathic complications for patients with demonstrated hypothermia.[20] Many strategies have been developed and instituted in the care of the acutely injured patient, and centers are encouraged to implement protocols to prevent hypothermia, incorporating both passive and active rewarming. With increasing severity of hypothermia, more aggressive interventions should be initiated, including fluid and forced air rewarming, heating pads, and humidified and heated ventilation.[21] Profound hypothermia will require even more drastic options, including heated body cavity lavage, extracorporeal warming via extracorporeal membrane oxygenation or hemodialysis circuits,[21] or active intravascular rewarming catheters.[22]

Permissive Hypotension

Although prehospital interventions are discussed elsewhere in this issue, the use of damage control resuscitation, or permissive hypotension, has been shown to be superior to older, more liberal resuscitation strategies. A goal systolic blood pressure of 90 mm Hg is sufficient for adequate organ perfusion in most injured patients[23] and crystalloid resuscitation should be limited as much as feasible. Fluid resuscitation in 250- to 500-mL aliquots can be used to maintain appropriate systolic blood pressure or the presence of a radial pulse.[24] Theoretically, the reduction in crystalloid utilization prevents worsening of coagulation via dilution of clotting factors, exacerbation of hypothermia and acidosis, and increased bleeding from hydrostatic pressure on forming clots. Exceptions to permissive hypotension include elderly patients, head injuries, pregnancy, and prolonged evacuation or transport times[17] due to clear harms from ongoing hypotension in these groups. This strategy should be implemented until definitive control of bleeding can be achieved,[25] or until an alternative cause for shock has been identified.

The use of permissive hypotension was shown to improve outcomes and reduce fluid resuscitation initially in penetrating injuries at an urban center.[23] There has been some difficulty in demonstrating a clear benefit when extrapolating these data to the general population or to other traumatic mechanisms.[24,26] Trauma centers outside of an urban center with long transport times or populations different from an urban population should consider these limitations before implementing a resuscitation strategy focused on permissive hypotension.

In addition, the use of permissive hypotension is contraindicated specifically in TBI, where hypotension is known to be associated with worse neurologic outcomes.[27] In this scenario, management should focus on the protection of injured but recoverable brain tissue, and some hypertension should be tolerated to avoid further neurologic injury. At very high systolic blood pressure, hydrostatic forces may worsen vasogenic cerebral edema and should be controlled with agents that do not increase the cerebral vasodilation, with preference given to beta-blockers over nitrates or calcium channel blockers[27–29]

Pulselessness

Resuscitative thoracotomy

Despite careful evaluation of resuscitative thoracotomy (RT) as a salvage maneuver, there remains significant controversy regarding its use. Current guidelines are focused primarily on mechanism and time since injury with clear consensus that the procedure is beneficial in penetrating injuries with a short transport time. This intervention is less clearly beneficial following blunt trauma because survival is dismal in this group and risk to both providers and resource utilization is high.[29,30] No specific recommendations exist regarding patient age, although pediatric thoracotomy appears to have similar survival rates to adult,[29] and geriatric thoracotomy is disfavored. In addition, new diagnostics, including US[31] and end tidal CO_2, are probably useful in the determination of candidacy. Use of these modalities has not yet appeared in major society guidelines,[32] although many trauma surgeons report using them to determine candidacy for RT.

Resuscitative endovascular balloon occlusion of the aorta

Resuscitative endovascular balloon occlusion of the aorta (REBOA) is gaining traction as a potential alternative to RT in select patients, with proponents citing similar time to aortic cross-clamping and significantly less morbidity,[33] whereas opponents argue that a lack of institutional experience and clear guidelines currently limit its use. REBOA is probably not an effective modality for control of hemorrhage in the chest, but its use for the profoundly hypotensive patient with abdominal or pelvic injuries may prove to be an effective alternative to RT.[34] Reduced catheter sizes and increasing experience are encouraging for this technology that is likely to find its role in the prearrest and periarrest trauma patient.[35]

Conceptually, REBOA is similar to open cross-clamping of the aorta. Arterial access is obtained at the femoral artery, preferably with the aid of US. Proceduralist preference and the availability of equipment will dictate sheath size, with some catheters usable with an initial 7-Fr sheath and others requiring upsizing to a larger catheter. In the acute trauma setting, proceduralists should be familiar with placement by external landmarks because imaging may not be available. REBOA placement is defined by zones (**Fig. 1**), with zone 1 extending from the left subclavian artery to the celiac artery, zone 2 extending from the celiac to the renal arteries, and zone 3 extending from the

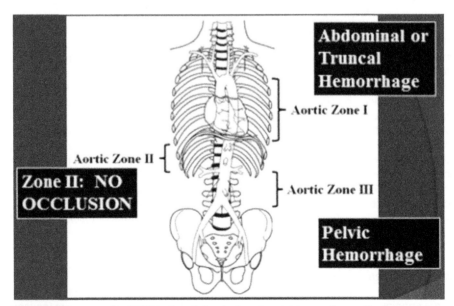

Fig. 1. Aortic zones for REBOA. For abdominal or truncal hemorrhage, the balloon is inflated in aortic zone I; for pelvic hemorrhage, the balloon is inflated in zone III. The balloon should not be used in zone II. (*Adapted from* Napolitano LM. Resuscitative endovascular balloon occlusion of the aorta: indications, outcomes, and training. Crit Care Clin 2017;33(1):57; with permission.)

renal arteries to the bifurcation of the aorta. In comparison with open cross-clamping, zone 1 should be considered similar to supraceliac cross-clamping and zone 3 considered similar to infrarenal cross-clamping. REBOA balloons are not typically placed in zone 2. When imaging is not available, the balloon can be placed just above the xiphoid process for zone 1 and just above the umbilicus for zone 3.[35]

Indications for REBOA have not been clearly defined. The patients most likely to benefit from its use are the profoundly hypotensive patients with injuries below the diaphragm. In these patients, placement will be determined by the likelihood of hemorrhage in the abdomen. In the setting of blunt trauma and transient or no response to resuscitation, REBOA should be placed in zone 1 for all patients with a positive focused assessment with sonography for trauma (FAST) and in zone 3 for patients with pelvic fractures and a negative FAST. Penetrating injuries to the abdomen are less clear, but REBOA may be helpful if placement is possible. It should be noted that REBOA is contraindicated in patients with potential injuries to the great vessels or above the balloon site or in patients with symptomatic blunt cardiac injury.[36]

REBOA should not be seen as synonymous with RT, because RT is most effective in patients that would be contraindicated to receive REBOA. It is these authors' opinion that pulseless patients who meet criteria should undergo RT. In patients who are profoundly hypotensive, REBOA is a helpful adjunct for resuscitation until hemorrhage can be controlled, such as severe blunt trauma. In addition, there may be a role for REBOA in patients who do not meet criteria for RT due to age or injury pattern but continue to have signs of life.

CAVITARY TRIAGE

With increased recognition of the harm of negative or surveillance operations, an important role in the initial assessment and resuscitation of the acutely injured patient is cavitary triage.[37] The provider should recognize not only which body cavities require intervention but also which ones may be at risk in the event of hemodynamic changes. Several adjunctive imaging studies are available to the clinician for cavitary triage and may be included in the trauma evaluation as part of the primary or secondary survey. The goal of cavitary triage is to identify all *hemodynamically significant* injuries, and ideal imaging and diagnostic modalities will have a high sensitivity for these. Less significant injuries can be identified with many other modalities once the patient's life-threatening injuries have been identified and managed. With increasing clinician comfort with US, initial triage of all major body cavities is now possible before leaving the trauma bay, and any major source of bleeding should be identifiable in the hemodynamically unstable patient. Imaging to identify hemodynamically significant injuries is reviewed in later discussion.

Chest Imaging

Chest Radiograph
Chest radiograph (CXR) should be obtained as primary triage of the chest, but is ineffective in demonstrating small hemothoraces and can often miss even substantial anterior pneumothoraces.[38] Although upright films may demonstrate blunting of the costophrenic angle with as little as 400 cc of hemothorax, supine films are substantially more limited and may require as much as 1 L before significant changes occur.[38,39] Often, however, the CXR may be the only efficiently available imaging modality in the acute setting, and even with these limitations, can effectively identify immediately life-threatening injuries.

Ultrasonography

Although limited in its ability to identify bony injuries to the chest, US has emerged as a reliable diagnostic test for both pneumothorax and hemothorax, with sensitivities ranging from 60% to greater than 90%, and is often superior to plain radiographs.[40] When compared with CT, US is significantly faster,[40] although slightly inferior to CT in the diagnosis of pneumothorax. Although not directly addressed in studies, the sensitivity of US for tension pneumothorax would be expected to be remarkably high, and diagnosis of this disorder is likely to be faster to obtain with US than with plain radiographs or CT.

Computed tomography

CT has a remarkable sensitivity for the acute injury to the chest, although some investigators have argued that this sensitivity may be too high,[41] with many nonclinically significant pulmonary contusions and occult pneumothoraces being identified. As such, it continues to be considered the gold standard for triage in the stable patient. Because of time constraints and need for transport to the radiology department, CT imaging should generally only be used for stable or fluid-responsive patients.

Abdominal Diagnostic Modalities

Focused abdominal sonography for trauma

FAST has become the standard of care for rapid diagnosis of intraabdominal hemorrhage and should be used for all unstable patients at risk for abdominal injury. With experience, as little as 200 cc of hemoperitoneum can be reliably identified within as little as 3 minutes without leaving the trauma bay.[42] Sensitivity for hemoperitoneum is 73% to 88%.[42] As a diagnostic modality for cavitary triage, injuries with less than 200 cc of bleeding are unlikely to be the cause of hemodynamic instability and can be identified easily on CT in the stable patient. FAST is known to be unreliable for hollow viscus injury and cannot grade solid organ injury,[42] and as such, is not beneficial to the stable trauma patient, although its use is often encouraged to improve operator speed and reliability. In addition, in the setting of penetrating injury, FAST will identify hemodynamically significant sources of hemorrhage, but will not identify trajectory or hollow viscus injury.

Computed tomography

Just as in chest trauma, CT remains the gold-standard imaging modality for the stable trauma patient and is increasingly being used in penetrating trauma to establish trajectory and rule out retroperitoneal injury.[42] Sensitivity for any intraabdominal injury is between 92% and 97.6%, with multicenter trial data demonstrating a negative predictive value as high as 99.6%.[37]

Diagnostic peritoneal lavage

Use of diagnostic peritoneal lavage (DPL) has dropped dramatically since the advent of FAST and increasing availability of CT. The negative predictive value of DPL is significantly higher than FAST alone, with accuracy as high as 92% to 98%,[42] and is more sensitive than CT for mesenteric injury.[43] However, DPL is limited by a known high rate of false positive results, especially in the setting of pelvic fracture. Some centers advocate continued use of DPL because of speed and convenience in the trauma bay, although it has largely been supplanted by a combination of CT, FAST, and selective use of observation as necessary.

Pelvic and Femur Fractures

Pelvic fractures representing hemodynamically significant injury are typically identifiable on plain radiograph. Cadaver studies have shown that 5-cm pubis diastasis results in a 20% increase in pelvic volume, whereas a 10-cm diastasis leads to 40% increase, indicating a large potential space for blood loss with associated injury to the pelvic veins. The use of pelvic binders has become commonplace in an attempt to quickly reduce pelvic volume and decrease transfusion needs.[44,45] FAST will identify some retroperitoneal injury, but should not be regarded as specific enough to rule out these injuries. In the hemodynamically unstable patient with pelvic fracture, DPL may be warranted to exclude intraabdominal hemorrhage as a source, whereas a stable patient may undergo CT scan with IV contrast to determine a source of ongoing bleeding.

Patients with contrast extravasation, regardless of pelvic fracture pattern, on CT scan should undergo angioembolization.[46] In addition, pelvic hematomas that are more that 500 cc are associated with an almost 5 times relative risk of having a concomitant arterial injury and should also be evaluated with angiography. Delay to angiography in hemodynamically unstable patients with pelvic fractures has been associated with increased mortality.

Retroperitoneal packing is often reserved for patients who require exploratory laparotomy in addition to intervention for ongoing retroperitoneal hemorrhage or for whom angiography cannot be accomplished expeditiously due to the need to mobilize resources.[47,48] Although some centers that use it preferentially for pelvic bleeding, common availability of angiography has largely replaced this procedure.

Femur fractures can also be a source of significant blood loss, with one retrospective study of isolated femur fractures estimating blood loss at an average of more than 1200 cc.[49] Physical examination coupled with plain radiograph of the thigh will be sufficient to rule out hemodynamically significant femur injury for the sake of cavitary triage. For patients who do not have other more life-threatening injuries, it is recommended that they undergo fixation within 24 hours to reduce ongoing blood loss as well as improve orthopedic outcomes.[50]

SUMMARY

The initial assessment of the trauma patient involves coordination of a multidisciplinary team with the goal of identifying life-threatening injuries, intervening on those deemed critical, and then prioritizing a care plan for the patient. It is an intense period of treatment and triage as the team initiates resuscitation and calls upon appropriate resources to reduce morbidity and mortality. In order to best care for the patient, the clinician must know what resources are available and be facile in mobilizing the care team in an efficient manner. This expeditious coordination of care requires training and practice with the ultimate goal of saving lives during the golden hour of resuscitation.

REFERENCES

1. American College of Surgeons. Advanced trauma life support: ATLS; student course manual. 9th edition. Chicago: American College of Surgeons; 2012.
2. Tsang B, McKee J, Engels PT, et al. Compliance to advanced trauma life support protocols in adult trauma patients in the acute setting. World J Emerg Surg 2013; 8(1):39.

3. Young J, Gondek S, Kahn S, et al. Challenging IV access in the patient with septic shock. In: Diaz JJ, Efron DT, editors. Complications in acute care surgery: the management of difficult clinical scenarios. 2017. Available at: http://lib.myilibrary.com?id=971614. Accessed March 14, 2017.

4. Bradley M. Brief report: systemic vascular access and resuscitation via corpus cavernosum. Mil Med 2016;181(11):e1491–4.

5. Mayglothling J, Duane TM, Gibbs M, et al. Emergency tracheal intubation immediately following traumatic injury: an Eastern Association for the Surgery of Trauma practice management guideline. J Trauma Acute Care Surg 2012;73(5 Suppl 4):S333–40.

6. Sise MJ, Shackford SR, Sise CB, et al. Early intubation in the management of trauma patients: indications and outcomes in 1,000 consecutive patients. J Trauma 2009;66(1):32–9, 40.

7. Como JJ, Sutton ERH, McCunn M, et al. Characterizing the need for mechanical ventilation following cervical spinal cord injury with neurologic deficit. J Trauma 2005;59(4):912–6 [discussion: 916].

8. Hassid VJ, Schinco MA, Tepas JJ, et al. Definitive establishment of airway control is critical for optimal outcome in lower cervical spinal cord injury. J Trauma 2008; 65(6):1328–32.

9. Velmahos GC, Toutouzas K, Chan L, et al. Intubation after cervical spinal cord injury: to be done selectively or routinely? Am Surg 2003;69(10):891–4.

10. Zeiler FA, Teitelbaum J, West M, et al. The ketamine effect on ICP in traumatic brain injury. Neurocrit Care 2014;21(1):163–73.

11. Neto AS, Simonis FD, Barbas CSV, et al. Lung-protective ventilation with low tidal volumes and the occurrence of pulmonary complications in patients without acute respiratory distress syndrome: a systematic review and individual patient data analysis. Crit Care Med 2015;43(10):2155–63.

12. Ferguson ND. Low tidal volumes for all? JAMA 2012;308(16):1689–90.

13. Fuller BM, Ferguson IT, Mohr NM, et al. Lung-protective ventilation initiated in the emergency department (LOV-ED): a quasi-experimental, before-after trial. Ann Emerg Med 2017. [Epub ahead of print].

14. Schroeder E, Valdez C, Krauthamer A, et al. Average chest wall thickness at two anatomic locations in trauma patients. Injury 2013;44(9):1183–5.

15. Inaba K, Lustenberger T, Recinos G, et al. Does size matter? A prospective analysis of 28-32 versus 36-40 French chest tube size in trauma. J Trauma Acute Care Surg 2012;72(2):422–7.

16. Gentilello LM, Jurkovich GJ, Stark MS, et al. Is hypothermia in the victim of major trauma protective or harmful? A randomized, prospective study. Ann Surg 1997; 226(4):439–47, 449.

17. Sharrock AE, Midwinter M. Damage control - trauma care in the first hour and beyond: a clinical review of relevant developments in the field of trauma care. Ann R Coll Surg Engl 2013;95(3):177–83.

18. Lier H, Krep H, Schroeder S, et al. Preconditions of hemostasis in trauma: a review. The influence of acidosis, hypocalcemia, anemia, and hypothermia on functional hemostasis in trauma. J Trauma 2008;65(4):951–60.

19. Peng RY, Bongard FS. Hypothermia in trauma patients. J Am Coll Surg 1999; 188(6):685–96.

20. Shafi S, Elliott AC, Gentilello L. Is hypothermia simply a marker of shock and injury severity or an independent risk factor for mortality in trauma patients? Analysis of a large national trauma registry. J Trauma 2005;59(5):1081–5.

21. Perlman R, Callum J, Laflamme C, et al. A recommended early goal-directed management guideline for the prevention of hypothermia-related transfusion, morbidity, and mortality in severely injured trauma patients. Crit Care 2016; 20(1):107.

22. Kiridume K, Hifumi T, Kawakita K, et al. Clinical experience with an active intravascular rewarming technique for near-severe hypothermia associated with traumatic injury. J Intensive Care 2014;2(1):11.

23. Bickell WH, Wall MJ, Pepe PE, et al. Immediate versus delayed fluid resuscitation for hypotensive patients with penetrating torso injuries. N Engl J Med 1994; 331(17):1105–9.

24. Dutton RP, Mackenzie CF, Scalea TM. Hypotensive resuscitation during active hemorrhage: impact on in-hospital mortality. J Trauma 2002;52(6):1141–6.

25. Duchesne JC, McSwain NE, Cotton BA, et al. Damage control resuscitation: the new face of damage control. J Trauma 2010;69(4):976–90.

26. Stahel PF, Smith WR, Moore EE. Current trends in resuscitation strategy for the multiply injured patient. Injury 2009;40(Suppl 4):S27–35.

27. Chesnut RM, Marshall LF, Klauber MR, et al. The role of secondary brain injury in determining outcome from severe head injury. J Trauma 1993;34(2):216–22.

28. Helmy A, Vizcaychipi M, Gupta AK. Traumatic brain injury: intensive care management. Br J Anaesth 2007;99(1):32–42.

29. Burlew CC, Moore EE, Moore FA, et al. Western Trauma Association critical decisions in trauma: resuscitative thoracotomy. J Trauma Acute Care Surg 2012;73(6): 1359–63.

30. Seamon MJ, Haut ER, Van Arendonk K, et al. An evidence-based approach to patient selection for emergency department thoracotomy: a practice management guideline from the Eastern Association for the Surgery of Trauma. J Trauma Acute Care Surg 2015;79(1):159–73.

31. Ferrada P, Wolfe L, Anand RJ, et al. Use of limited transthoracic echocardiography in patients with traumatic cardiac arrest decreases the rate of nontherapeutic thoracotomy and hospital costs. J Ultrasound Med 2014;33(10):1829–32.

32. Dennis BM, Medvecz AJ, Gunter OL, et al. Survey of trauma surgeon practice of emergency department thoracotomy. Am J Surg 2016;212(3):440–5.

33. Brenner ML, Moore LJ, DuBose JJ, et al. A clinical series of resuscitative endovascular balloon occlusion of the aorta for hemorrhage control and resuscitation. J Trauma Acute Care Surg 2013;75(3):506–11.

34. Biffl WL, Fox CJ, Moore EE. The role of REBOA in the control of exsanguinating torso hemorrhage. J Trauma Acute Care Surg 2015;78(5):1054–8.

35. DuBose JJ, Scalea TM, Brenner M, et al. The AAST prospective aortic occlusion for resuscitation in trauma and acute care surgery (AORTA) registry: data on contemporary utilization and outcomes of aortic occlusion and resuscitative balloon occlusion of the aorta (REBOA). J Trauma Acute Care Surg 2016;81(3): 409–19.

36. Napolitano LM. Resuscitative endovascular balloon occlusion of the aorta: indications, outcomes, and training. Crit Care Clin 2017;33(1):55–70.

37. Livingston DH, Lavery RF, Passannante MR, et al. Admission or observation is not necessary after a negative abdominal computed tomographic scan in patients with suspected blunt abdominal trauma: results of a prospective, multi-institutional trial. J Trauma 1998;44(2):273–80, 282.

38. Velmahos GC, Demetriades D. Early thoracoscopy for the evacuation of undrained haemothorax. Eur J Surg 1999;165(10):924–9.

39. Mowery NT, Gunter OL, Collier BR, et al. Practice management guidelines for management of hemothorax and occult pneumothorax. J Trauma 2011;70(2): 510–8.

40. Soldati G, Testa A, Pignataro G, et al. The ultrasonographic deep sulcus sign in traumatic pneumothorax. Ultrasound Med Biol 2006;32(8):1157–63.

41. Kwon A, Sorrells DL, Kurkchubasche AG, et al. Isolated computed tomography diagnosis of pulmonary contusion does not correlate with increased morbidity. J Pediatr Surg 2006;41(1):78–82, 82.

42. Como JJ, Bokhari F, Chiu WC, et al. Practice management guidelines for selective nonoperative management of penetrating abdominal trauma. J Trauma 2010; 68(3):721–33.

43. Ceraldi CM, Waxman K. Computerized tomography as an indicator of isolated mesenteric injury. A comparison with peritoneal lavage. Am Surg 1990;56(12): 806–10.

44. Baqué P, Trojani C, Delotte J, et al. Anatomical consequences of "open-book" pelvic ring disruption: a cadaver experimental study. Surg Radiol Anat 2005; 27(6):487–90.

45. Krieg JC, Mohr M, Ellis TJ, et al. Emergent stabilization of pelvic ring injuries by controlled circumferential compression: a clinical trial. J Trauma 2005;59(3): 659–64.

46. Stephen DJ, Kreder HJ, Day AC, et al. Early detection of arterial bleeding in acute pelvic trauma. J Trauma 1999;47(4):638–42.

47. Evers BM, Cryer HM, Miller FB. Pelvic fracture hemorrhage. Priorities in management. Arch Surg 1989;124(4):422–4.

48. Cothren CC, Osborn PM, Moore EE, et al. Preperitonal pelvic packing for hemodynamically unstable pelvic fractures: a paradigm shift. J Trauma 2007;62(4): 834–9, 842.

49. Lieurance R, Benjamin JB, Rappaport WD. Blood loss and transfusion in patients with isolated femur fractures. J Orthop Trauma 1992;6(2):175–9.

50. Gandhi RR, Overton TL, Haut ER, et al. Optimal timing of femur fracture stabilization in polytrauma patients: a practice management guideline from the Eastern Association for the Surgery of Trauma. J Trauma Acute Care Surg 2014;77(5): 787–95.

Balanced Resuscitation in Trauma Management

Paul M. Cantle, MD, MBT, FRCSC, Bryan A. Cotton, MD, MPH, FACS*

KEYWORDS

- Balanced resuscitation • Trauma • Coagulopathy • Hemorrhagic shock
- Damage control

KEY POINTS

- Crystalloid, once considered central to the resuscitation of traumatic hemorrhagic shock, leads to numerous complications and increases patient morbidity and mortality.
- Trauma-induced coagulopathy is frequent in injured patients at the time of hospital presentation and is worsened by aggressive crystalloid use.
- Balanced resuscitation minimizes coagulopathy through permissive hypotension, restrictive crystalloid use, and high ratios of plasma and platelet to red blood cell transfusion.
- Balanced resuscitation with plasma, platelets, and red blood cells in a 1:1:1 ratio improves outcomes and should be initiated early, including prehospital, when possible.
- Balanced resuscitation can be achieved through the use of preplanned, matured massive transfusion protocols, specifically designed to be continued until actively turned off.

INTRODUCTION

As the leading global cause of death among youth and young adults, the impact of trauma on years of productive life lost cannot be overstated.[1] With only brain injury as a larger cause of overall mortality, hemorrhage is the leading cause of preventable trauma death.[2–6] Rates of mortality in injured patients requiring a massive blood transfusion in the late 1980s were greater than 80%. Prehospital strategies considered standard of care at the time included early intravenous (IV) access with 2 large-bore cannulas and aggressive administration of crystalloid, regardless of patient physiology. In the civilian setting, in which blunt trauma predominates, paramedical, emergency, and surgical trauma providers loyally performed these same resuscitation strategies for several decades. Until recently, they continued to be taught on a global scale. The Advanced Trauma Life Support Course, used as a benchmark international trauma reference and teaching tool, and last updated in 2012, still promotes these

Disclosures: Nothing to disclose.

Division of Acute Care Surgery, Department of Surgery, McGovern Medical School, University Professional Building, Memorial Hermann Hospital, University of Texas, at Houston, 6431 Fannin, MSB 4.286 Houston, TX 77030, USA

* Corresponding author.

E-mail address: Bryan.A.Cotton@uth.tmc.edu

resuscitation strategies.[7,8] As a result, over the last 30 years, the initial resuscitation of patients with trauma had changed very little. At the start of the new millennium, despite many significant advances, those patients with significant hemorrhage continued to have a mortality of more than 50%.[9]

However, the last decade has witnessed the birth of a new paradigm in early trauma resuscitation. This radical shift emphasizes balanced resuscitation, using ratios of plasma, platelets, and red blood cells (RBCs) that approximate whole blood as early as possible in a patient's care. It has become understood that aggressive crystalloid resuscitation worsens coagulopathy through dilution, contributes to acidosis through pH alteration, and exacerbates hypothermia via infusion of large volumes of cold solution. To address this, a central tenet of balanced resuscitation is to limit early crystalloid use in an attempt to attenuate the predictable metabolic derangements that are associated with this traditional approach. With the addition of permissive hypotension, the third pillar of balanced resuscitation, current mortalities in hemorrhaging patients have decreased to as low as 20% (**Fig. 1**).[10] This article focuses on the balanced resuscitation portion of trauma management. The aim is to understand the motives behind the long-standing use of crystalloid resuscitation, review the advantages and disadvantages of various resuscitative agents, and present the compelling evidence that exists for balanced resuscitation in the management of trauma.

THE HISTORY OF WHOLE-BLOOD AND COMPONENT THERAPY

At the outset of World War 1 (WW1), the British military thought that blood transfusions caused harm and were instead focused on using crystalloids for resuscitation.[11] Concurrently, significant advancements in the tools and techniques necessary for blood typing, anticoagulation, and storage were being made. As a result, by the end of WW1, many casualties were being resuscitated with whole blood and this quickly became the standard of care in several military hospitals. Knowledge of whole blood–based resuscitation continued to evolve during both World War II (WWII) and the Korean War. The British had a functional blood transfusion system in place at the outset of WWII and the United States military shortly followed suit. By the end of WWII, the American military was mobilizing massive volumes of blood for transfusion. The American Red Cross drew more than 13 million units of whole blood from

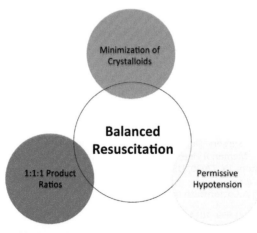

Fig. 1. The 3 tenets of balanced resuscitation.

donors during this war.[11] However, product waste was common. For example, during both the Korean War and the Vietnam War product waste was estimated at greater than 50%. Although fractionated products, including fresh frozen plasma (FFP), became available during the Vietnam War, going forward the United States military focused primarily on the procurement, transport, and storage of large volumes of RBCs. Despite this, fresh whole blood remained a useful tool because it could be readily procured from front-line soldiers and avoided the limitation of physical storage needed for component products. Furthermore, colloids, such as hydroxyethyl starch, with their significant ability to increase circulating volume and their reduced weight compared with crystalloids, were being developed and were touted as advantageous for the transport needs required in the conflict environment.[12]

In the civilian setting, in which concerns about the volume and weight of fluids used for resuscitation are minimal, storage of large quantities of product in centralized blood banks and dedicated care centers is efficient and practical. Whole blood, depending on the anticoagulant used, can be refrigerated and stored on average for 4 weeks. Using component separation, RBCs can be stored at 2°C to 6°C for 6 weeks while still maintaining viability, and FFP (plasma that has been frozen within 8 hours of collection) can be stored at −18°C for 1 year or at −65°C for 7 years.[13,14] Plasma separation from whole blood therefore significantly extends its useful lifespan. Once thawed, plasma can be kept refrigerated at 1°C to 6°C for a further 5 days while still retaining useful levels of coagulation factors.[15] In the United States, platelets are stored at room temperature for 5 days, at which point they must be discarded secondary to possible bacterial contamination.[16] Fractionation also provides the advantage of targeting components for specific clinical use, including those outside of trauma and resuscitation, for which individual components rather than whole blood may be desired (**Fig. 2**).

Although early work studying transfusion in trauma suggested that component therapy was not necessary to supplement whole blood, once the fractionation of products occurred, RBCs (and large volumes of crystalloid) alone became the standard to resuscitate bleeding patients.[11,17] The contribution of plasma and platelets to trauma

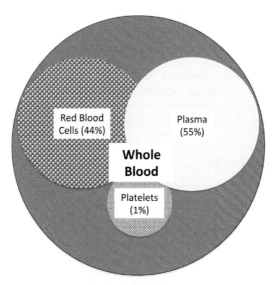

Fig. 2. The 3 primary components of whole blood.

resuscitation was discounted and a strategy of crystalloid first then RBCs later took hold.

THE CRYSTALLOID ADVANTAGE?

Because patients with trauma arrived in the emergency department (ED) without a type and screen and away from the centralized blood bank, early crystalloid therapy provided a means to rapidly resuscitate these patients while blood was being prepared.[18] With this in mind, crystalloid use in trauma resuscitation had several theoretic advantages. Most notably, it was seen as an inexpensive resource that was readily accessible and easily stored. It could be kept in the resuscitation bay or the operating room in quantities limited only by the physical storage space available. It did not require a refrigerator and small volumes could be kept in a warmer and readily replaced. Furthermore, it had an extremely long shelf life, could be mass produced by industry, rarely required being discarded secondary to expiration, and was cheap to restock.

Crystalloids were also familiar agents, used on a daily basis by most nurses and physicians. They required little adaptation for implementation in the resuscitation bay and did not require monitoring for transfusion reactions. Furthermore, crystalloids did not require testing for pathogens, such as human immunodeficiency virus (HIV) and hepatitis, did not pose a risk of blood-borne exposure to either health care workers or patients, and did not need to be typed or cross-matched. An ongoing crystalloid infusion, for the most part, did not require special IV lines or filters. Crystalloids could also be easily implemented in the prehospital setting, in which the advantages were similar, including ease of use, storage, and longevity. Patients could arrive at a resuscitation bay and have the same fluid bag continued while the primary survey was initiated and while improved IV or central venous access was obtained.

In contrast, blood products cannot be mass produced, require complex collection, sensitive screening for blood-borne pathogens, and careful means of transport and storage. They require processing and separation into components and close monitoring for transfusion reactions, both early and delayed. To infuse a blood product, there is a potential delay in order to check the blood band. Their high cost and short shelf life also mean that their use in the prehospital setting is limited, expensive, and potentially wasteful. In many countries, there is a history of significant fear of blood transfusion because of the previous use of tainted products and the infection of many recipients with hepatitis C and, later, HIV in the 1970s and early 1980s.[19,20] This stigma likely further contributed to health care workers' trepidation with transfusions and probably increased their favor for crystalloids. Blood product use decreased in trauma care from 54% of patients receiving product in 1991 to 42% in 1995.[21] The overall number of units being transfused between these 2 time points also decreased significantly.

CRYSTALLOID RESUSCITATION

What was the evidence behind using crystalloid in trauma resuscitation? Clinical experience with the use of crystalloid in elective and emergency surgical patients expanded rapidly in the 1980s and 1990s, and many physicians thought that this resuscitation knowledge was applicable to patients with trauma in hemorrhagic shock. However, the use of these fluids leads to a decrease in osmotic pressure and an increase in capillary permeability. A significant portion of the infused volume is lost from the intravascular space into the interstitium. When considering fluid resuscitation in major surgical operations, Shires and colleagues[22] showed that, with tissue injury, extracellular volume was lost, independent of blood loss. The degree of extracellular volume loss and internal redistribution seemed to be related to the extent of tissue injury. It was realized that, despite providing intravascular volume, fluid inherently moved out of the intravascular and intracellular spaces and into the extracellular space during tissue trauma, in the form of surgery, and that postoperative extracellular volume was directly related to the amount of intraoperative fluid administered.[23] The focus, therefore, became to maintain or even expand the extracellular volume throughout a major operation, even beyond the fluid volumes that were thought to be necessary for maintenance.[24] This observation of the contraction of extracellular fluid in surgical patients suggested that replacement with balanced salt solutions might be of benefit in trauma resuscitation as well.

Moore and Shires,[25] in a 1967 editorial entitled "Moderation," attempted to stop these aggressive resuscitation strategies before they became standard practice. The investigators raised concern about the use of crystalloid solutions to maximize the intravascular volume and to maintain excess volume in the interstitium so that patients had the necessary volume to replace any potential losses from bleeding. This approach was being used to such an extreme that patients were often receiving more than an entire blood volume equivalent of crystalloid during any major abdominal surgery. Moore and Shires[25] recommended that "replacement during operation should be carefully estimated and limited" and that blood "should still be replaced during major operative surgery as it is lost." The use of balanced salt solutions, they added, "appears to be a physiological adjunct to surgical trauma, not a substitute for blood." What is often lost, and is critical to remember, is that these cautions were coming during a time when the blood being used for trauma and major surgery was whole blood, not simply fractioned components such as RBCs.

Despite this caution, the use of crystalloids for replacement of lost blood gained momentum. Focus became placed on the prophylactic optimization of defined physiologic parameters through intensive, and often invasive, monitoring.[26] These invasive catheters and monitors provided new numbers (cardiac index, pulmonary artery pressures, central venous pressures, and mixed venous oxygen tension) and new laboratory values (lactate level, base deficit) to measure. It was no longer considered enough to simply maintain normal heart rate, blood pressure, and urine output.[27] Establishing and prophylactically maintaining normal patient parameters for each of these criteria in the critically ill population became the norm, even if extremely aggressive resuscitation was required to achieve these supraphysiologic results. At this same time, the idea of the damage-control laparotomy was emerging. This abbreviated laparotomy was initially described to help manage patients with severe physiologic disturbances by leaving them open to return for closure once stable.[28,29] However, surgeons increasingly found that they struggled to close fascia at subsequent explorations and the resultant sequelae of abdominal compartment syndrome began to be seen and treated as a new and accepted entity.[30,31]

The complications of aggressive crystalloid resuscitation were also being recognized to extend well beyond that of abdominal compartment syndrome. Both normal saline and lactated Ringer in large volumes have been shown to contribute to various forms of acidosis. Normal saline leads to a hyperchloremic metabolic acidosis that in turn leads to decreased cardiac contractility, decreased renal perfusion, and less ionotropic response, whereas large volumes of lactated Ringer contribute to a compensatory respiratory acidosis.[32–34] An overloaded fluid status has been shown to increase mortality from postoperative pulmonary edema.[35] Studies assessing fluid management strategies in acute lung injury and acute respiratory distress syndrome have found that a conservative use of fluid leads to more ventilator-free days, shorter intensive care unit (ICU) stays, and improved lung function without increasing failure rates of other organ systems.[36] Although, at small doses, fluid may improve cardiac performance in some populations, aggressive saline resuscitation can further compromise cardiac performance, driving many critically ill surgical patients and patients with trauma off their optimal Starling curve.[37,38] Postoperative patients receiving greater than 3 L of crystalloid at normal saline concentrations have been shown to have delayed gastric emptying time, delayed return of bowel function, prolonged hospital stay, and more perioperative complications compared with a restrictive fluid strategy.[39] Overall, it seems that the downsides of crystalloids are extensive, and, despite their convenience in the trauma bay, they likely do more harm than good in resuscitation for hemorrhagic shock.

COLLOIDS

The advantage of colloids for resuscitation was thought to be that they could significantly and rapidly expand circulating volume. Synthetic options including dextran, starch-based solutions such as hydroxyethyl starch, and plasma-derived albumin all contain large molecules that exert a significant osmotic effect on the surrounding tissue. They effectively draw fluid into the intravascular space from the interstitial and intracellular spaces, resulting in both a maintenance and expansion of the circulating volume in patients with trauma.[40,41] Commonly referred to as plasma expanders, as larger molecule liquids they stay in the intravascular space for a longer period of time and are able to expand intravascular volume more effectively than crystalloids. However, in addition to higher cost of colloids, there are several other downsides compared with crystalloids. There is an uncommon, but recognized, risk of hypersensitivity reaction to these solutions. Dextran is known to reduce platelet aggregation in some populations and has been used as an anticoagulant in the past.[42] Albumin, a byproduct of human blood fractionation, is expensive to produce. The starch-based colloid solutions have been associated with anaphylactoid reactions and with renal failure.[43] Importantly, hydroxyethyl starches have been shown to cause coagulopathy.[44] They reduce maximal clot firmness and reduce all coagulation factor activities, with the greatest impact on fibrinogen and factor II, XIII, and X activity. They are so effective at this that they are used to create dilutional coagulopathy in studies evaluating the efficacy of hemostatic adjuncts.[45]

PLASMA AS THE OPTIMAL RESUSCITATION FLUID

Plasma has long been recognized as an excellent buffer solution.[46] It has been shown to be a 50-fold better buffer than crystalloids and 5-fold better than albumin. This ability, secondary to its high citrate content, makes it ideal for the resuscitation of patients in a state of severe acidosis from shock. In addition to containing all necessary clotting factors and countless microparticles, plasma contains up to 500 mg of fibrinogen per unit.[47] Like colloids, plasma provides the additional benefit of being an excellent volume expander by leading to a significant increase in osmotic pressure. As a result, it increases intravascular volume both directly and indirectly by drawing interstitial and intracellular volume into circulation. Furthermore, plasma has been shown in animal models to have a positive impact on endothelial vascular integrity by stabilizing the endothelial glycocalyx and inhibiting permeability by as much as 10-fold.[48]

So why has its use not been universally adopted? In addition to availability, transfusion-related events, including ABO incompatibility, transfusion reactions, and transmission of infections, have been reported. Plasma also has a high cost of procurement, testing, and storage. Opponents of aggressive plasma resuscitation cite data that suggest that it leads to a higher incidence of transfusion-related acute lung injury.[49] However, newer, compelling evidence argues that the development of moderate to severe hypoxemia after trauma is more likely to be caused by a patients age, extent of lung injury, and the use of crystalloid resuscitation and shows no relationship with product use, whether it be RBCs, plasma, or platelets transfused.[50] Animal model evidence exists that plasma may mitigate the lung injury sustained from shock compared with crystalloid.[51] Acute lung injury after trauma is much more likely to be caused by hemorrhagic shock and crystalloid resuscitation than by plasma transfusion. Plasma transfusion is likely to be beneficial in this scenario.

THE BALANCED RESUSCITATION STRATEGY

In the setting of hemorrhage, balanced (or damage control) resuscitation refers to the strategy adopted by the US military to improve outcomes of patients undergoing an abbreviated laparotomy or other procedure because of grossly disturbed physiology. As an adjunct to the care of these critically injured patients, its early implementation focused on delivering higher ratios of plasma and platelets, along with other strategies to prevent "popping the clot." Its 3 basic tenets are permissive hypotension, minimizing the use of crystalloid before surgical control of bleeding, and transfusion of blood products in a ratio approximating whole blood.[52] Ideally, this process begins in the prehospital setting, continues through early trauma bay/emergency room resuscitation, and is completed in the operating room or the ICU, as needed.

As massive transfusion protocols (MTPs) developed, studies began to explore outcomes from different product ratios given to patients who ended up requiring more than 10 units of RBCs within a 24-hour period. Work on determining both the ideal plasma to RBC and platelet to RBC ratios was pursued. Examining different MTPs used by different trauma centers and organizations, Malone and colleagues[53] suggested that preemptive treatment of coagulopathy with a 1:1:1 product ratio seems to be associated with improved outcomes and provides the additional benefit of ease of use. Ho and colleagues[54] made a similar argument for this strategy with the aim of transfusing patients with trauma with factors equivalent to whole blood in a timely fashion. In 2008, Holcomb and colleagues[55] published data from 16 civilian trauma centers showing that plasma/RBC and platelet/RBC ratios of greater than 1:2 improved early and late survival, primarily through a reduction in rates of truncal hemorrhage. They concluded that MTPs should target an ideal ratio of 1:1:1. Gunter and colleagues[56] showed that both higher plasma to RBC and higher platelet to RBC ratios each individually improved the 30-day mortality of patients with MT trauma. These data formed the basis for the landmark (The Pragmatic, Randomized Optimal Platelet and Plasma Ratios trial) PROPPR trial. Investigators directly compared the mortality of patients with trauma (predicted to receive MT) randomized to a ratio of 1:1:1 versus 1:1:2.[10] Although the 2 groups did not have a significant difference in 24-hour or 30-day mortality, the 1:1:1 group had fewer deaths caused by bleeding and improved rates of achieving hemostasis. These findings led to the recent Eastern Association for the Surgery of Trauma's (EAST) recommendation for transfusion of equal amounts of RBC, plasma, and platelets during the early, empiric phase of resuscitation.[57]

The role of fibrinogen (concentrate or cryoprecipitate) in the resuscitation of patients with hemorrhagic shock remains unclear. Cryoprecipitate acts as a concentrated source of fibrinogen and other coagulation proteins; however, its transfusion is often delayed for several hours in patients with trauma. Transfusion of cryoprecipitate within 90 minutes of patient arrival has undergone preliminary study that suggests that it is feasible to administer and possibly affects mortality.[58] As a result, a United

Kingdom–funded, multicenter, randomized trial comparing early cryoprecipitate transfusion with standard blood transfusion therapy in severely bleeding patients with trauma is currently underway (CRYOSTAT-2).

PREHOSPITAL RESUSCITATION

In 2011, Haut and colleagues[59] showed, in a review of the National Trauma Data Bank, that patients with trauma who received prehospital IV lines had significantly higher mortality than those who did not. Given the resuscitation and transfusion trends of the time period during which these patient data were collected (2001–2005), it is highly likely that the patients receiving prehospital IV fluid were receiving crystalloid only resuscitation. They were almost certainly not receiving blood products. In the development of guidelines for prehospital fluid administration, EAST found insufficient data to support the administration of prehospital fluids to severely injured patients as well as insufficient data to recommend one type of resuscitation fluid rather than another.[60] In 2015, a randomized study from the Resuscitation Outcomes Consortium compared a standard resuscitation protocol of 2 L of fluid plus additional boluses as needed to maintain a systolic blood pressure of 110 mm Hg or greater against a controlled resuscitation protocol using 250-mL boluses to maintain a radial pulse or a systolic blood pressure of 70 mm Hg or greater.[61] Simultaneously examining 2 of the tenets of hemostatic resuscitation (permissive hypotension and limited crystalloid use), the investigators found that the controlled resuscitation strategy offered an early survival advantage. In the military setting, this concept had previously been proposed by both Cannon and colleagues[62] and Beecher.[63,64] Cannon and colleagues[62] in 1918 reported that the "injection of a fluid that will increase blood pressure has dangers in itself." They argued that, in hemorrhage, if the blood pressure is "raised before the surgeon is ready to check any bleeding that may take place, blood that is sorely needed may be lost." Beecher,[64] just after WWII, wrote that, before surgical control of bleeding, "elevation of his systolic blood pressure to about 85 mm Hg is all that is, necessary... and when profuse internal bleeding is occurring, it is wasteful of time and blood to attempt to get the patient's blood pressure up to normal."

As emphasis has moved away from prehospital crystalloid use, several recent studies evaluating blood product transfusion (both plasma and RBC) in the prehospital setting have shown that these products are associated with improved early outcomes, with little, if any, wastage.[65] In addition, patients receiving these products arrive with improved acid-base status and a lower incidence of coagulopathy.[65–67] Several centers have since developed and matured their protocols with prehospital products whereby the flight team (nurses and paramedics) may initiate transfusion based on field variables. Both the Mayo Clinic and University of Texas–Houston initiate plasma and RBC transfusion based on the prehospital Assessment of Blood Consumption (ABC) score (**Table 1**).[68,69] Others have recommended the prehospital shock index to guide blood product use.[70]

TRAUMA BAY RESUSCITATION

There is increasing evidence that patients should not be aggressively resuscitated in the prehospital environment and that blood products are of benefit in this setting, so the question becomes how should clinicians resuscitate these patients once they arrive at the trauma center, where definitive hemorrhage control can be attempted and achieved? The data in this setting are more robust, older, and more convincing than the evolving prehospital literature. As early as 1994, the concept of a possible benefit from delayed resuscitation was being considered.

Table 1
Assessment of blood consumption score for the prediction of massive transfusion

Variable	Yes or No? (Yes = 1, No = 0)
1. Penetrating mechanism	Yes/no
2. Positive FAST	Yes/no
3. HR $\geq$ 120 bpm	Yes/no
4. SBP $\leq$ 90 mm Hg	Yes/no
Total out of 4	If $\geq$2 = yes, initiate MTP

Abbreviations: bpm, beats per minute; FAST, focused assessment with sonography for trauma; HR, heart rate; SBP, systolic blood pressure.

Bickell and colleagues[71] reported that patients with penetrating torso injuries who were randomized to delayed fluid resuscitation (no fluid until operating room arrival) had improved survival, shorter hospital stays, and fewer complications than those randomized to immediate crystalloid resuscitation from the scene and during their ED stays. In 2002, Dutton and colleagues[72] reported that the resuscitation of patients presenting with severe hemorrhage to a systolic pressure of greater than 110 mm Hg was not superior to allowing for permissive hypotension with a systolic goal of 70 mm Hg. Mortality was similar between these groups, and permissive hypotension had the potential to allow better control of bleeding with fewer transfusions than the higher target.

As in the prehospital setting, early recognition of the need for MT is important and can be facilitated by scores designed for the prediction of MT, such as the ABC score.[68,73] For balanced resuscitation to be effective, blood products, including plasma and platelets, should be as readily available as RBCs. Ideally, universal thawed plasma is on hand at the time of patient arrival and, to accomplish this, some centers have begun stocking their trauma bays/EDs with plasma, which significantly reduces the time it takes for plasma to be delivered to patients in hemorrhage. Radwan and colleagues[74] showed that having thawed (or liquid) plasma available in the ED was associated with fewer transfusions of RBC, plasma, and platelets in the first 24 hours and was an independent predictor of reduced 30-day mortality in this population. The strategy should therefore be to have thawed AB plasma available in the resuscitation bay to be used until type-specific plasma can be thawed and becomes available from the blood bank. However, to have plasma immediately available is challenging in many centers. If thawed AB plasma in the ED is not feasible or practical, one solution is to use liquid (never frozen) plasma. Liquid plasma has a hemostatic profile that is superior to thawed plasma and it can viably be stored in a refrigerated setting for up to 26 days.[75] The hemostatic ability of this product, and its long refrigerator storage potential, suggest that it may be the ideal product to be kept within the trauma bay where it is close at hand for the resuscitation of hemorrhaging patients with trauma. In addition, although less than 5% of donors are AB blood group, at least 40% of donors are type A and many of them have low enough titers of anti-B that it can be safely given as a universal product. Therefore, liquid AB and low-titer A plasma should be strongly conserved for ED use.

OPERATING ROOM RESUSCITATION

In evaluating all components of damage control resuscitation, including permissive hypotension, limitation of crystalloids, and delivering high ratios of plasma and platelets, Cotton and colleagues[76] found that those patients with trauma undergoing damage control laparotomy had a significant increase in 30-day survival when this resuscitation strategy was implemented. Morrison and colleagues[77] published randomized data that suggested that the hypotensive resuscitation strategy should potentially extend beyond the trauma bay and into the operating room. They reported that patients with trauma requiring urgent operative intervention required less fluid and blood product when an intraoperative MAP target of 50 mm Hg was used, as opposed to an MAP target of 65 mm Hg, but these patients also had lower rates of early postoperative mortality and a trend toward lower overall mortality. They were also less likely to develop early coagulopathy, less likely to have a severe coagulopathy, and less likely to die from bleeding. The investigators concluded that a hypotensive resuscitation strategy is safe in trauma. Duke and colleagues[78] showed that, as part of a damage control resuscitation strategy, restrictive fluid use in patients with trauma, compared with standard fluid use, led to lower rates of intraoperative mortality and shorter lengths of hospital stay. In addition, the PROPPR trial noted that, compared with patients receiving 1:1:2 ratio, those receiving a 1:1:1 ratio more rapidly achieved clinical hemostasis, had their MTP discontinued sooner, and had lower bleeding-related mortality.[10] Continuing a balanced resuscitation strategy intraoperatively is critical.

One of the intrinsic benefits of an MTP is to provide the resuscitation team with the ability to transfuse patients without having to track product ratios closely during an intense operation and resuscitation. Each MTP pack should be designed to contain a balanced ratio of product and each patient should receive 1 complete pack before moving onto the next. This system compels the resuscitation team to provide a balanced ratio of product, rather than transfusing based on delayed laboratory results or personal sentiment. In addition to ensuring that patients receive hemostatic ratios, this strategy removes a responsibility from the numerous demands already placed on resuscitation teams as they multitask through the resuscitations, providing a secondary benefit to patients by allowing the teams to focus instead on other important tasks.

INTENSIVE CARE UNIT RESUSCITATION

In general, hemorrhage sufficient to warrant an MT requires ICU admission. Arrival of these patients to the ICU marks an important checkpoint or node in the patient's care and should prompt a review of the resuscitative efforts so far and a plan and direction for further care. In addition to addressing factors that exacerbate coagulopathy, including hypothermia, acidosis, and hypocalcemia, clinicians should ask whether the patient is still receiving MTP or whether the patient has been transitioned to laboratory-directed resuscitation. An appropriate laboratory-directed algorithm should be in place, and care at this point should be guided according to these assays. If an active MTP is still required, clinicians should ask whether the patient warrants a return to the operating room. If not, blood pressures targets may be returned to normal and supportive or maintenance fluids begun. However, should the patient's abdomen remain open, substituting hypertonic saline for maintenance fluids (rather than standard crystalloids) should be considered to reduce bowel wall and mesenteric edema.[79]

With respect to continued high ratios of plasma and platelets, the PROMMTT (Prospective, Observational, Multicenter, Major Trauma Transfusion) study provided answers to this question.[80] This prospective cohort study found that higher (1:1:1) ratios of plasma and platelet to RBC decreased patient mortality during the first

6 hours. However, the investigators noted that, after 6 hours (and continuing through 30 days), although higher ratios were not associated with increased complications they were also of no benefit.

RETURN TO WHOLE BLOOD

The reasons for a shift away from whole-blood transfusion were many. With advances in blood banking, fractionation provided a means by which components specific to the needs of the patient, including patients without trauma, could be provided without having to administer whole blood. Furthermore, blood banking provided a means by which some components could be stored for extended durations, thereby decreasing concerns about a limited and time-sensitive supply. As a result, whole blood was removed as an available product. However, this was done without consideration of whether whole blood was more or less superior to component therapy in the resuscitation of hemorrhaging patients. In 2013, Cotton and colleagues[81] challenged the assumption that component therapy was equal to whole blood by completing a pilot randomized controlled trial. They discovered that the use of modified whole blood did not decrease transfusion volumes compared with component therapy. However, when patients with severe brain injuries were excluded, the remaining patients receiving modified whole blood required less volume of transfusion than those receiving component therapy. Of note, the modified whole-blood group required the additional transfusion of platelets at a ratio equivalent to the component therapy group. This work suggests that the use of whole blood may lead to similar survival outcomes as component therapy but with a decrease in the volume of transfusion required to achieve this goal. Further work by the Early Whole Blood Investigators has found that patients transfused with modified whole blood compared with component therapy showed improved thrombin potential and platelet aggregation.[82] This area requires further study. The use of fresh whole blood is likely to continue in the military setting because it has been found to be convenient, safe, and effective.[83]

SUMMARY

Balanced resuscitation has become a key tenet in the care of patients with trauma. The implementation of this central strategy has been associated with reduced death from major bleeding, decreasing reported mortalities from more than 60% in 2007 to as low as 20% currently. During this time, clinicians have begun to appreciate that aggressive crystalloid resuscitation leads to significant clinical complications and harm and that massive fluid resuscitation should be avoided. The use of crystalloids and colloids should be as thoughtful and careful as with any medication. When the limitation of crystalloid resuscitation is combined with permissive hypotension, prevention of hypothermia, and the transfusion of component blood into ratios that match the composition of whole blood early in the care of patients with trauma, outcomes are significantly improved. Balanced resuscitation provides an early means to treat trauma-induced coagulopathy, leads to an overall decrease in the use of blood products, and improves patient survival. Although further advances in the resuscitation strategies used to treat patients with trauma will be made and improvements in patient-specific targeting of transfusions will be developed, there is little doubt that balanced resuscitation using modern MTPs is likely here to stay. Bleeding needs blood to stop bleeding.

REFERENCES

1. Cothren CC, Moore EE, Hedegaard HB, et al. Epidemiology of urban trauma deaths: a comprehensive reassessment 10 years later. World J Surg 2007; 31(7):1507–11.
2. Centers for Disease Control and Prevention. Web-based injury statistics query and reporting system. Atlanta (GA): US Department of Health and Human Services, CDC, National Center for Injury Prevention and Control; 2003.
3. Sauaia A, Moore FA, Moore EE, et al. Epidemiology of trauma deaths: a reassessment. J Trauma 1995;38(2):185–93.
4. Acosta JA, Yang JC, Winchell RJ, et al. Lethal injuries and time to death in a level I trauma center. J Am Coll Surg 1998;186(5):528–33.
5. Rhee P, Joseph B, Pandit V, et al. Increasing trauma deaths in the United States. Ann Surg 2014;260(1):13–21.
6. Tieu BH, Holcomb JB, Schreiber MA. Coagulopathy: its pathophysiology and treatment in the injured patient. World J Surg 2007;31(5):1055–64.
7. American College of Surgeons Committee on Trauma. ATLS, advanced trauma life support student course manual. 9th edition. Chicago: American College of Surgeons; 2012.
8. ATLS Subcommittee, American College of Surgeons' Committee on Trauma, International ATLS Working Group. Advanced trauma life support (ATLS®): the ninth edition. J Trauma 2013;74(5):1363–6.
9. Cinat ME, Wallace WC, Nastanski F, et al. Improved survival following massive transfusion in patients who have undergone trauma. Arch Surg 1999;134(9): 964–8.
10. Holcomb JB, Tilley BC, Baraniuk S, et al. Transfusion of plasma, platelets, and red blood cells in a 1:1:1 vs a 1:1:2 ratio and mortality in patients with severe trauma: the PROPPR randomized clinical trial. JAMA 2015;313(5):471–82.
11. Hess JR, Thomas MJ. Blood use in war and disaster: lessons from the past century. Transfusion 2003;43(11):1622–33.
12. Holcomb JB. Fluid resuscitation in modern combat casualty care: lessons learned from Somalia. J Trauma 2003;54(5S):S46–51.
13. Sullivan MT, Cotten R, Read EJ, et al. Blood collection and transfusion in the United States in 2001. Transfusion 2007;47(3):385–94.
14. Dumont LJ, AuBuchon JP. Evaluation of proposed FDA criteria for the evaluation of radiolabeled red cell recovery trials. Transfusion 2008;48(6):1053–60.
15. Downes KA, Wilson E, Yomtovian R, et al. Serial measurement of clotting factors in thawed plasma stored for 5 days. Transfusion 2001;41(4):570.
16. Hess JR. Conventional blood banking and blood component storage regulation: opportunities for improvement. Blood Transfus 2010;8(S3):S9–15.
17. Counts RB, Haisch C, Simon TL, et al. Hemostasis in massively transfused trauma patients. Ann Surg 1979;190(1):91–9.
18. Carrico CJ, Canizaro PC, Shires GT. Fluid resuscitation following injury: rationale for the use of balanced salt solutions. Crit Care Med 1976;4(2):46–54.
19. Picard A. The gift of death: confronting Canada's tainted-blood tragedy. Toronto: HarperCollins; 1995.
20. Meier, B. Blood, money and aids: haemophiliacs are split; liability cases bogged down in disputes. The New York Times. June 11, 1996.
21. Farion KJ, McLellan BA, Boulanger BR, et al. Changes in red cell transfusion practice among adult trauma victims. J Trauma 1998;44(4):583–7.

22. Shires T, Williams J, Brown F. Acute change in extracellular fluids associated with major surgical procedures. Ann Surg 1961;154(5):803–10.
23. Virtue RW, LeVine DS, Aikawa JK. Fluid shifts during the surgical period: RISA and s^{35} determinations following glucose, saline or lactate infusion. Ann Surg 1966;163(4):523–8.
24. Nielsen OM, Engell HC. The importance of plasma colloid osmotic pressure for interstitial fluid volume and fluid balance after elective abdominal vascular surgery. Ann Surg 1986;203(1):25–9.
25. Moore FD, Shires GT. Moderation. Ann Surg 1967;166(2):300–1.
26. Shoemaker WC, Appel P, Bland R. Use of physiologic monitoring to predict outcome and to assist in clinical decisions in critically ill postoperative patients. Am J Surg 1983;146(1):43–50.
27. Abramson D, Scalea TM, Hitchcock R, et al. Lactate clearance and survival following injury. J Trauma 1993;35(4):584–8.
28. Stone HH, Strom PR, Mullins RJ. Management of the major coagulopathy with onset during laparotomy. Ann Surg 1983;197(5):532–5.
29. Rotondo MF, Schwab CW, McGonigal MD, et al. 'Damage control': an approach for improved survival in exsanguinating penetrating abdominal injury. J Trauma 1993;35(3):375–82.
30. Fietsam R Jr, Villalba M, Glover JL, et al. Intra-abdominal compartment syndrome as a complication of ruptured abdominal aortic aneurysm repair. Am Surg 1989; 55(6):396–402.
31. Bendahan J, Coetzee CJ, Papagianopoulos C, et al. Abdominal compartment syndrome. J Trauma 1995;38(1):152–3.
32. Scheingraber S, Rehm M, Sehmisch C, et al. Rapid saline infusion produces hyperchloremic acidosis in patients undergoing gynecologic surgery. Anesthesiology 1999;90(5):1265–70.
33. Williams EL, Hildebrand KL, McCormick SA, et al. The effect of intravenous lactated Ringer's solution versus 0.9% sodium chloride solution on serum osmolality in human volunteers. Anesth Analg 1999;88(5):999–1003.
34. Takil A, Eti Z, Irmak P, et al. Early postoperative respiratory acidosis after large intravascular volume infusion of lactated ringer's solution during major spine surgery. Anesth Analg 2002;95(2):294–8.
35. Arieff AI. Fatal postoperative pulmonary edema: pathogenesis and literature review. Chest 1999;115(5):1371–7.
36. Wiedemann HP, Wheeler AP, Bernard GR, et al, National Heart, Lung, and Blood Institute Acute Respiratory Distress Syndrome (ARDS) Clinical Trials Network. Comparison of two fluid-management strategies in acute lung injury. N Engl J Med 2006;354(24):2564–75.
37. Richard C, Warszawski J, Anguel N, et al, French Pulmonary Artery Catheter Study Group. Early use of the pulmonary artery catheter and outcomes in patients with shock and acute respiratory distress syndrome: a randomized controlled trial. JAMA 2003;290(20):2713–20.
38. Sandham JD, Hull RD, Brant RF, et al, Canadian Critical Care Clinical Trials Group. A randomized, controlled trial of the use of pulmonary-artery catheters in high-risk surgical patients. N Engl J Med 2003;348(1):5–14.
39. Lobo DN, Bostock KA, Neal KR, et al. Effect of salt and water balance on recovery of gastrointestinal function after elective colonic resection: a randomised controlled trial. Lancet 2002;359(9320):1812–8.
40. Lamke LO, Liljedahl SO. Plasma volume expansion after infusion of 5%, 20% and 25% albumin solutions in patients. Resuscitation 1976;5(2):85–92.

41. Tønnessen T, Tølløfsrud S, Kongsgaard UE, et al. Colloid osmotic pressure of plasma replacement fluids. Acta Anaesthesiol Scand 1993;37(4):424–6.
42. Robless P, Okonko D, Mikhailidis DP, et al. Dextran 40 reduces in vitro platelet aggregation in peripheral arterial disease. Platelets 2004;15(4):215–22.
43. Zarychanski R, Abou-Setta AM, Turgeon AF, et al. Association of hydroxyethyl starch administration with mortality and acute kidney injury in critically ill patients requiring volume resuscitation: a systematic review and meta-analysis. JAMA 2013;309(7):678–88.
44. Fenger-Eriksen C, Tønnesen E, Ingerslev J, et al. Mechanisms of hydroxyethyl starch-induced dilutional coagulopathy. J Thromb Haemost 2009;7(7):1099–105.
45. Schramko AA, Suojaranta-Ylinen RT, Kuitunen AH, et al. Rapidly degradable hydroxyethyl starch solutions impair blood coagulation after cardiac surgery: a prospective randomized trial. Anesth Analg 2009;108(1):30–6.
46. Traverso LW, Medina F, Bolin RB. The buffering capacity of crystalloid and colloid resuscitation solutions. Resuscitation 1985;12(4):265–70.
47. Ketchum L, Hess JR, Hiippala S. Indications for early fresh frozen plasma, cryoprecipitate, and platelet transfusion in trauma. J Trauma 2006;60(6S):S51–8.
48. Pati S, Matijevic N, Doursout MF, et al. Protective effects of fresh frozen plasma on vascular endothelial permeability, coagulation, and resuscitation after hemorrhagic shock are time dependent and diminish between days 0 and 5 after thaw. J Trauma 2010;69(S1):S55–63.
49. Khan H, Belsher J, Yilmaz M, et al. Fresh-frozen plasma and platelet transfusions are associated with development of acute lung injury in critically ill medical patients. Chest 2007;131(5):1308–14.
50. Robinson BR, Cotton BA, Pritts TA, et al. Application of the Berlin definition in PROMMTT patients: the impact of resuscitation on the incidence of hypoxemia. J Trauma 2013;75(1S):S61–7.
51. Kozar RA, Peng Z, Zhang R, et al. Plasma restoration of endothelial glycocalyx in a rodent model of hemorrhagic shock. Anesth Analg 2011;112(6):1289–95.
52. Holcomb JB, Jenkins D, Rhee P, et al. Damage control resuscitation: directly addressing the early coagulopathy of trauma. J Trauma 2007;62(2):307–10.
53. Malone DL, Hess JR, Fingerhut A. Massive transfusion practices around the globe and a suggestion for a common massive transfusion protocol. J Trauma 2006;60(6 Suppl):S91–6.
54. Ho AM, Karmakar MK, Dion PW. Are we giving enough coagulation factors during major trauma resuscitation? Am J Surg 2005;190(3):479–84.
55. Holcomb JB, Wade CE, Michalek JE, et al. Increased plasma and platelet to red blood cell ratios improves outcome in 466 massively transfused civilian trauma patients. Ann Surg 2008;248(3):447–58.
56. Gunter OL Jr, Au BK, Isbell JM, et al. Optimizing outcomes in damage control resuscitation: identifying blood product ratios associated with improved survival. J Trauma 2008;65(3):527–34.
57. Cannon JW, Khan MA, Raja AS, et al. Damage control resuscitation in patients with severe traumatic hemorrhage: a practice management guideline from the Eastern Association for the Surgery of Trauma. J Trauma 2017;82(3):605–17.
58. Curry N, Rourke C, Davenport R, et al. Early cryoprecipitate for major haemorrhage in trauma: a randomised controlled feasibility trial. Br J Anaesth 2015;115(1):76–83.
59. Haut ER, Kalish BT, Cotton BA, et al. Prehospital intravenous fluid administration is associated with higher mortality in trauma patients: a National Trauma Data Bank analysis. Ann Surg 2011;253(2):371–7.

60. Cotton BA, Jerome R, Collier BR, et al, Eastern Association for the Surgery of Trauma Practice Parameter Workgroup for Prehospital Fluid Resuscitation. Guidelines for prehospital fluid resuscitation in the injured patient. J Trauma 2009;67(2):389–402.

61. Schreiber MA, Meier EN, Tisherman SA, et al, ROC Investigators. A controlled resuscitation strategy is feasible and safe in hypotensive trauma patients: results of a prospective randomized pilot trial. J Trauma 2015;78(4):687–95.

62. Cannon WB, Fraser J, Cowell EM. The preventive treatment of wound shock. JAMA 1918;70:618–21.

63. Beecher HK. Preparation of battle casualties for surgery. Ann Surg 1945;21: 769–92.

64. Beecher HK. Resuscitation and anesthesia for wounded men. Springfield (IL): Banerstone House; 1949.

65. Holcomb JB, Donathan DP, Cotton BA, et al. Prehospital transfusion of plasma and red blood cells in trauma patients. Prehosp Emerg Care 2015;19(1):1–9.

66. Kim BD, Zielinski MD, Jenkins DH, et al. The effects of prehospital plasma on patients with injury: a prehospital plasma resuscitation. J Trauma 2012;73(2 Suppl 1):S49–53.

67. Brown JB, Sperry JL, Fombona A, et al. Pre-trauma center red blood cell transfusion is associated with improved early outcomes in air medical trauma patients. J Am Coll Surg 2015;220(5):797–808.

68. Nunez TC, Voskresensky IV, Dossett LA, et al. Early prediction of massive transfusion in trauma: simple as ABC (assessment of blood consumption)? J Trauma 2009;66(2):346–52.

69. Goodman MD, Hawes HG, Pommerening MJ, et al. Prehospital ABC score accurately triages patients who will require immediate resource utilization. Presented at the 72nd Annual Meeting of AAST and Clinical Congress of Acute Care Surgery. San Francisco, CA, September 18–21, 2013.

70. Parimi N, Hu PF, Mackenzie CF, et al. Automated continuous vital signs predict use of uncrossed matched blood and massive transfusion following trauma. J Trauma 2016;80(6):897–906.

71. Bickell WH, Wall MJ Jr, Pepe PE, et al. Immediate versus delayed fluid resuscitation for hypotensive patients with penetrating torso injuries. N Engl J Med 1994; 331(17):1105–9.

72. Dutton RP, Mackenzie CF, Scalea TM. Hypotensive resuscitation during active hemorrhage: impact on in-hospital mortality. J Trauma 2002;52(6):1141–6.

73. Cantle PM, Cotton BA. Prediction of massive transfusion in trauma. Crit Care Clin 2017;33(1):71–84.

74. Radwan ZA, Bai Y, Matijevic N, et al. An emergency department thawed plasma protocol for severely injured patients. JAMA Surg 2013;148(2):170–5.

75. Matijevic N, Wang YW, Cotton BA, et al. Better hemostatic profiles of never-frozen liquid plasma compared with thawed fresh frozen plasma. J Trauma 2013;74(1): 84–90.

76. Cotton BA, Reddy N, Hatch QM, et al. Damage control resuscitation is associated with a reduction in resuscitation volumes and improvement in survival in 390 damage control laparotomy patients. Ann Surg 2011;254(4):598–605.

77. Morrison CA, Carrick MM, Norman MA, et al. Hypotensive resuscitation strategy reduces transfusion requirements and severe postoperative coagulopathy in trauma patients with hemorrhagic shock: preliminary results of a randomized controlled trial. J Trauma 2011;70(3):652–63.

78. Duke MD, Guidry C, Guice J, et al. Restrictive fluid resuscitation in combination with damage control resuscitation: time for adaptation. J Trauma 2012;73(3): 674–8.

79. Harvin JA, Mims MM, Duchesne JC, et al. Chasing 100%: the use of hypertonic saline to improve early, primary fascial closure after damage control laparotomy. J Trauma 2013;74(2):426–30.

80. Holcomb JB, del Junco DJ, Fox EE, et al, PROMMTT Study Group. The Prospective, Observational, Multicenter, Major Trauma Transfusion (PROMMTT) study: comparative effectiveness of a time-varying treatment with competing risks. JAMA Surg 2013;148(2):127–36.

81. Cotton BA, Podbielski J, Camp E, et al, Early Whole Blood Investigators. A randomized controlled pilot trial of modified whole blood versus component therapy in severely injured patients requiring large volume transfusions. Ann Surg 2013;258(4):527–32.

82. Rahbar E, Cardenas JC, Matijevic N, et al, Early Whole Blood Investigators. Trauma, time, and transfusions: a longitudinal analysis of coagulation markers in severely injured trauma patients receiving modified whole blood or component blood products. Shock 2015;44(5):417–25.

83. Kauvar DS, Holcomb JB, Norris GC, et al. Fresh whole blood transfusion: a controversial military practice. J Trauma 2006;61(1):181–4.

Acute Management of Traumatic Brain Injury

Michael A. Vella, MD, MBA[a,b], Marie L. Crandall, MD, MPH[c],
Mayur B. Patel, MD, MPH[d,e],*

KEYWORDS

- Traumatic brain injury • Intracranial hypertension • Secondary injury
- Hyperosmolar therapy • Barbiturate coma • Decompressive craniectomy

KEY POINTS

- Traumatic brain injury (TBI) is a leading cause of death and disability in patients with trauma with a significant economic impact.
- The acute management of TBI focuses on the prevention of secondary injury through the avoidance of hypotension and hypoxia and maintenance of appropriate cerebral perfusion pressure and, by extension, cerebral blood flow.
- Mass lesions may require operative intervention based on imaging characteristic, examination findings, and measurements of intracranial pressure (ICP).
- Increased ICP can be managed in an algorithmic fashion using a combination of simple bedside maneuvers, hyperosmolar therapy, cerebrospinal fluid drainage, pentobarbital coma, and decompressive craniectomy.
- Other important considerations in patients with TBI include venous thromboembolism, stress ulcer, and seizure prophylaxis, as well as nutrition and metabolic optimization.

Disclosures and funding: M.B. Patel is supported by National Institutes of Health (Bethesda, MD) NHLBI R01 HL111111 and NIGMS R01 GM120484. This work was also supported by REDCap UL1 TR000445 from NCATS/NIH. The authors have no other disclosures relevant to this article.
[a] Department of Surgery, Section of Surgical Sciences, Vanderbilt University Medical Center, Medical Center North, CCC-4312, 1161 21st Avenue South, Nashville, TN 37232-2730, USA; [b] Division of Traumatology, Surgical Critical Care, and Emergency Surgery, Department of Surgery, University of Pennsylvania, Philadelphia, PA 19104, USA; [c] Division of Acute Care Surgery, Department of Surgery, University of Florida, Jacksonville, 655 West 8th Street, Jacksonville, FL 32209, USA; [d] Division of Trauma, Surgical Critical Care, and Emergency General Surgery, Department of Surgery, Section of Surgical Sciences, Center for Health Services Research, Vanderbilt Brain Institute, Vanderbilt University Medical Center, 1211 21st Avenue South, Medical Arts Building, Suite 404, Nashville, TN 37212, USA; [e] Surgical Services, Nashville Veterans Affairs Medical Center, Tennessee Valley Healthcare System, 1310 24th Avenue South, Nashville, TN 37212, USA

* Corresponding author. Division of Trauma, Surgical Critical Care, and Emergency General Surgery, Department of Surgery, Section of Surgical Sciences, Center for Health Services Research, Vanderbilt Brain Institute, Vanderbilt University Medical Center, 1211 21st Avenue South, Medical Arts Building, Suite 404, Nashville, TN 37212.
E-mail address: mayur.b.patel@vanderbilt.edu

EPIDEMIOLOGY

Trauma is the leading cause of death in individuals aged 1 to 45 years, with traumatic brain injury (TBI) responsible for most these deaths; more than 50,000 deaths per year in the United States.[1-3] TBI can be clinically stratified into mild, moderate, and severe based on the Glasgow Coma Scale (GCS) score, with associated permanent disability rates of 10%, 60%, and 100%, respectively, and overall mortalities of 20% to 30%.[3,4] The economic impact is more than $80 billion in the United States alone according to the most recent US Centers for Disease Control and Prevention data.[3,5] This article focuses on the prehospital, emergency department, and intensive care unit (ICU) management of TBI.

MECHANISM AND PATHOPHYSIOLOGY

Traumatic brain injuries can result from both blunt and penetrating mechanisms. Falls (35%) and motor vehicle collisions (17%) are the most common, with motor vehicle collisions leading most fatalities. Gunshot wounds to the head are the most lethal of injuries, but, because of overall incidence, result in fewer total deaths.[3,4]

The primary insult to the brain cannot be undone and results in brain tissue damage, impaired cerebral blood flow (CBF) regulation, and alterations in brain metabolism with upregulation of inflammatory mediators, oxidative stress, and vasospasm. These processes ultimately lead to cell death and generalized brain edema.[6]

The Monro-Kellie hypothesis holds that the total intracranial volume is made up of brain tissue, cerebral spinal fluid (CSF), venous blood, and arterial blood. CBF remains constant under normal conditions via cerebral autoregulatory mechanisms over a range of blood pressures. When one compartment is increased, by a hematoma for example, there must be a compensatory decrease in another compartment in order to prevent intracranial hypertension. Cerebral perfusion pressure (CPP) is a surrogate for CBF. CPP is defined as mean arterial pressure (MAP) minus intracranial pressure (ICP). A decrease in CPP implies a decrease in CBF, although this association is not perfect. Decreased CBF ultimately leads to ischemia and hypoxia and worsening of the initial brain insult.[2,5] The goal of TBI management is to prevent this secondary insult.

AVOIDANCE OF SECONDARY INJURY

At present, the initial insult causing a TBI cannot be reversed, and this is referred to as the primary injury. Hypotension, previously defined as systolic blood pressure (SBP) less than 90 mm Hg, and hypoxia, defined as a Pao_2 less than or equal to 60 mm Hg, have been associated with doubling of mortality in patients with head injuries.[7,8] Early studies from the 1970s showed an association between systemic insults (mainly hypotension, hypoxia, and hypercarbia) and increased mortality, suggesting an important role for trauma center transfer in patients with severe TBI.[9] Management strategies must therefore focus on the prevention of secondary injury (ie, hypoxia, hypotension) through maintenance of adequate CBF and prevention of hypoxia.

PREHOSPITAL MANAGEMENT

Consistent with all phases of TBI management, prehospital strategies should focus on preventing secondary brain injury. In one study, patients with moderate to severe TBI transferred to level I trauma centers via helicopter and who had secondary insults (either SBP<90 mm Hg or Spo_2<92%) had a 28% mortality, compared with 20% of patients without such insults. Prehospital hypoxia in these same patients was associated with a significant increase in mortality, and there was no difference in hypoxic episodes between patients intubated versus those not intubated in the field.[10] Similarly, prehospital rapid-sequence intubation performed by paramedics in patients with head injuries with GCS less than 9 was associated with an increase in mortality. This result may be associated with the transient hypoxia during the prehospital procedures, excessive overventilation causing hypocarbia, vasoconstriction, impaired CBF, and longer scene times.[11] This body of work implies a need for rapid transfer to definitive care and a focus on more basic airway strategies to maintain oxygenation in patients with head injuries.

Several studies have also evaluated the use of hypertonic saline in the prehospital arena as a means to improve CPP by decreasing ICP and increasing MAP. In a 2004 study by Cooper and colleagues,[12] patients with severe TBI (GCS<9) and hypotension (SBP<100 mm Hg) were assigned to either rapid administration of 7.5% saline or a similar bolus of Ringer lactate by paramedics. Neurologic function at 6 months did not differ between the two groups, although mean sodium level in the treatment group was only 149 mEq/L. A multicenter randomized clinical trial in 2010 by Bulger and colleagues[13] studied patients with severe TBI (GCS<9) not in hypovolemic shock. Patients were administered either 7.5% saline/6% dextran 70, 7.5% saline alone, or 0.9% saline. Neurologic outcome at 6 months and survival did not differ among groups. At this time, prehospital use of hypertonic saline cannot be recommended.

EMERGENCY DEPARTMENT MANAGEMENT

The initial management of patients with TBI is identical to that of all patients with trauma, focusing on the Advanced Trauma Life Support (ATLS) principles of management of airway, breathing, and circulation, followed by a rapid neurologic examination and exposure of the patient with prevention of hypothermia.[14]

The airway should be secured according to local protocols. Induction agents such as propofol should be carefully used, possibly in conjunction with induction inotropes, given the risk of systemic hypotension with impaired CBF. Ketamine is an attractive agent in patients with trauma, given its favorable hemodynamic profile. Despite theoretic risks, a systematic review of ketamine use in TBI suggests that ketamine does not increase ICP[15]

Breathing should be optimized to maintain oxygenation and prevent ventilatory dysfunction, because extremes in CO_2 levels can lead to cerebral vasoconstriction and vasodilatation, and have been shown to be predictors of morbidity and mortality.[8] Hyperventilation is used by some providers to acutely decrease ICP through hypocarbic vasoconstriction, despite evidence showing an association between even brief periods of hyperventilation and increased levels of mediators of secondary brain injury in areas adjacent to injured brain tissue as well as local reductions in cerebral perfusion.[16–18] This strategy should be used with caution, and perhaps only to acutely combat signs of active herniation while initiating more definitive treatment.

Circulation should be maintained to prevent hypotension and maintain CBF. There is a known coagulopathy related to head injury likely related to tissue factor release coupled with hypoperfusion, which may be exacerbated by a pure crystalloid resuscitation. A balanced blood product resuscitation has been shown to be beneficial in patients with trauma,[19–21] and may be extended to patients with TBI. Non–cross-matched packed red blood cells are an initial resuscitative fluid choice that is often used in hypotensive patients with trauma, with a goal to maintain SBP at greater than or equal to 90 mm Hg in patients suspected of having a TBI. The concept of permissive hypotension does not apply to patients with known or suspected TBI, and normal physiologic blood pressure parameters should be targeted in this population.

During the disability component of the primary survey, a rapid neurologic evaluation is performed. The evaluation focuses on the pupillary examination, assesses for lateralizing signs suggesting a mass lesion with increased ICP, and calculates a GCS score to stratify the TBI severity. The patient should then be exposed to evaluate for injury and rapidly covered to prevent hypothermia. A more detailed examination is performed during the secondary survey. Agents such as hypertonic saline and/or mannitol (discussed in more detail later) can be given during this initial resuscitation if physical examination findings suggest a neurologic decline, significant head injury, or lateralizing neurologic examination.

Following the initial resuscitation, patients suspected of having a TBI usually undergo a noncontrasted head computed tomography (CT) scan, depending on the presence of other injuries that require more urgent attention. Recent level II recommendations from the Eastern Association for the Surgery of Trauma (EAST) suggest obtaining a head CT scan in patients who present with suspected brain injury in the acute setting if it is available. If rapid CT scanning is not available, providers can consider using one of the various criteria for determining need for additional imaging, such as the Canadian CT Head Rule and the New Orleans Criteria.[22,23]

OPERATIVE MANAGEMENT OF MASS LESIONS

Recent guidelines recommend surgical evacuation for epidural hematomas (EDHs) larger than 30 cm^3 regardless of GCS. Surgical evacuation should be considered for patients with EDH and GCS less than 9, clot thickness greater than 15 mm, midline shift greater than 5 mm, or focal neurologic deficits. EDHs less than 30 cm^3, less than 15 mm thick, with less than 5 mm shift in patients with GCS greater than 8 and no focal deficits can be watched with close observation and serial imaging (with repeat scan 6–8 hours after the previous scan).[24] Evacuation should be considered for subdural hematomas (SDHs) larger than 1 cm or those associated with midline shift greater than 5 mm, a GCS less than 8 with rapid decline, or ICP less than 20 mm Hg.[25] Patients with parenchymal lesions and progressive neurologic decline, mass effect, refractory intracranial hemorrhage (ICH), GCS scores of 6 to 8 with frontal or temporal contusions greater than 20 cm^3, midline shift of at least 5 mm and/or compression of cisterns, or lesion volume greater than 50 cm^3 should be considered for decompression.[26] Early studies found a significant mortality benefit if evacuation was performed within 4 hours from injury.[27,28] The STITCH (Trauma) trial (Surgical Trial in Traumatic Intracerebral Hemorrhage), which compared 6-month outcomes in patients with trauma with intraparenchymal hemorrhage randomized to early operative evacuation (<12 hours) with conservative management, was stopped early at 170 patients because of recruitment issues but showed a mortality benefit in patients who underwent early operative intervention.[29]

INTENSIVE CARE UNIT CIRCULATORY CONSIDERATIONS

SBP should be maintained a greater than or equal to 90 mm Hg through use of fluids and pressors, although the Brain Trauma Foundation (BTF) provides level III recommendations for higher thresholds, depending on age.[30,31] The ideal fluid for patients with TBI is unknown, although fluids should be administered judiciously and hypotonic fluids avoided to prevent volume overload and potential worsening of cerebral edema. In a post-hoc analysis of patients with head injuries in the SAFE (Saline vs Albumin Fluid Evaluation) study, those who received albumin had higher mortalities compared with those who received saline.[32] Although packed red blood cells are often used as the initial fluid in traumatically injured patients, transfusing to a hemoglobin level greater than 10 g/dL has been associated with more adverse events and no improvement in 6-month neurologic outcome in patients with TBI compared with those transfused to a restrictive threshold of 7 g/dL.[33]

Brain-injured patients may require reversal of anticoagulant and antiplatelet agents, because the prehospital use of these medications may increase mortality after TBI.[34–36] The most recent EAST guideline suggests that all elderly patients on prehospital systemic anticoagulation who are suspected of having a head injury should undergo rapid head CT evaluation.[37] It is also recommended that patients with head injuries on warfarin should undergo rapid (within 2 hours of presentation) reversal of warfarin with fresh frozen plasma (FFP) and vitamin K.[37,38] McMillian and Rogers[39] propose a simple algorithm for management of patients on aspirin, clopidogrel, and warfarin who are suspected of having a head injury. If intracranial hemorrhage is identified on an immediate head CT scan in a patient on warfarin, 4 units of type-specific FFP and 10 mg of intravenous (IV) vitamin K are administered with a goal International Normalized Ratio (INR) of less than 1.6. If the patient is on an antiplatelet agent, a 10 pack of type-specific platelets is administered. Prothrombin complex concentration (PCC) and desmopressin can also be considered to reverse warfarin anticoagulation and antiplatelet agents, respectively.[40–42] Novel anticoagulants, both direct thrombin inhibitors (dabigatran) and factor Xa inhibitors (rivaroxaban, apixaban, edoxaban), pose a unique challenge given a lack of reversal options. Readers are referred to a review article from 2013 that suggests an approach to the management of bleeding patients on novel anticoagulants, which may be extrapolated to patients with head injuries. In addition to treating coagulopathies with FFP and platelets when appropriate, 4-factor or activated PCC can be administered, and dialysis can be considered for patients on dabigatran if feasible.[43] Idarucizumab, a monoclonal antibody fragment, has been found to rapidly reverse the effects of dabigatran in patients with serious bleeding and may have a role in patients with trauma.[44] Early administration of tranexamic acid (TXA), an antifibrinolytic agent, has been shown to reduce all-cause mortality and death caused by bleeding in patients with trauma with significant bleeding.[45] The CRASH-2 (Clinical Randomisation of an Antifibrinolytic in Significant Haemorrhage 2) intracranial bleeding study showed that neither moderate benefits nor moderate harmful effects of TXA can be excluded in bleeding patients with trauma with TBI.[46] The CRASH-3 trial is designed to quantify the effects of early administration of TXA on death and disability in patients with TBI and is currently underway.[47]

INTENSIVE CARE UNIT MANAGEMENT OF INTRACRANIAL HYPERTENSION

Fig. 1 presents a simple algorithm for the management of patients with severe TBI used at the authors' institution and focuses mainly on the management of increased ICP. The neurosurgical service is consulted on identification of a TBI, and mass lesions are evacuated if indicated. Basic laboratory tests are ordered to evaluate for coagulopathy and seizure prophylaxis is started (discussed later). Patients with moderate to severe TBI are admitted to the ICU for ongoing resuscitation and prevention of secondary brain injury. A 2013 study found that acute care surgeons can effectively manage patients with mild TBI without neurosurgical evaluation, although this cannot be firmly extrapolated to patients with moderate or severe TBI, and the authors suggest neurosurgical consultation for any ICH, irrespective of neurologic function.[48]

As noted in **Fig. 1**, patients admitted to the ICU should have optimization of oxygen, ventilation, and SBP. Simple maneuvers like loosening of the cervical collar, raising the head of bed to greater than 30° or maintaining a reverse Trendelenburg position (if no contraindication), and optimizing sedation and analgesia can decrease ICP, although some of these may not improve CBF or CPP.[49] Blood products can be given to keep

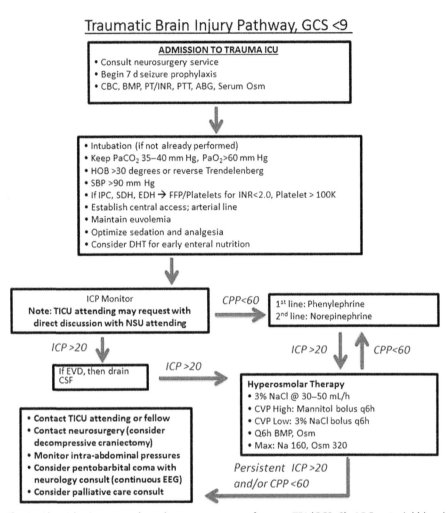

Traumatic Brain Injury Pathway, GCS <9

ADMISSION TO TRAUMA ICU
- Consult neurosurgery service
- Begin 7 d seizure prophylaxis
- CBC, BMP, PT/INR, PTT, ABG, Serum Osm

- Intubation (if not already performed)
- Keep $PaCO_2$ 35–40 mm Hg, PaO_2>60 mm Hg
- HOB >30 degrees or reverse Trendelenberg
- SBP >90 mm Hg
- If IPC, SDH, EDH → FFP/Platelets for INR<2.0, Platelet > 100K
- Establish central access; arterial line
- Maintain euvolemia
- Optimize sedation and analgesia
- Consider DHT for early enteral nutrition

ICP Monitor
Note: TICU attending may request with direct discussion with NSU attending

CPP<60 → 1st line: Phenylephrine / 2nd line: Norepinephrine

ICP >20

If EVD, then drain CSF

ICP >20

Hyperosmolar Therapy
- 3% NaCl @ 30–50 mL/h
- CVP High: Mannitol bolus q6h
- CVP Low: 3% NaCl bolus q6h
- Q6h BMP, Osm
- Max: Na 160, Osm 320

ICP >20   *CPP<60*

- Contact TICU attending or fellow
- Contact neurosurgery (consider decompressive craniectomy)
- Monitor intra-abdominal pressures
- Consider pentobarbital coma with neurology consult (continuous EEG)
- Consider palliative care consult

Persistent ICP >20 and/or CPP <60

Fig. 1. Algorithmic approach to the management of severe TBI (GCS<9). ABG, arterial blood gas; BMP, basic metabolic panel; CBC, complete blood count; CVP, central venous pressure; DHT, Dobhoff tube; EEG, electroencephalogram; EVD, extraventricular drain; HOB, head of bed; IPC, intraparenchymal contusion; NSU, neurosurgery unit; Osm, osmolality; PT, prothrombin time; PTT, partial thromboplastin time; Q, every; TICU, trauma ICU.

INR less than 1.5 and platelets greater than or equal to 100,000/µL to prevent further intracranial bleeding, although these are arbitrary hemostatic thresholds and may be influenced by preinjury antiplatelet/anticoagulants, availability of thromboelastography, neurologic changes, imaging changes, and/or institutional culture.

INTRACRANIAL PRESSURE MONITORING

Consideration should be given to placement of an ICP monitor in patients with severe TBI. External ventricular drains (EVDs), which are placed in the lateral ventricle and connected to a pressure monitor, can also be used for continuous or intermittent drainage of CSF as a means to decrease ICP. Open or continuous EVDs have been associated with better ICP reduction than intermittent or closed EVDs, although EVD monitors have not been shown to be superior to intraparenchymal ICP monitors. Intraparenchymal monitors are placed directly into brain tissue but may not accurately measure pressure in the CSF because of pressure gradients that occur after TBI.[50–52] Both device types measure ICP, and the calculated CPP is used as a surrogate for CBF, and, by extension, brain oxygenation and metabolic supply.

The BTF recommends (level IIB) ICP monitoring in patients with severe TBI (GCS<9) and abnormal CT scan to reduce 2-week and in-hospital mortality. It is also recommended that CSF drainage be considered to reduce ICP in patients with a GCS less than 6 within the first 12 hours of injury. General goals are to maintain an ICP less than 20 mm Hg and CPP between 50 and 70 mm Hg, depending on autoregulatory status. Values higher have been associated with respiratory complications and poor outcomes.[30,53]

In a study evaluating compliance with the third edition of the BTF ICP monitoring guidelines, patients who underwent ICP monitoring had less in-hospital mortality and less herniation-related mortality but longer ICU and hospital lengths of stay compared with patients who did not undergo ICP monitoring.[54] In 2134 patients with severe TBI, those treated with a protocol-based ICP monitoring algorithm had significantly less mortality compared with patients treated without an ICP monitor (19% vs 33%), although no mention is made regarding goal ICP/CPP or the treatment modalities used to reduce ICP.[55] In contrast, the Benchmark Evidence from South American Trials: Treatment of Intracranial Pressure (BEST:TRIP) multicenter randomized clinical trial from 6 hospitals and 324 ICU patients with severe TBI, ICP monitoring was not superior to care based on imaging and physical examination.[56]

CPP and ICP are inexact surrogates for CBF given the heterogeneity of TBI and an unknown optimal CPP for a given patient, suggesting a role for more multimodal monitoring.[57,58] Transcranial Doppler ultrasonography is a noninvasive technique that measures CBF velocity, and uses differences in CBF velocity to estimate differences in CBF. Jugular bulb monitoring of arteriovenous oxygen content difference ($AVDo_2$) uses a central line placed in the jugular bulb and a peripheral arterial line. The difference in oxygen content between blood entering and leaving the brain can be calculated to provide a global picture of supply and demand. Cerebral microdialysis is a technique in which a catheter is placed in the penumbra, or area adjacent to the traumatized brain, and used to evaluate the local biochemical environment. Brain tissue oxygen tension can be measured with a parenchymal probe but is highly dependent on placement, provides a very focal measurement of oxygenation, and may not be an appropriate surrogate for global perfusion.[52] Given lack of sufficient data, routine use of novel neuromonitoring strategies is not common at this time. In its most recent guidelines, the BTF provides level III recommendations for measurement of $AVDo_2$, the optimization of which has been associated with favorable outcomes 6 months after injury. It is recommended to avoid $AVDo_2$ less than 50%.[30,59–61]

As noted in **Fig. 1**, patients undergo EVD placement if criteria are met and the procedure is technically feasible. If ICP remains increased, continuous CSF drainage is used. If the CPP remains low, MAP is increased using a combination of volume expansion and pressors, as discussed later.

HYPEROSMOLAR THERAPY

Intracranial hypertension can be managed with hyperosmolar therapy, although there is no strong evidence about the appropriate agent, administration (ie, continuous vs bolus), or timing. Hypertonic saline (HTS) of various concentrations and mannitol are the primary pharmacologic agents used to reduce ICP, perhaps through reduction in blood viscosity, improved microcirculatory flow, and decreased cerebral blood volume.

A BTF class II retrospective study using data from the BTF's Database evaluated patients treated with a single agent for ICP reduction. HTS administrations were typically 3% concentrations, and mannitol administrations were 20% concentrations. Bolus HTS therapy was more effective at reducing ICP and ICU length of stay. There was no statistically significant difference in 2-week mortality.[62]

The 2016 BTF guidelines indicate that there is insufficient evidence on clinical outcomes to support recommendations on the use or type of hyperosmolar therapy.[30] Our protocol as noted in **Fig. 1** is to use 3% saline at 30 to 50 mL/h and 250-mL to 500-mL intermittent boluses every 4 to 6 hours with laboratory draws to maintain serum sodium level at 145 to 160 mEq/L and osmolality less than 320 mOsm/L. Mannitol is used as a second-line agent and/or considered when hypervolemia is present. If CPP remains less than 60 mm Hg, MAP can be increased with a combination of fluid resuscitation and pressors, with phenylephrine often used.[31]

BARBITURATE COMA

Patients without mass lesions amenable to intervention and refractory ICP greater than 20 mm Hg can be treated with barbiturates. In one multicenter study, patients with severe TBI refractory to basic maneuvers, hyperosmolar therapy, and intraventricular catheter drainage were treated with a continuous pentobarbital drip with electroencephalogram (EEG) monitoring. Pentobarbital coma effectively improved CPP. Forty percent of patients survived to discharge and 68% of patients had good functional outcomes in 1 year or more after injury.[63] Other investigators question the benefit of pentobarbital therapy, especially in light of systemic effects like hypotension.[64] Ultimately, the 2016 BTF guidelines do not advocate barbiturate therapy as prophylaxis against intracranial hypertension. However, when treating refractory intracranial hypertension with barbiturates, avoiding hemodynamic instability is recommended.[30]

The authors suggest that patients with ICP 21 to 29 mm Hg for at least 30 minutes, 30 to 39 mm Hg for at least 15 minutes, or 40 mm Hg or more for 1 minute who have met sodium and osmolality thresholds (ie, on maximal hyperosmolar therapy) are candidates for pentobarbital coma. Pentobarbital is bolused at 10 mg/kg over 30 minutes, followed by a 5 mg/kg/h infusion for 3 hours, after which time it is titrated to 1 mg/kg/h and adjusted as needed with an EEG burst suppression goal of 2 to 5 bursts per minute while monitoring for significant side effects (ie, hypotension).[65]

DECOMPRESSIVE CRANIECTOMY

Decompressive craniectomy (DC) has been shown to reduce ICP and can be considered if ICP is refractory to other measures, although some clinicians consider it earlier in the treatment algorithm.[24,26,66,67] In the DECRA (Decompressive Craniectomy in Diffuse Traumatic Brain Injury) randomized clinical trial, bifrontotemporoparietal DC in patients with diffuse TBI and refractory ICH resulted in lower ICP and shorter ICU length of stay. However, DC was associated with unfavorable long-term neurologic function, as measured by the Extended Glasgow Outcome Scale (GOSE), and similar mortality at 6 months compared with patients receiving standard treatment.[68]

The most recent 2016 guidelines from the BTF do not recommend bifrontal DC as a means to improve neurologic outcomes based on these results, although they do recommend a large frontoparietal DC rather than a smaller one.[30] This BTF recommendation was released before the results of the more recently published RESCUEicp study (Randomized Evaluation of Surgery with Craniectomy for Uncontrollable Elevation of Intracranial Pressure). In the RESCUEicp randomized clinical trial, patients with refractory ICP greater than 25 mm Hg for 1 to 12 hours despite multimodal therapy were assigned to either DC or standard management. The primary outcome was the 6-month GOSE. Patients undergoing DC had higher rates of vegetative state but lower rates of mortality, severe disability, and upper severe disability. Compared with the DECRA trial, patients in this most recent study underwent DC as the last tier in the algorithm for management of refractory ICH. Patients with mass lesions were included as well as those who underwent unilateral decompression. Similar to the DECRA RCT, the RESCUEicp showed increased disability among survivors.[69]

ABDOMINAL DECOMPRESSION

The differential for intracranial hypertension should also include intra-abdominal hypertension or abdominal compartment syndrome, in particular in patients subject to large volume resuscitations and/or patients with polytrauma.[70] Monitoring serial bladder pressures with possible paralysis may assist with the diagnosis. Abdominal decompression in patients with increased ICP refractory to medical management with concomitant intra-abdominal hypertension has been shown to be efficacious in reducing ICP and should be considered in this patient group.[71,72]

HYPOTHERMIA

Hypothermia has been investigated as a means of neuroprotection following TBI. A systemic review of randomized controlled trials of hypothermia in TBI found that hypothermia was associated with reduced mortality and improvements in neurologic function.[73] Other investigators question the benefits of hypothermia in TBI, citing poor-quality trials.[74] The BTF currently recommends against the routine use of early, short-term prophylactic hypothermia in patients with diffuse TBI.[30]

INTENSIVE CARE UNIT MANAGEMENT: VENOUS THROMBOEMBOLISM PROPHYLAXIS

Patients with TBI are at risk for venous thromboembolic disease given venous stasis, venous injury, and potential coagulopathy associated with TBI. Pharmacologic agents are often withheld in the initial postinjury period because of concerns for worsening of an intracranial bleed. A study from 2011 by Scudday and colleagues[75] investigated 812 patients with head injuries, about half of whom received pharmacologic prophylaxis (most with heparin). Forty percent of patients received prophylaxis within 48 hours, with an average start time of 96 hours after hospital arrival. Patients who received pharmacologic prophylaxis had a lower incidence of venous thromboembolism (VTE) compared with those who did not (1% vs 3%). There was also a trend toward lower incidence of worsening hemorrhage in the treatment group, although VTE diagnosis in that study was based on clinical symptoms and asymptomatic VTE may have been more prevalent.

A review by Phelan[76] in 2012 presents a protocol whereby patients with low-risk TBI can be started on enoxaparin within 24 hours postinjury, those with moderate-risk TBI based on specified imaging characteristics can be started after 72 hours, and those with high-risk TBI should undergo inferior vena cava (IVC) filter placement. The BTF recommends pharmacologic deep vein thrombosis prophylaxis if the injury is stable and the benefits of prophylaxis outweigh the risks of hemorrhage progression. There are no recommendations regarding timing, dose, or agent.[30] Local culture along with input from neurosurgery colleagues may help to dictate the approach to anticoagulation in these patients as well.

INTENSIVE CARE UNIT MANAGEMENT: STRESS ULCER PROPHYLAXIS

Head injury has been associated with increased gastric acid secretion. Both proton pump inhibitors (PPIs) and histamine-2 receptor antagonists (H$_2$) have been shown to reduce the incidence of upper gastrointestinal bleeding in patients with trauma and receiving neurocritical care.[77–79] In a review of the literature involving neurologic and neurosurgical ICU patients, H$_2$ blockers were found to be associated with increased rates of pneumonia, drug interactions, and coagulopathy, calling into question the role of these agents in patients with TBI.[78] In one recent study of mechanically ventilated critical care patients, including a small number of patients with ICH, PPIs were associated with increased rates of pneumonia, *Clostridium difficile* infection, and gastrointestinal hemorrhage.[80] These data suggest a role for future prospective studies evaluating the ideal prophylaxis in patients with severe TBI.

INTENSIVE CARE UNIT MANAGEMENT: SEIZURE PROPHYLAXIS

Early studies showed the benefit of phenytoin in the prevention of early posttraumatic seizures (ie, seizures within the first week after injury). However, early prophylaxis with antiepileptics has not been showed to improve late posttraumatic seizures (ie, >7 days postinjury), mortality, or neurologic function.[81] The 2016 BTF guidelines recommend phenytoin to decrease early posttraumatic seizures when the risk/benefit ratio favors treatment.[30]

Studies comparing levetiracetam and phenytoin have shown that levetiracetam is as effective at reducing early seizures and is an attractive alternative given that it does not require serum monitoring, is less expensive, and has fewer drug-drug interactions.[82–84] Although the BTF currently outlines insufficient evidence to recommend levetiracetam rather than phenytoin, our practice is to use levetiracetam (1000mg IV bolus followed by 500 mg IV/by mouth twice a day for 7 days with renal adjustment if needed) for patients with any structural intracranial injury on cross-sectional imaging. We also consider omission of seizure prophylaxis if patients are older than 65 years with good neurologic function.

NUTRITION

Early enteral nutrition (EN) has been shown to have a beneficial effect in many patient populations, including those with TBI. A study by Hartle and colleagues[85] found that patients who were not fed within the first week after TBI had significant increases in mortality, even when controlled for other factors known to affect outcome. Early enhanced EN, in which goal feeds are reached on day 1 of injury, has also showed benefit compared with more traditional EN in terms of infectious and overall complications and possibly even longer term outcomes out to 3 months postinjury.[86] Other studies have shown that EN within 48 hours is associated with improved survival and neurologic outcome in patients with severe head injuries.[87] There is some evidence that transpyloric feeding is associated with a decreased incidence of pneumonia and is more efficacious than the gastric route in patients with TBI.[88] Achieving adequate caloric intake by day 7 and transgastric jejunal feeding is currently supported by the BTF guidelines.

INTENSIVE CARE UNIT MANAGEMENT: OTHER THERAPIES

Results of the CRASH trial do not support use of corticosteroids in patients with head injuries.[89,90] Intensive insulin therapy (80–120 mg/dL) in patients with TBI has been associated with fewer infectious complications and shorter ICU length of stay compared with a less aggressive strategy (<220 mg/dL), but was associated with more hypoglycemia and similar outcomes and infectious complications and has not generated strong clinical enthusiasm.[91] In 2 large multicenter randomized clinical trials, administration of IV progesterone also failed to show a clinical benefit in humans.[92,93] Previous work has shown an association between beta-blockade and improvement in mortality after TBI in humans and improvement in CBF in mice.[94,95] There are currently trials underway to assess the effect of adrenergic and sympathetic blockade on outcomes after TBI (NCT01322048 and NCT02957331).[96,97]

SUMMARY

TBI is a leading cause of death and disability in patients with trauma. The rapid transfer of patients with TBI to trauma centers and the avoidance of secondary insults such as hypotension and hypoxia are paramount. Increased ICP should be managed in an algorithmic fashion using simple beside maneuvers, hyperosmolar agents, ventricular drainage, barbiturates, and operative intervention when appropriate. Nutritional status should be optimized and clinicians should focus on prophylaxis against stress ulceration, early seizures, and VTEs. The role of novel techniques to measure CBF and oxygenation is still being elucidated.

REFERENCES

1. Langlois JA, Rutland-Brown W, Wald MM. The epidemiology and impact of traumatic brain injury: a brief overview. J Head Trauma Rehabil 2006;21(5):375–8.
2. Stocchetti N, Maas AI. Traumatic intracranial hypertension. N Engl J Med 2014; 371(10):972.
3. Traumatic Brain Injury & Concussion; TBI: Get the Facts. Available at https://www.cdc.gov/traumaticbraininjury/get_the_facts.html. Accessed July 8, 2017.
4. Crandall M, Rink RA, Shaheen AW, et al. Patterns and predictors of follow-up in patients with mild traumatic brain injury. Brain Inj 2014;28(11):1359–64.
5. Patel MB, Guillamondegui OD. Severe Traumatic Brain Injury: Medical and Surgical Management. Section: Head Injury. In: Papadakos P, Gestring M, editors. Encyclopedia of Trauma Care. Heidelberg, Berlin: Springer-Verlag; 2015. p. 1711–6.
6. Werner C, Engelhard K. Pathophysiology of traumatic brain injury. Br J Anaesth 2007;99(1):4–9.
7. Chesnut RM, Marshall LF, Klauber MR, et al. The role of secondary brain injury in determining outcome from severe head injury. J Trauma 1993;34(2):216–22.
8. Jeremitsky E, Omert L, Dunham CM, et al. Harbingers of poor outcome the day after severe brain injury: hypothermia, hypoxia, and hypoperfusion. J Trauma 2003;54(2):312–9.
9. Miller JD, Sweet RC, Narayan R, et al. Early insults to the injured brain. JAMA 1978;240(5):439–42.
10. Chi JH, Knudson MM, Vassar MJ, et al. Prehospital hypoxia affects outcome in patients with traumatic brain injury: a prospective multicenter study. J Trauma 2006;61(5):1134–41.

11. Davis DP, Hoyt DB, Ochs M, et al. The effect of paramedic rapid sequence intubation on outcome in patients with severe traumatic brain injury. J Trauma 2003; 54(3):444–53.
12. Cooper DJ, Myles PS, McDermott FT, et al. Prehospital hypertonic saline resuscitation of patients with hypotension and severe traumatic brain injury: a randomized controlled trial. JAMA 2004;291(11):1350–7.
13. Bulger EM, May S, Brasel KJ, et al. Out-of-hospital hypertonic resuscitation following severe traumatic brain injury: a randomized controlled trial. JAMA 2010;304(13):1455–64.
14. Chapter 6: Head Trauma. ATLS Advanced Trauma Life Support for Doctors - Student Course Manual: Ninth Edition. Chicago, IL: American College of Surgeons Committee on Trauma; 2012. p. 148–69.
15. Zeiler FA, Teitelbaum J, West M, et al. The ketamine effect on ICP in traumatic brain injury. Neurocrit Care 2014;21(1):163–73.
16. Imberti R, Bellinzona G, Langer M. Cerebral tissue PO_2 and $SjvO_2$ changes during moderate hyperventilation in patients with severe traumatic brain injury. J Neurosurg 2002;96(1):97–102.
17. Marion DW, Puccio A, Wisniewski SR, et al. Effect of hyperventilation on extracellular concentrations of glutamate, lactate, pyruvate, and local cerebral blood flow in patients with severe traumatic brain injury. Crit Care Med 2002;30(12):2619–25.
18. Thomas SH, Orf J, Wedel SK, et al. Hyperventilation in traumatic brain injury patients: inconsistency between consensus guidelines and clinical practice. J Trauma 2002;52(1):47–52 [discussion: 52–3].
19. Cohen MJ, Brohi K, Ganter MT, et al. Early coagulopathy after traumatic brain injury: the role of hypoperfusion and the protein C pathway. J Trauma 2007; 63(6):1254–61 [discussion: 1261–2].
20. Holcomb JB, Tilley BC, Baraniuk S, et al. Transfusion of plasma, platelets, and red blood cells in a 1:1:1 vs a 1:1:2 ratio and mortality in patients with severe trauma: the PROPPR randomized clinical trial. JAMA 2015;313(5):471–82.
21. Stein SC, Smith DH. Coagulopathy in traumatic brain injury. Neurocrit Care 2004; 1(4):479–88.
22. Barbosa RR, Jawa R, Watters JM, et al. Evaluation and management of mild traumatic brain injury: an Eastern Association for the Surgery of Trauma practice management guideline. J Trauma Acute Care Surg 2012;73(5 Suppl 4):S307–14.
23. Smits M, Dippel DW, de Haan GG, et al. External validation of the Canadian CT Head Rule and the New Orleans Criteria for CT scanning in patients with minor head injury. JAMA 2005;294(12):1519–25.
24. Bullock MR, Chesnut R, Ghajar J, et al. Surgical management of acute epidural hematomas. Neurosurgery 2006;58(3 Suppl):S7–15 [discussion: Si–iv].
25. Cameron John L, Cameron Andrew M. Chapter 205: The Management of Traumatic Brain Injury in Current Surgical Therapy, 12th Edition. USA: Elsevier; 2017.
26. Bullock MR, Chesnut R, Ghajar J, et al. Surgical management of traumatic parenchymal lesions. Neurosurgery 2006;58(3 Suppl):S25–46 [discussion: Si–iv].
27. Seelig JM, Becker DP, Miller JD, et al. Traumatic acute subdural hematoma: major mortality reduction in comatose patients treated within four hours. N Engl J Med 1981;304(25):1511–8.
28. Wilberger JE Jr, Harris M, Diamond DL. Acute subdural hematoma: morbidity, mortality, and operative timing. J Neurosurg 1991;74(2):212–8.
29. Mendelow AD, Gregson BA, Rowan EN, et al. Early surgery versus initial conservative treatment in patients with traumatic intracerebral hemorrhage (STITCH [Trauma]): the first randomized trial. J Neurotrauma 2015;32(17):1312–23.

30. Carney N, Totten AM, O'Reilly C, et al. Guidelines for the management of severe traumatic brain injury, fourth edition. Neurosurgery 2016;80(1):6–15.
31. Feinstein AJ, Patel MB, Sanui M, et al. Resuscitation with pressors after traumatic brain injury. J Am Coll Surg 2005;201(4):536–45.
32. SAFE Study Investigators, Australian and New Zealand Intensive Care Society Clinical Trials Group, Myburgh J, Cooper DJ, Finfer S, et al. Saline or albumin for fluid resuscitation in patients with traumatic brain injury. N Engl J Med 2007; 357(9):874–84.
33. Robertson CS, Hannay HJ, Yamal JM, et al. Effect of erythropoietin and transfusion threshold on neurological recovery after traumatic brain injury: a randomized clinical trial. JAMA 2014;312(1):36–47.
34. Grandhi R, Harrison G, Voronovich Z, et al. Preinjury warfarin, but not antiplatelet medications, increases mortality in elderly traumatic brain injury patients. J Trauma Acute Care Surg 2015;78(3):614–21.
35. Mina AA, Knipfer JF, Park DY, et al. Intracranial complications of preinjury anticoagulation in trauma patients with head injury. J Trauma 2002;53(4):668–72.
36. Pieracci FM, Eachempati SR, Shou J, et al. Degree of anticoagulation, but not warfarin use itself, predicts adverse outcomes after traumatic brain injury in elderly trauma patients. J Trauma 2007;63(3):525–30.
37. Calland JF, Ingraham AM, Martin N, et al. Evaluation and management of geriatric trauma: an Eastern Association for the Surgery of Trauma practice management guideline. J Trauma Acute Care Surg 2012;73(5 Suppl 4):S345–50.
38. Ivascu FA, Howells GA, Junn FS, et al. Rapid warfarin reversal in anticoagulated patients with traumatic intracranial hemorrhage reduces hemorrhage progression and mortality. J Trauma 2005;59(5):1131–7 [discussion: 1137–9].
39. McMillian WD, Rogers FB. Management of prehospital antiplatelet and anticoagulant therapy in traumatic head injury: a review. J Trauma 2009;66(3):942–50.
40. Matsushima K, Benjamin E, Demetriades D. Prothrombin complex concentrate in trauma patients. Am J Surg 2015;209(2):413–7.
41. Joseph B, Hadjizacharia P, Aziz H, et al. Prothrombin complex concentrate: an effective therapy in reversing the coagulopathy of traumatic brain injury. J Trauma Acute Care Surg 2013;74(1):248–53.
42. Beynon C, Hertle DN, Unterberg AW, et al. Clinical review: traumatic brain injury in patients receiving antiplatelet medication. Crit Care 2012;16(4):228.
43. Siegal DM, Cuker A. Reversal of novel oral anticoagulants in patients with major bleeding. J Thromb Thrombolysis 2013;35(3):391–8.
44. Pollack CV Jr, Reilly PA, Eikelboom J, et al. Idarucizumab for dabigatran reversal. N Engl J Med 2015;373(6):511–20.
45. CRASH-2 trial collaborators, Shakur H, Roberts I, Bautista R, et al. Effects of tranexamic acid on death, vascular occlusive events, and blood transfusion in trauma patients with significant haemorrhage (CRASH-2): a randomised, placebo-controlled trial. Lancet 2010;376(9734):23–32.
46. Crash-2 Collaborators IBS. Effect of tranexamic acid in traumatic brain injury: a nested randomised, placebo controlled trial (CRASH-2 Intracranial Bleeding Study). BMJ 2011;343:d3795.
47. Dewan Y, Komolafe EO, Mejia-Mantilla JH, et al. CRASH-3-tranexamic acid for the treatment of significant traumatic brain injury: study protocol for an international randomized, double-blind, placebo-controlled trial. Trials 2012;13:87.
48. Joseph B, Aziz H, Sadoun M, et al. The acute care surgery model: managing traumatic brain injury without an inpatient neurosurgical consultation. J Trauma Acute Care Surg 2013;75(1):102–5 [discussion: 105].

49. Feldman Z, Kanter MJ, Robertson CS, et al. Effect of head elevation on intracranial pressure, cerebral perfusion pressure, and cerebral blood flow in head-injured patients. J Neurosurg 1992;76(2):207–11.

50. Kasotakis G, Michailidou M, Bramos A, et al. Intraparenchymal vs extracranial ventricular drain intracranial pressure monitors in traumatic brain injury: less is more? J Am Coll Surg 2012;214(6):950–7.

51. Nwachuku EL, Puccio AM, Fetzick A, et al. Intermittent versus continuous cerebrospinal fluid drainage management in adult severe traumatic brain injury: assessment of intracranial pressure burden. Neurocrit Care 2014;20(1):49–53.

52. Tisdall MM, Smith M. Multimodal monitoring in traumatic brain injury: current status and future directions. Br J Anaesth 2007;99(1):61–7.

53. Juul N, Morris GF, Marshall SB, et al. Intracranial hypertension and cerebral perfusion pressure: influence on neurological deterioration and outcome in severe head injury. The Executive Committee of the International Selfotel Trial. J Neurosurg 2000;92(1):1–6.

54. Talving P, Karamanos E, Teixeira PG, et al. Intracranial pressure monitoring in severe head injury: compliance with Brain Trauma Foundation guidelines and effect on outcomes: a prospective study. J Neurosurg 2013;119(5):1248–54.

55. Farahvar A, Gerber LM, Chiu YL, et al. Increased mortality in patients with severe traumatic brain injury treated without intracranial pressure monitoring. J Neurosurg 2012;117(4):729–34.

56. Chesnut RM, Temkin N, Carney N, et al. A trial of intracranial-pressure monitoring in traumatic brain injury. N Engl J Med 2012;367(26):2471–81.

57. Bouzat P, Sala N, Payen JF, et al. Beyond intracranial pressure: optimization of cerebral blood flow, oxygen, and substrate delivery after traumatic brain injury. Ann Intensive Care 2013;3(1):23.

58. Prabhakar H, Sandhu K, Bhagat H, et al. Current concepts of optimal cerebral perfusion pressure in traumatic brain injury. J Anaesthesiol Clin Pharmacol 2014;30(3):318–27.

59. Robertson CS, Gopinath SP, Goodman JC, et al. SjvO$_2$ monitoring in head-injured patients. J Neurotrauma 1995;12(5):891–6.

60. Stocchetti N, Canavesi K, Magnoni S, et al. Arterio-jugular difference of oxygen content and outcome after head injury. Anesth Analg 2004;99(1):230–4.

61. Robertson C. Desaturation episodes after severe head injury: influence on outcome. Acta Neurochir Suppl (Wien) 1993;59:98–101.

62. Mangat HS, Chiu YL, Gerber LM, et al. Hypertonic saline reduces cumulative and daily intracranial pressure burdens after severe traumatic brain injury. J Neurosurg 2015;122(1):202–10.

63. Marshall GT, James RF, Landman MP, et al. Pentobarbital coma for refractory intra-cranial hypertension after severe traumatic brain injury: mortality predictions and one-year outcomes in 55 patients. J Trauma 2010;69(2):275–83.

64. Roberts I, Sydenham E. Barbiturates for acute traumatic brain injury. Cochrane Database Syst Rev 2012;(12):CD000033.

65. Eisenberg HM, Frankowski RF, Contant CF, et al. High-dose barbiturate control of elevated intracranial pressure in patients with severe head injury. J Neurosurg 1988;69(1):15–23.

66. Bor-Seng-Shu E, Figueiredo EG, Amorim RL, et al. Decompressive craniectomy: a meta-analysis of influences on intracranial pressure and cerebral perfusion pressure in the treatment of traumatic brain injury. J Neurosurg 2012;117(3):589–96.

67. Weiner GM, Lacey MR, Mackenzie L, et al. Decompressive craniectomy for elevated intracranial pressure and its effect on the cumulative ischemic burden and therapeutic intensity levels after severe traumatic brain injury. Neurosurgery 2010;66(6):1111–8 [discussion: 1118–9].
68. Cooper DJ, Rosenfeld JV, Murray L, et al. Decompressive craniectomy in diffuse traumatic brain injury. N Engl J Med 2011;364(16):1493–502.
69. Hutchinson PJ, Kolias AG, Timofeev IS, et al. Trial of decompressive craniectomy for traumatic intracranial hypertension. N Engl J Med 2016;375(12):1119–30.
70. Kirkpatrick AW, Roberts DJ, De Waele J, et al. Intra-abdominal hypertension and the abdominal compartment syndrome: updated consensus definitions and clinical practice guidelines from the World Society of the Abdominal Compartment Syndrome. Intensive Care Med 2013;39(7):1190–206.
71. Dorfman JD, Burns JD, Green DM, et al. Decompressive laparotomy for refractory intracranial hypertension after traumatic brain injury. Neurocrit Care 2011;15(3): 516–8.
72. Joseph DK, Dutton RP, Aarabi B, et al. Decompressive laparotomy to treat intractable intracranial hypertension after traumatic brain injury. J Trauma 2004;57(4): 687–93.
73. McIntyre LA, Fergusson DA, Hebert PC, et al. Prolonged therapeutic hypothermia after traumatic brain injury in adults: a systematic review. JAMA 2003;289(22): 2992–9.
74. Sydenham E, Roberts I, Alderson P. Hypothermia for traumatic head injury. Cochrane Database Syst Rev 2009;(2):CD001048.
75. Scudday T, Brasel K, Webb T, et al. Safety and efficacy of prophylactic anticoagulation in patients with traumatic brain injury. J Am Coll Surg 2011;213(1): 148–53 [discussion: 153–4].
76. Phelan HA. Pharmacologic venous thromboembolism prophylaxis after traumatic brain injury: a critical literature review. J Neurotrauma 2012;29(10):1821–8.
77. Halloran LG, Zfass AM, Gayle WE, et al. Prevention of acute gastrointestinal complications after severe head-injury: a controlled trial of cimetidine prophylaxis. Am J Surg 1980;139(1):44–8.
78. Schirmer CM, Kornbluth J, Heilman CB, et al. Gastrointestinal prophylaxis in neurocritical care. Neurocrit Care 2012;16(1):184–93.
79. Lasky MR, Metzler MH, Phillips JO. A prospective study of omeprazole suspension to prevent clinically significant gastrointestinal bleeding from stress ulcers in mechanically ventilated trauma patients. J Trauma 1998;44(3):527–33.
80. MacLaren R, Reynolds PM, Allen RR. Histamine-2 receptor antagonists vs proton pump inhibitors on gastrointestinal tract hemorrhage and infectious complications in the intensive care unit. JAMA Intern Med 2014;174(4):564–74.
81. Temkin NR, Dikmen SS, Wilensky AJ, et al. A randomized, double-blind study of phenytoin for the prevention of post-traumatic seizures. N Engl J Med 1990; 323(8):497–502.
82. Inaba K, Menaker J, Branco BC, et al. A prospective multicenter comparison of levetiracetam versus phenytoin for early posttraumatic seizure prophylaxis. J Trauma Acute Care 2013;74(3):766–71.
83. Jones KE, Puccio AM, Harshman KJ, et al. Levetiracetam versus phenytoin for seizure prophylaxis in severe traumatic brain injury. Neurosurg Focus 2008; 25(4):E3.
84. Szaflarski JP, Sangha KS, Lindsell CJ, et al. Prospective, randomized, single-blinded comparative trial of intravenous levetiracetam versus phenytoin for seizure prophylaxis. Neurocrit Care 2010;12(2):165–72.

85. Hartl R, Gerber LM, Ni Q, et al. Effect of early nutrition on deaths due to severe traumatic brain injury. J Neurosurg 2008;109(1):50–6.

86. Taylor SJ, Fettes SB, Jewkes C, et al. Prospective, randomized, controlled trial to determine the effect of early enhanced enteral nutrition on clinical outcome in mechanically ventilated patients suffering head injury. Crit Care Med 1999;27(11):2525–31.

87. Chiang YH, Chao DP, Chu SF, et al. Early enteral nutrition and clinical outcomes of severe traumatic brain injury patients in acute stage: a multi-center cohort study. J Neurotrauma 2012;29(1):75–80.

88. Acosta-Escribano J, Fernandez-Vivas M, Grau Carmona T, et al. Gastric versus transpyloric feeding in severe traumatic brain injury: a prospective, randomized trial. Intensive Care Med 2010;36(9):1532–9.

89. Edwards P, Arango M, Balica L, et al. Final results of MRC CRASH, a randomised placebo-controlled trial of intravenous corticosteroid in adults with head injury-outcomes at 6 months. Lancet 2005;365(9475):1957–9.

90. Roberts I, Yates D, Sandercock P, et al. Effect of intravenous corticosteroids on death within 14 days in 10008 adults with clinically significant head injury (MRC CRASH trial): randomised placebo-controlled trial. Lancet 2004;364(9442):1321–8.

91. Bilotta F, Caramia R, Cernak I, et al. Intensive insulin therapy after severe traumatic brain injury: a randomized clinical trial. Neurocrit Care 2008;9(2):159–66.

92. Skolnick BE, Maas AI, Narayan RK, et al. A clinical trial of progesterone for severe traumatic brain injury. N Engl J Med 2014;371(26):2467–76.

93. Wright DW, Yeatts SD, Silbergleit R, et al. Very early administration of progesterone for acute traumatic brain injury. N Engl J Med 2014;371(26):2457–66.

94. Cotton BA, Snodgrass KB, Fleming SB, et al. Beta-blocker exposure is associated with improved survival after severe traumatic brain injury. J Trauma 2007;62(1):26–33 [discussion: 33–5].

95. Ley EJ, Scehnet J, Park R, et al. The in vivo effect of propranolol on cerebral perfusion and hypoxia after traumatic brain injury. J Trauma 2009;66(1):154–9 [discussion: 159–61].

96. Patel MB, McKenna JW, Alvarez JM, et al. Decreasing adrenergic or sympathetic hyperactivity after severe traumatic brain injury using propranolol and clonidine (DASH After TBI Study): study protocol for a randomized controlled trial. Trials 2012;13:177.

97. Alali AS, Mukherjee K, McCredie VA, et al. Beta-Blockers and Traumatic Brain Injury: A Systematic Review, Meta-analysis, and Eastern Association for the Surgery of Trauma Guideline. Ann Surg 2017. [Epub ahead of print].

Trauma: Spinal Cord Injury

Matthew J. Eckert, MD[a],*, Matthew J. Martin, MD[a,b]

KEYWORDS

- Spine • Spine trauma • Spinal cord injury • Spinal cord syndromes • Spinal shock
- Spine immobilization

KEY POINTS

- Hypotension following trauma should be considered secondary to hemorrhage until proven otherwise, even in patients with early suspicion of spinal injury. Neurogenic shock and spinal shock are separate, important entities that must be understood.
- Hypoxia and hypotension should be aggressively corrected because they lead to secondary spinal cord injury, analogous to traumatic brain injury. Critical care support of multiple organ systems is frequently required early after injury.
- Early spinal decompression may lead to improved neurologic outcomes in select spinal cord injuries, and prompt consultation with spine surgeons is recommended.
- Computed tomography (CT) is the gold-standard screening study for evaluation of the spine after trauma and has significantly greater sensitivity and specificity compared with plain radiographs.
- High-quality CT imaging without evidence of cervical spine injury may be adequate for removal of the cervical immobilization collar in obtunded patients.

INTRODUCTION

Traumatic spine and spinal cord injury (SCI) occurred in roughly 17,000 US citizens in 2016, with an estimated prevalence of approximately 280,000 injured persons.[1] Although the injury has historically been a disease of younger adult men, a progressive increase in SCI incidence among the elderly has been reported over the last few decades.[2] Upwards of 70% of SCI patients suffer multiple injuries concomitant with spinal cord trauma, contributing to the high rates of associated complications during the acute and long-term phases of care.[3] SCI is associated with significant reductions in life expectancy across the spectrum of injury and age at time of insult.[1]

Patients who survive the initial injury face significant risks of medical complications throughout the rest of their lives. More than half of all SCI patients will develop complications during the initial hospital stay, with higher rates corresponding to increased

[a] Department of Surgery, General Surgery, Madigan Army Medical Center, 9040-A Jackson Avenue, Tacoma, WA 98431, USA; [b] Trauma and Emergency Surgery Service, Legacy Emanuel Medical Center, 501 N. Graham Street, #580, Portland OR 97227, USA
* Corresponding author.
E-mail address: Matthew.j.eckert.mil@mail.mil

injury severity, the presence of associated traumatic brain injury, and cerebrovascular damage occurring with cervical spine injury.[4,5] SCI may result in numerous multisystem complications particularly during the acute phase of care with long-term complications often related to infectious morbidity (**Table 1**). For the trauma/acute care surgeon managing SCI patients during the acute phase of injury, respiratory compromise and shock are of primary concern, as discussed later.

During the initial presentation and evaluation of SCI patients, almost all other injuries should take precedent in both evaluation and management, unless the SCI is impeding the airway (cervical spine) or the hemodynamics (neurogenic shock). No emergent imaging of the spine is required before a laparotomy or other life-saving surgical intervention. Spinal immobilization is adequate for initial prevention of further injury while addressing sources of hemorrhage. Prevention of hypotension and hypoxia is also critical to mitigating further neurologic injury. Even if one of the rare spinal cord emergencies is encountered, such as a progressively worsening examination with cord compression that requires surgical decompression, your job will be to stabilize the patient and address any other life-threatening injury before intervention by a spine surgeon. Hypotension in the setting of a suspected acute traumatic SCI should always be first assumed to be due to hypovolemia/hemorrhage, until ruled out.

ASSESSMENT OF SPINAL CORD INJURIES

The critical step in early evaluation of patients with possible SCI is recognition of patients at risk and a focused, yet thorough neurologic examination. Too often the

Table 1	
Organ system complications following spinal cord injury	
Organ System	**Complications**
Cardiovascular	Bradycardia/dysrhythmia Cardiac arrest Cardiogenic pulmonary edema
Pulmonary	Hypoventilation/respiratory failure Poor secretion control Acute respiratory distress syndrome Aspiration Pneumonia
Gastrointestinal	Gastric dysmotility Adynamic ileus Gastritis and ulceration Pancreatitis
Hematologic	Venothromboembolism
Neurologic	Neurogenic shock Depression Posttraumatic stress disorder Anxiety Autonomic dysreflexia
Genitourinary	Bladder dysfunction Urinary tract infection Priapism
Integument	Pressure ulceration

Adapted from Stricsek G, Ghobrial G, Wilson J, et al. Complications in the management of patients with spine trauma. Neurosurg Clin N Am 2017;28:150–2; with permission.

steps of physical examination are deferred to the all-knowing computed tomographic (CT) scanner. This delay can slow recognition of SCI and establishment of baseline function and delay consultation of appropriate specialists and the initiation of preventive measures avoiding further secondary injury. The performance of such an examination is frequently overlooked in busy trauma bays. The main points are that in addition to global neurologic disability (Glasgow Coma Scale and pupil examination), the secondary survey of the patient should include sensory and motor testing in upper and lower extremity muscle groups as well as an anorectal examination for tone and sensation. **Table 2** lists the key muscle groups and their corresponding motor level that should be checked to determine the motor level of the injury. Both upper and lower extremities and the right and left sides should be tested, because certain syndromes may cause "skip" patterns or have unilateral asymmetric deficits (eg, central cord syndrome, Brown-Séquard). Both the motor and the sensory level should be clearly documented in the neurologic portion of the admission history and physical examination as well as communicated to any consulting spine provider.

The distinction of complete and incomplete cord injury should be made because this may influence operative decision making such as decompressive laminectomy or removal of bone fragments that are compressing the spinal cord. A "complete" injury is an injury pattern in which there is absolutely no spine-mediated neurologic function below the level of the injury. An "incomplete" injury is one in which there is *any* function below the level of injury, typically in the form of intact sensation (such as perineal) or slight distal motor function. Sacral root sparing, which may allow some residual anal sphincter function or sensation or slight movement of a great toe, is an indication that the injury is incomplete and carries a better prognosis for recovery of some degree of neurologic function.

The American Spinal Injury Association (ASIA) International Standards for Neurological Classification of SCI is the most frequently used and studied spinal injury severity assessment score.[6] ASIA injury scoring is dependent on the presence or absence of motor function and sacral nerve root sparing below the level of injury (**Fig. 1**). Knowledge of which muscle group is fired by each spinal cord level and a more thorough checking for neurologic function distal to the apparent spinal cord level (including

Table 2
Muscle function tested on physical examination and the corresponding motor level

Motor Level	Muscle Function
C5	Elbow flexion
C6	Wrist extension
C7	Elbow extension
C8	Finger flexion
T1	Finger abduction
L2	Hip flexion
L3	Knee extension
L4	Ankle dorsiflexion
L5	Great toe extension
S1	Ankle dorsiflexion

Adapted from Branco F, Cardenas DD, Svircev JN. Spinal cord injury: a comprehensive review. Phys Med Rehabil Clin N Am 2007;18(4):651–79; v; with permission.

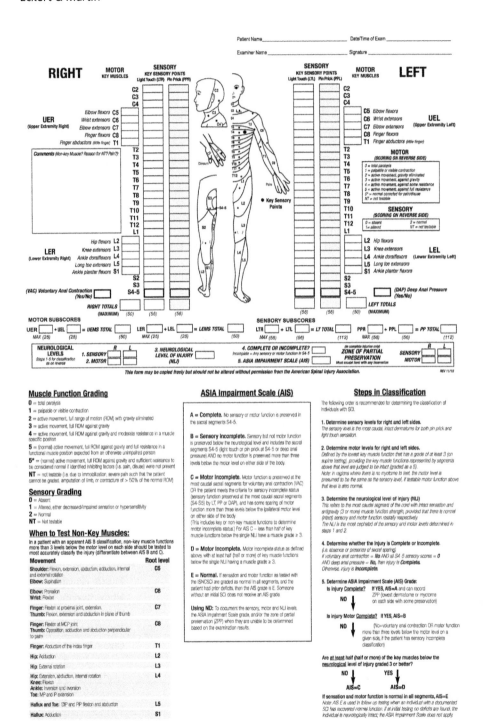

Fig. 1. ASIA SCI evaluation and scoring sheet. (*From* the American Spinal Injury Association (ASIA). Available at: www.asia-spinalinjury.org/information/downloads. Accessed February 1, 2017; with permission.)

rectal examination) can help identify patients with incomplete injuries who may benefit from more urgent operative intervention. In addition, such an examination may help identify the possible injury location in order to better immobilize and prevent iatrogenic extension of the neurologic deficit. If spinal shock is present, it cannot be determined whether the injury is complete or incomplete until 24 to 48 hours after the shock period resolves.

Although imaging of the spine is often thought of as being primarily about the bony structures, it is important to remember that complete assessment for spine injury and spinal stability requires assessment of the bone, the ligaments, and the spinal cord itself. Traditional plain radiograph imaging of the spine only evaluates the bony component and has essentially been replaced by the widespread availability and efficiency of modern multidetector CT imaging. Although the utility of plain radiograph screening of the cervical spine in select low-risk patients has been extensively studied, numerous studies have demonstrated the superiority of CT versus plain radiograph for screening acutely injured patients with suspected or at risk for spine injury.[7–9] Negative predictive values approaching 100% have been reported in several trials, particularly with relation to the presence of a clinically unstable injury or injury requiring intervention.[10–12] Although CT is ideal for screening identification of bony injury and suggestion of alignment abnormalities, the diagnostic accuracy of CT for spinal cord, ligamentous, and soft tissue injury is exceeded by MRI.[13,14] Patients with deficits on examination, CT findings suggestive of injury to the cord, disks, ligaments, or nerve roots, or unexplained neurologic examination may benefit from early MRI for diagnostic and therapeutic decisions.

SPINAL SHOCK VERSUS NEUROGENIC SHOCK

The terms "spinal shock" and "neurogenic shock" are often both used inappropriately or incorrectly, or are confused for one another in the clinical setting. Neurogenic shock is the hemodynamic consequence of the SCI, classically characterized by hypotension due to vasodilation and increased perfusion of the lower extremities (also known as "warm shock"). In cases of higher SCI (cervical spine), hypotension may often be accompanied by paradoxical bradycardia. This pattern is a relatively unique and specific hemodynamic pattern to SCI and should prompt immediate evaluation and interventions. Cervical spine and high thoracic spine injuries may result in loss of sympathetic cardiac stimulation (bradycardia) and vasomotor tone in the lower body (hypotension) that will benefit from early initiation of vasopressor medication along with standard trauma resuscitation to restore intravascular volume status.

Although neurogenic shock refers to a hemodynamic pattern, spinal shock refers to the neurologic examination findings that may be seen after an acute SCI. The diagnosis of spinal shock is made in the presence of complete loss of reflexes below the level of injury, including the monosynaptic pathways. If spinal shock is present, this means that it is not yet known what the ultimate amount of functional recovery will be. You will have to wait until the spinal shock period is over. If spinal shock is not present, or it has resolved, then whatever neurologic deficits you have at that time are likely to be fixed and permanent. Thus, for the patient presenting with paralysis in spinal shock, an unknown amount of functional recovery may still occur. Spinal shock is diagnosed through evaluation of the bulbocavernosus and/or cremasteric reflexes. If these reflexes are absent, then the patient is in spinal shock, and when they return, the shock period has ended.[15] Once the period of spinal shock has ended and the bulbocavernosus and/or cremasteric reflexes have returned, then the neurologic examination at that time likely reflects what the permanent level and degree of deficits will be.

MANAGEMENT OF ACUTE SPINAL CORD INJURY

The management of SCI begins with spine precautions (logrolling, cervical collar) and protection from further injury. Spinal immobilization precautions do not mean lying flat and motionless once the initial trauma evaluation has been completed. Reverse Trendelenburg position up to 30° will greatly benefit, and participatory pulmonary toilet should begin if they are not intubated. Ensure adequate pain control to maximize tidal volumes. Have a low threshold for nasogastric decompression because gastric ileus often accompanies SCI with paraplegia or quadriplegia. Similarly, bladder dysfunction is common, and a urinary catheter should be placed if not already present. Begin management of pressure points with padding and frequent patient repositioning immediately for paralyzed patients. Do not forget the psychological and emotional aspects of these injuries, particularly in young acutely injured patients. Early mental health professional and/or chaplain consultation to begin helping the patient deal with the almost uniform depression and grieving over the loss of bodily function that accompanies these injuries is essential.

Similar to studies of traumatic brain injury, avoidance of hypotension (systolic blood pressure <90 mm Hg) and hypoxia is critical to avoiding further secondary SCI.[16,17] Neurogenic shock may manifest as hypotension, which is poorly responsive to fluid resuscitation but responds briskly to vasopressor agents. In pure neurogenic shock, there is no associated tachycardia; the extremities may be warm and dry rather than cold and clammy, and typically, the patient has a significant cervical SCI. Treatment involves judicious volume resuscitation and the use of vasopressors to support blood pressure. A purely peripheral vasoconstrictor such as Neo-Synephrine is often used, but in the multitrauma patient or the patient with associated bradycardia, a balanced vasopressor such as norepinephrine is a better choice. Maintaining the mean arterial pressure greater than 85 mm Hg for up to 7 days after injury has been associated with improved ASIA scores and is recommended in current guidelines.[18,19] The concept of spinal cord perfusion pressure monitoring through direct measure of intraspinal pressure (ISP) after placement of an intradural catheter has demonstrated significant promise. Small trials have demonstrated safety and efficacy of monitoring ISP at the site of maximal cord edema for up to 1 week after injury.[20–22]

Controversy persists over the utility of high-dose systemic steroids following blunt SCI. The series of National Acute Spinal Cord Injury Studies (NASCIS) I-III trials failed to demonstrate any difference in neurologic outcomes after high-dose methylprednisolone.[23–25] Post hoc subgroup analyses in the later NASCIS trials showed a 5-point (ASIA) motor scoring improvement across 15 muscle groups but did not correlate with any measure of functional improvement or effect upon disability. In contrast, patients receiving high-dose steroids consistently suffered increased rates of infectious complications, gastric ulceration, venothromboembolic events, wound complications, and trended toward increased mortality related to pulmonary complications. Numerous additional trials confirmed the NASCIS outcomes with similar complication profiles.[26,27] The use of high-dose steroids after penetrating SCI has consistently shown poor outcomes.[28–30] Previous guidelines had recommended intravenous steroid bolus and infusion for all patients with blunt SCI and no contraindication to treatment. However, this approach has now been widely abandoned because of the highly questionable clinical benefit identified in the NASCIS trials as well as more recent data indicating no benefit to steroid use. Recent evidence-based management guidelines recommend against the use of high-dose steroids for all acute SCI.[31] There may be a role for steroid use in highly select or atypical types of spinal cord trauma and injury, and this decision should be at the discretion of the managing spine surgeon.

Not infrequently, the examination of an injured patient will suggest neurologic deficit without any obvious supporting radiographic findings. These SCI without radiographic abnormalities (SCIWORA) represent a challenging group because limited evidence and support for treatment have been established. Unfortunately, the ultimate neurologic outcome in SCIWORA patients appears correlated with the initial deficits on examination similar to those patients with radiographic abnormalities and neurologic deficits.[32] MRI appears particularly useful in identifying subtle intraneural and extraneural abnormalities that may be associated with the neurologic deficits and correlate with outcomes.[33] Supportive care is similar to that described previously for those patients with neurologic injury and radiographic abnormalities. Despite increased reports on populations of SCIWORA patients, limited high-quality data are available, and no randomized controlled trials of management have been conducted.

The timing of surgical spinal decompression in the setting of compressive phenomena, such as epidural hematoma, cord edema or hemorrhage, or impinging bony fragments and foreign bodies, has been extensively studied. Preclinical models have demonstrated that the extent and duration of cord compression correlate with ultimate neurologic deficit.[34,35] Human series have suggested that early decompression in the first 8 to 24 hours after injury in those patients with incomplete SCI is associated with improved neurologic outcomes. In the Surgical Timing in Acute Spinal Cord Injury Study, patients with cervical SCI that underwent decompression in the first 24 hours after injury had a significant improvement in ASIA grade.[36] Additional studies have confirmed the benefits of early decompression for these incomplete patients; however, not all trials of time to decompression have shown neurologic improvement with early intervention.[37] Early surgical decompression is also associated with decreased pulmonary morbidity and duration of mechanical ventilation as well as decreased intensive care unit and hospital length of stay.[38,39] Unfortunately, surgical decompression in patients presenting with ASIA A complete injury has not shown significant improvements in neurologic outcomes.[40,41]

As previously noted, one of the early measures in the assessment and stabilization of a suspected SCI patient is the prevention of future mechanical injury due to instability of the spinal column. Although logroll precautions, maintenance of axial alignment, pressure point management, and attentive nursing care are generally adequate for thoracolumbar spinal protection, the cervical spine is generally protected with specialized cervical immobilization devices, or "c-collars." Controversy persists regarding the actual effectiveness and necessity of these devices to maintain proper alignment and prevent skeletal motion.[42-45] In addition, these hard devices may be associated with development of pressure ulceration in upwards of 30% of patients.[46] For the obtunded trauma patient with associated brain injury or critical illness in whom the cervical spine cannot be cleared by standard imaging and physical examination, a particular challenge arises. Traditionally, these patients were left in a hard cervical collar until examinable or until an MRI or other imaging adjunct demonstrated no evidence of injury. Recent studies from multiple centers have demonstrated the safety of cervical collar removal after a negative high-quality CT given negative predictive values of 100% for unstable injuries.[12] As a result of these studies, practice patterns are changing with expected decreased utilization of MRI resources and prevention of complications of hard cervical immobilization devices.

MANAGEMENT OF PENETRATING SPINE TRAUMA

Penetrating SCI is most commonly secondary to gunshot wounds and typically results in complete SCI due to direct trauma to the cord and associated blast effect as well as secondary hemorrhage and ischemia.[47] In civilian trauma centers, the thoracolumbar spine is the region most frequently injured. The management options for open spine trauma are not much different than those for closed spine trauma, even in patients with open vertebral column fractures. The wound must be managed with irrigation and debridement of all nonviable tissues and early antibiotic coverage. The choice of antibiotics is generally the same as for patients with open extremity fractures, and there are no good data on recommended duration of therapy (ranges of 48 hours to 10 days reported). Patients with associated intestinal injuries, particularly if those injuries communicate with the spinal column injury, may require broader coverage. These devastating injuries will obviously require multidisciplinary care for optimal outcomes.

Incomplete SCI, cauda equina syndrome, or evidence of cord compression after penetrating injury due to hematoma or bony fragments may benefit from surgical decompression.[48] In addition, surgical stabilization of unstable vertebral column injuries is necessary in any patient likely to survive the acute phase of care. Exploration of the injuries may be required for debridement, neurologic deterioration due to cord compression, or persistent cerebrospinal fluid leak. Wound infection, spinal column instability, and cerebrospinal fluid leaks were the most common complications in a series of penetrating SCI.[49] These penetrating injuries are frequently managed conservatively as outcomes have been shown to be equivocal or even more favorable in nonoperative management.[50]

AIRWAY MANAGEMENT

The need for appropriate airway management is of particular importance for patients with cervical SCIs. Most patients with high cervical SCIs will present with quadriplegia and respiratory distress or arrest and clearly require intubation. The difficult patient population is the lower cervical spine injury (C5-C7) and upper thoracic spine (T1-T6), who frequently present with no obvious respiratory distress due to the ability to continue shallow breathing. Be wary of these patients: previous reports have demonstrated that up to 50% will slowly decompensate and require a delayed emergent airway intervention.[51,52] This can result in secondary SCI due to hypoxia and trauma from manipulation during emergent intubation attempts. Over a period of several hours to days, the shallow breathing will result in progressive atelectasis, pulmonary consolidation or pneumonia, and finally, acute hypoxic decompensation. The insidious airway collapse in this setting can be severely harmful or even fatal and should be anticipated. A low threshold for intubating these patients semi-electively for the initial hospital period or before transfer may be prudent, because up to 30% will require intubation in the first 24 hours after cervical SCI.[53] Factors suggestive of early intubation include higher level of injury (above C5), complete paralysis, the presence of associated injuries (particularly chest wall or intrathoracic), and low lung volumes on chest radiograph. If you have the capability to measure and follow vital capacity, then this may be a useful adjunct to identify the patient progressing to respiratory failure.

Numerous publications discuss the methods for intubation in the patient with a cervical spine injury and the potential impact on spinal mobility. Direct laryngoscopy with manual in-line stabilization of the cervical spine during the procedure has been shown to be safe and effective in 2 large studies.[54,55] If available, fiberoptic intubation is safe and avoids significant spinal motion but requires manual stabilization during the procedure as well if the collar is released. Finally, a surgical airway is always an option and may be necessary for patients who will require long-term mechanical ventilation and/or pulmonary toilet. Consideration should be given to potential incision location for anterior cervical spine surgical stabilization if indicated. Although the definitions of what constitutes "early" tracheostomy vary in the literature, those patients who require or are projected to require mechanical ventilation for more than 2 weeks after injury certainly may benefit from tracheostomy. Improved secretion control, enhanced facilitation of mechanical ventilation weaning, patient comfort, ability to participate in rehabilitation, and possibly reduced risks of pneumonia and resource utilization have been associated with tracheostomy in SCI patients.[56–58]

SPINAL CORD SYNDROMES

Although simple complete traumatic SCI is relatively straightforward, with a dense and complete neurologic deficit below the level of injury, there are several spinal cord syndromes involving injuries to an isolated segment that have a much more varied and subtle presentation. These syndromes can be easily missed or misdiagnosed if a thorough neurologic examination and appropriate differential diagnosis are not performed. **Table 3** reviews the cause, diagnosis, and management for the common spinal syndromes. Although relatively uncommon, these syndromes have very characteristic presentations and common etiologic/mechanistic factors that

Table 3
Cause, diagnosis, and management for the common spinal syndromes

Syndrome	Cause	Examination Findings	Management
Central cord	Hyperflexion or extension, usually elderly with existing spinal stenosis; most common syndrome	Motor weakness of arms > legs with sacral sensory sparing	No proven benefit of prolonged immobilization Course of steroids may benefit Physical therapy and rehabilitation Spinal decompression
Brown-Séquard (cord hemisection)	Spinal hemisection, often gunshot or knife wound	Ipsilateral loss of motor and proprioception; contralateral loss of pain and temperature sensation	Spinal stabilization if unstable Course of steroids Physical therapy
Anterior cord	Damage to anterior 2/3 of cord, usually direct injury or ischemia from anterior spinal artery injury	Loss of motor function and pain/temperature with preserved proprioception and light touch sensation	Worst prognosis with low chance of muscle recovery Physical and occupational therapy
Conus medullaris	Injury to sacral cord and lumbar nerve roots, upper lumbar (L1) fractures, disk herniation, tumors	Bowel, bladder, and sexual dysfunction with areflexia, normal leg motor function, bulbocavernosus present with high lesion	Emergent surgical decompression Course of steroids GM1 ganglioside (100 mg) intravenous (IV) Bowel/bladder training
Cauda equina	Injury to lumbar/sacral nerve roots, lumbar (L2 or lower), or sacral fractures, also pelvic fractures, herniated disk, tumors	Weakness or flaccid leg paralysis, high lesions spare bowel/bladder, bulbocavernosus absent	Emergent surgical decompression Course of steroids GM1 ganglioside (100 mg) IV Bowel/bladder training

the managing physician should be aware of. Central cord syndrome is almost always a flexion/extension injury in an elderly patient with preexisting spinal stenosis. Although spinal immobilization is often maintained in these patients because of the presence of neurologic deficits, it is typically not an unstable spine injury, and there is no proven benefit of immobilization with a cervical collar. Brown-Séquard (or "cord hemisection") is extremely uncommon and typically only seen after direct penetrating injury to the spinal cord that results in different unilateral and contralateral deficits. Anterior cord syndrome is typically a vascular cause related to injury or interruption of flow through the anterior spinal artery. For all of the spinal cord syndromes presenting with fixed and established defects, management is usually expectant and aimed at treating symptoms and pain.[59,60] However, for any patient with a progressively worsening neurologic deficit, emergent consultation with a spine surgeon for possible decompression should be a priority.

VENOUS THROMBOEMBOLISM AFTER SPINAL CORD INJURY

Venous thromboembolism (VTE) events and appropriate prophylaxis are major concerns in the acute and long-term management of SCI patients. A recent large population study of roughly 48,000 SCI patients found an approximately 2.5-fold increased risk of deep venous thrombosis (DVT) and 1.6-fold increased risk of pulmonary embolism compared with controls. The risks were greatest within the first 3 months following injury and with increasing age.[61] Additional studies confirm the heightened risk in the early period after injury and with increased patient age, pointing to the significance of falls in older patients.[62,63] Overall incidence of VTE after SCI in recent publications suggests an incidence of approximately 3% to 5%, with associated early mortality of 7.5%, but up to 20% in patients greater than 70 years of age.[2,63] For unclear reasons, the location of SCI along the spine may also be associated with VTE risk. Maung and colleagues[64] found upper thoracic SCI to be associated with a higher rate of VTE compared with other spinal level injury. Variation in reported incidence of VTE is likely due to the timing and modality of screening methods. Duplex and Doppler ultrasonography are the most frequently and conveniently used screening modalities today.[65] There is no clear consensus on the timing or schedule for screening after acute SCI; however, the systematic review by Furlan and Fehlings[66] suggests that weekly screening for asymptomatic DVT in the early high-risk period following SCI may be appropriate.

In recognizing the increased risk of VTE following SCI, optimal preventive measures are an important facet of care for these patients. Until recently, controversy persisted regarding the optimal treatment with mechanical and/or chemoprophylaxis. A series of studies has confirmed the superior efficacy of low-molecular-weight heparin (LMWH) versus unfractionated subcutaneous heparin for the prevention of VTE and a lower associated bleeding risk.[67,68] Optimal dosing of LMWH remains controversial. Studies suggest that standard daily or twice daily enoxaparin dosing may not achieve therapeutic anti-Xa levels in trauma patients; however, no consensus for dose adjustment currently exists.[69,70] Combined preventive therapy with gradient elastic stockings or sequential pneumatic compression devices of the lower extremities and LMWH may offer an even greater reduction in VTE risk after SCI.[71] Early initiation of chemoprophylaxis (<72 hours from injury) has been associated with a significant reduction in the incidence of VTE after SCI (2% vs 26%) and recommended in at least one consensus guideline.[72,73] For patients with contraindications to chemoprophylaxis or VTE despite treatment, retrievable vena cava filter placement may be appropriate. However, outside these unique situations, studies suggest empiric filter placement offers no benefit over routine mechanical/chemoprophylaxis for acute SCI.[74–76]

SUMMARY

The impact of a SCI in any trauma patient can range from a minor nuisance to devastating paralysis, and unfortunately, the full spectrum of these injuries is frequently seen after trauma. Although much of the damage is done at the time of presentation and irreversible immediately, adherence to comprehensive supportive care aimed at treating the injury and preventing secondary injury may make a significant difference in the patient's ultimate functional outcome. Every physician should be able to perform a quick but thorough neurologic examination and understand the implications of significant examination findings such as spinal shock.

REFERENCES

1. National Spinal Cord Injury Statistical Center. Facts and figures at a glance. Birmingham (AL): University of Alabama; 2016.
2. Jain NB, Ayers GD, Peterson EN, et al. Traumatic spinal cord injury in the United States, 1993-2012. JAMA 2015;313(22):2236–43.
3. Herbert JS, Burnham RS. The effect of polytrauma in persons with traumatic spine injury. A prospective database of spine fractures. Spine (Phila Pa 1976) 2000;25(1):55–60.
4. Kushner DS, Alvarez G. Dual diagnosis: traumatic brain injury with spinal cord injury. Phys Med Rehabil Clin N Am 2014;25(3):681–96.
5. Silva Santos E, Santos Filho W, Possatti L, et al. Clinical complications in patients with severe cervical spine trauma: a ten-year prospective study. Arq Neuropsiquiatr 2012;70(7):524–8.
6. Kirshblum SC, Burns SP, Biering-Sorensen F, et al. International standards for neurological classification of spinal cord injury (revised 2011). J Spinal Cord Med 2011;34(6):535–46.
7. Ryken TC, Hadley MN, Walters BC, et al. Radiographic assessment. Neurosurgery 2013;72(Suppl 2):54–72.
8. Holmes JF, Akkinepalli R. Computed tomography versus plain radiography to screen for cervical spine injury: a meta-analysis. J Trauma 2005;58(5):902–5.
9. Bailitz J, Starr F, Beecroft M, et al. CT should replace three-view radiographs as the initial screening test in patients at high, moderate, and low risk for blunt cervical spine injury: a prospective comparison. J Trauma 2009;66(6):1605–9.
10. Hogan GJ, Mirvis SE, Shanmuganathan K, et al. Exclusion of unstable cervical spine injury in obtunded patients with blunt trauma: is MR imaging needed when multi-detector row CT findings are normal? Radiology 2005;237(1):106–12.
11. Adams JM, Cockburn MI, Difazio LT, et al. Spinal clearance in the difficult trauma patient: a role or screening MRI of the spine. Am Surg 2006;72(1):101–5.
12. Patel MB, Humble SS, Cullinane DC, et al. Cervical spine collar clearance in the obtunded adult blunt trauma patient: a systematic review and practice management guideline from the Eastern Association for the Surgery of Trauma. J Trauma Acute Care Surg 2015;78(2):430–41.
13. Bozzo A, Marcoux J, Radhakrishna M, et al. The role of magnetic resonance imaging in the management of acute spinal cord injury. J Neurotrauma 2011;28(8): 1401–11.
14. Beers GJ, Raque GH, Wagner GG, et al. MR imaging in acute cervical spine trauma. J Comput Assist Tomogr 1988;12(5):755–61.

15. Ditunno JF, Little JW, Tessler A, et al. Spinal shock revisited: a four-phase model. Spinal Cord 2004;42(7):383–95.
16. Vale F, Burns J, Jackson A, et al. Combined medical and surgical treatment after acute spinal cord injury: results of a prospective pilot study to assess the merits of aggressive medical resuscitation and blood pressure management. J Neurosurg 1997;87:239–46.
17. Stevens R, Bhardwaj A, Kirsh J. Critical care and perioperative management in traumatic spinal cord injury. J Neurosurg Anesthesiol 2003;15:215–29.
18. Hamryluk G, Whetstone W, Saigal R, et al. Mean arterial blood pressure correlates with neurologic recovery after human spinal cord injury. J Neurotrauma 2015;32(24):1958–67.
19. Ryken T, Hurlbert R, Hadley M, et al. The acute cardiopulmonary management of patients with cervical spinal cord injuries. Neurosurgery 2013;77:84–92.
20. Werndle MC, Saadoun S, Phang I, et al. Monitoring of spinal cord perfusion pressure in acute spinal cord injury: initial findings of the injured spinal cord pressure evaluation study. Crit Care Med 2014;42(3):646–55.
21. Phang I, Zoumprouli A, Saadoun S, et al. Safety profile and probe placement accuracy of intraspinal pressure monitoring for traumatic spinal cord injury: injured spinal cord pressure evaluation study. J Neurosurg Spine 2016;25(3):398–405.
22. Varsos GV, Werndle MC, Czosnyka ZH, et al. Intraspinal pressure and spinal cord perfusion pressure after spinal cord injury: an observational study. J Neurosurg Spine 2015;23(6):763–71.
23. Bracken MB, Shepard MJ, Hellenberg KG, et al. Methylprednisolone and neurological function 1 year after spinal cord injury. Results of the National Acute Spinal Cord Injury Study. J Neurosurg 1985;63:704–13.
24. Bracken MB, Shepard MJ, Collins WF, et al. A randomized controlled trial of methylprednisolone or naloxone in the treatment of acute spinal-cord injury. Results of the Second National Acute Spinal Cord Injury Study. N Engl J Med 1990;322: 1405–11.
25. Bracken MH, Shepard MJ, Holford TR, et al. Administration of methylprednisolone for 24 or 48 hours or tirilazad mesylate for 48 hours in the treatment of acute spinal cord injury. Results of the Third National Acute Spinal Cord Injury Randomized Controlled Trial. National Acute Spinal Cord Injury Study. JAMA 1997;277: 1597–604.
26. Otani K, Abe H, Kadoya S, et al. Beneficial effect of methylprednisolone sodium succinate in the treatment of acute spinal cord injury. Sekitsui Sekizui 1994;7:633–47.
27. Petitjean ME, Pointillart V, Dixmerias F, et al. Medical treatment of spinal cord injury in the acute stage. Ann Fr Anesth Reanim 1998;17:114–22.
28. Prendergast MR, Saxe JM, Ledgerwood AM, et al. Massive steroids do not reduce the zone of injury after penetrating spinal cord injury. J Trauma 1994; 37:576–9.
29. Levy ML, Gans W, Wijesinghe HS, et al. Use of methylprednisolone as an adjunct in the management of patients with penetrating spinal cord injury: outcome analysis. Neurosurgery 1996;39:1141–8.
30. Heary RF, Vaccaro AR, Mesa JJ, et al. Steroids and gunshot wounds to the spine. Neurosurgery 1997;41:576–83.
31. Hurlbert RJ, Hadley MN, walters BC, et al. Pharmacological therapy for acute spinal cord injury. Neurosurgery 2015;76(Suppl 1):S71–83.
32. Wilson JR, Cadotte DW, Fehlings MG. Clinical predictors of neurologic outcome, functional status, and survival after traumatic spinal cord injury: a systematic review. J Neurosurg Spine 2012;17(Suppl 1):S11–26.

33. Boese CK, Lechler P. Spinal cord injury without radiographic abnormalities in adults: a systematic review. J Trauma Acute Care Surg 2013;75:320–30.

34. Dimar JR, Glassman SD, Raque GH, et al. The influence of spinal canal narrowing and timing of decompression on neurologic recovery after spinal cord contusion in a rat model. Spine (Phila Pa 1976) 1999;24(16):1623–33.

35. Batchelor PE, Willis TE, Skeers P, et al. Meta-analysis of pre-clinical studies of early decompression in acute spinal cord injury: a battle of time and pressure. PLoS One 2013;8(8):e72659.

36. Fehlings MG, Vaccaro A, Wilson JR, et al. Early versus delayed decompression for traumatic cervical spinal cord injury: results of the surgical timing in acute spinal cord injury study (STASCIS). PLoS One 2012;7(2):e32037.

37. Wilson JR, Singh A, Craven C, et al. Early versus late surgery for traumatic spinal cord injury: the results of a prospective Canadian cohort study. Spinal Cord 2012; 50(11):840–3.

38. Bourassa-Moreau E, Mac-Thiong JM, Feldman DE, et al. Complications in acute phase hospitalization of traumatic spinal cord injury: does surgical timing matter? J Trauma Acute Care Surg 2013;74(3):849–54.

39. Liu JM, Long XH, Zhou Y, et al. Is urgent decompression superior to delayed surgery for traumatic spinal cord injury? A meta-analysis. World Neurosurg 2016;87: 124–31.

40. Petitjean ME, Mousselard H, Pointillart V, et al. Thoracic spinal trauma and associated injuries: should early spinal decompression be considered? J Trauma 1995;39(2):368–72.

41. Bourassa-Moreau E, Mac-Thiong JM, Li A, et al. Do patients with complete spinal cord injury benefit from early surgical decompression? Analysis of neurological improvement in a prospective cohort study. J Neurotrauma 2016;33(3):301–6.

42. Clemency BM, Bart JA, Malhotra A, et al. Patient immobilized with a long spine board rarely have unstable thoracolumbar injuries. Prehosp Emerg Care 2016; 20(2):266–72.

43. Wampler DA, Pineda C, Polk J, et al. The long spine board does not reduce lateral spine motion during transport- a randomized healthy volunteer crossover trial. Am J Emerg Med 2016;34(4):717–21.

44. Horodyski M, DiPaola CP, Conrad BP, et al. Cervical collars are insufficient for immobilizing an unstable cervical spine injury. J Emerg Med 2011;41:513–9.

45. Lador R, Ben-Galim P, Hippa JA. Motion within the unstable cervical spine during patient maneuvering: the neck-pivot-shift phenomenon. J Trauma 2011;70: 247–50.

46. Ham W, Schoonhoven L, Schuurmans MJ, et al. Pressure ulcers from spinal immobilization in trauma patients: a systematic review. J Trauma Acute Care Surg 2014;76(4):1131–41.

47. Rosenfeld JV, Bell RS, Armonda R. Current concepts in penetrating and blast injury to the central nervous system. World J Surg 2015;39(6):1352–62.

48. Klimo P, Ragel BT, Rosner M, et al. Can surgery improve neurologic function in penetrating spinal injury? A review of the military and civilian literature and treatment recommendations for military neurosrgeons. Neurosurg Focus 2010; 28(5):E4.

49. Simpson RK, Venger BH, Narayan RK. Treatment of acute penetrating injuries of the spine: a retrospective analysis. J Trauma 1989;29(1):42–6.

50. Sidu GS, Ghag A, Prokuski V, et al. Civilian gunshot injuries of the spinal cord: a systematic review of the current literature. Clin Orthop Relat Res 2013;471: 3945–55.

51. Jackson AB, Grommers TE. Incidence of respiratory complications following SCI. Arch Phys Med Rehabil 1994;75:270–5.

52. Cotton BA, Pryor JP, Chinwilla I, et al. Respiratory complications and mortality risk associated with thoracic spine injury. J Trauma 2005;59:1400–9.

53. Gardner BP, Watt JW, Krishnan KR. The artificial ventilation of acute spinal cord damaged patients: a retrospective study of forty-four patients. Paraplegia 1986;24(4):208–20.

54. Grande CM, Barton CR, Stene JK. Appropriate techniques for the airway management of emergency patients with suspected spinal cord injury. Anesth Analg 1988;67(7):714–5.

55. Shatney CH, Brunner RD, Nguyen TQ. The safety of orotracheal intubation in patients with unstable cervical spine fracture or high spinal cord injury. Am J Surg 1995;170(6):676–9.

56. Como JJ, Sutton ER, McCunn M, et al. Characterizing the need for mechanical ventilation following cervical spinal cord injury with neurologic deficit. J Trauma 2005;59:912–6.

57. Harrop J, Sharan A, Scheid E, et al. Tracheostomy placement in patients with complete cervical spinal cord injuries: American Spinal Injury Association Grade A. J Neurosurg 2004;100:20–3.

58. Jaeger J, Littlewood K, Durbin C. The role of tracheostomy in weaning from mechanical ventilation. Respir Care 2002;47(4):469–80.

59. Brooks NP. Central cord syndrome. Neurosurg Clin N Am 2017;28(1):41–7.

60. Radcliff KE, Kepler CK, Delasota LA, et al. Current management review of thoracolumbar cord syndromes. Spine J 2011;11(9):884–92.

61. Chung WS, Lin CL, Chang SN, et al. Increased risk of deep vein thrombosis and pulmonary thromboembolism in patients with spinal cord injury: a nationwide cohort prospective study. Thromb Res 2014;133(4):579–84.

62. Giorgi PM, Donadini MP, Dentali F, et al. The short- and long-term risk of venous thromboembolism in patients with acute spinal cord injury: a prospective cohort study. Thromb Haemost 2013;109(1):34–8.

63. Jones T, Ugalde V, Franks P, et al. Venous thromboembolism after spinal cord injury: incidence, time course, and associated risk factors in 16,240 adults and children. Arch Phys Med Rehabil 2005;86(12):2240–7.

64. Maung AA, Schuster KM, Kaplan LJ, et al. Risk of venous thromboembolism after spinal cord injury: not all levels are the same. J Trauma Acute Care Surg 2011; 71(5):1241–5.

65. Zierler BK. Ultrasonography and diagnosis of venous thromboembolism. Circulation 2004;109(12 Suppl 1):I–9.

66. Furlan JC, Fehlings MG. Role of screening tests for deep venous thrombosis in asymptomatic adults with acute spinal cord injury: an evidence-based analysis. Spine (Phila Pa 1976) 2007;32(17):1908–16.

67. Spinal Cord Injury Thromboprophylaxis Investigators. Prevention of venous thromboembolism in the acute treatment phase after spinal cord injury: a randomized, multicenter trial comparing low-dose heparin plus intermittent pneumatic compression with enoxaparin. J Trauma Acute Care Surg 2003;54(6): 1116–24.

68. Teasell RW, Hsieh JT, Aubut JA, et al. Spinal cord injury rehabilitation evidence review research team. Venous thromboembolism after spinal cord injury. Arch Phys Med Rehabil 2009;90(2):232–45.

69. Rutherford EJ, Schooler WG, Sredzienski E, et al. Optimal dose of enoxaparin in critically ill trauma and surgical patients. J Trauma Acute Care Surg 2005;58(6): 1167–70.
70. Costantini TW, Min E, Box K, et al. Dose adjusting enoxaparin is necessary to achieve adequate venous thromboembolism prophylaxis in trauma patients. J Trauma Acute Care Surg 2013;74(1):128.
71. Aito S, Pieri A, D'Andrea M, et al. Primary prevention of deep venous thrombosis and pulmonary embolism in acute spinal cord injured patients. Spinal Cord 2002; 40(6):300.
72. Christie S, Thibault-Halman G, Casha S. Acute pharmacological DVT prophylaxis after spinal cord injury. J Neurotrauma 2011;28(8):1509–14.
73. Harrop JS, Tetreault L, Aarabi B, et al. Guidelines for the management of patients with spinal cord injury: efficacy, safety and timing of anticoagulation prophylaxis. Spine J 2016;16(10):S214.
74. Gorman PH, Qadri SF, Rao-Patel A. Prophylactic inferior vena cava (IVC) filter placement may increase the relative risk of deep venous thrombosis after acute spinal cord injury. J Trauma Acute Care Surg 2009;66(3):707–12.
75. Maxwell RA, Chavarria-Aguilar M, Cockerham WT, et al. Routine prophylactic vena cava filtration is not indicated after acute spinal cord injury. J Trauma Acute Care Surg 2002;52(5):902–6.
76. Cook AD, Gross BW, Osler TM, et al. Vena cava filter use in trauma and rates of pulmonary embolism, 2003-2015. JAMA Surg 2017. [Epub ahead of print].

Thoracic Trauma

Bradley M. Dennis, MD[a],*, Seth A. Bellister, MD[b],
Oscar D. Guillamondegui, MD, MPH[a]

KEYWORDS

- Chest trauma • Thoracic trauma • Pneumothorax • Hemothorax • VATS
- Rib fractures • Pulmonary contusion

KEY POINTS

- Management of chest wall injuries requires multidisciplinary approach highlighted by multimodal pain management and occasionally operative intervention.
- Rib fixation is an evolving field that require additional study to delineate the most appropriate candidates for this therapy.
- Pneumothorax should be treated immediately with tube thoracostomy if tension physiology is present. Otherwise, symptomatic or enlarging pneumothoraces or hemothoraces should be evacuated.
- Retained hemothoraces of more than 300 mL in volume should be preferentially treated with videoassisted thoracoscopic evacuation unless prohibitive operative candidate.
- Tracheobronchial injuries are definitively diagnosed bronchoscopically and should be treated by surgical repair, if possible, after securing the airway.

CHEST WALL INJURY

Chest wall injury is one of the most common in trauma, present in 10% or more of all trauma admissions.[1] It is also a significant marker of mortality, injury severity, and associated injuries.[1–3] In isolation, chest wall injury is a powerful predictor of pulmonary deterioration and complications.[3–5] The effect seems to be greatest in older populations with increased ventilator days, and pneumonia and acute respiratory distress syndrome rates compared with younger cohorts with similar injury patterns.[4–7]

Flail chest, most commonly defined as 3 or more consecutive ribs fractured in multiple locations, can significantly alter chest wall mechanics and result in serious respiratory complications. Flail segments can cause paradoxic chest wall motion, which

Disclosure Statement: The authors have nothing to disclose.
[a] Division of Trauma, Surgical Critical Care, and Emergency General Surgery, Department of Surgery, Vanderbilt University Medical Center, 1211 21st Avenue South, 404 Medical Arts Building, Nashville, TN 37212, USA; [b] Division of Trauma, Surgical Critical Care, and Emergency General Surgery, Department of Surgery, Vanderbilt University Medical Center, 1211 21st Avenue South, 404 Medical Arts Building, Nashville, TN 37212, USA
* Corresponding author.
E-mail address: Bradley.m.dennis@vanderbilt.edu

can effect respiratory mechanics throughout the respiratory cycle (**Fig. 1**).[8] The impact of this injury is significant. More than 80% of patients with flail chests require admission to the intensive care unit (ICU) and nearly 60% will require mechanical ventilation with a 20% tracheostomy rate. The injury has a significant effect on in-hospital complications because 20% will develop pneumonia and up to 7% will develop sepsis.[9]

This diagnosis is suspected in patients with chest wall pain after injury. Crepitus, chest wall asymmetry, paradoxic breathing, and dyspnea are often present. Chest radiographs can identify many rib fractures, particularly significantly displaced fractures. Sternal fractures and nondisplaced rib fractures are often only identified with computed tomography (CT) imaging.

The management of these injuries requires a multidisciplinary approach with 3 primary components: pain management, respiratory therapy, and mobility. Anesthesia, nursing, and respiratory and physical therapy all play significant roles in the successful management of patients with chest wall injury.

Pain management consists of 3 basic categories: nonregional analgesia, regional anesthetics, and surgical fixation. Surgical fixation will be discussed elsewhere in this review. Nonregional analgesia, primarily oral and intravenous analgesics, is often the initial therapy for pain management for mild to moderate chest wall injury. Because of the relative dearth of clinical research in this area, this initial approach is essentially an adaptation of postoperative pain control approaches. Recent emphasis on reducing opioid use has increased the push for multimodal analgesia. Multimodal analgesia is defined as simultaneous use of a combination of analgesics that each have different mechanisms of action and thus target different receptors in the peripheral and/or central nervous system.[10] A recent joint practice guideline from the Eastern Association for the Surgery of Trauma (EAST) and the Trauma Anesthesia Society noted very limited data describing multimodal analgesia in management of blunt thoracic trauma. However, they were able to conditionally recommend the use of

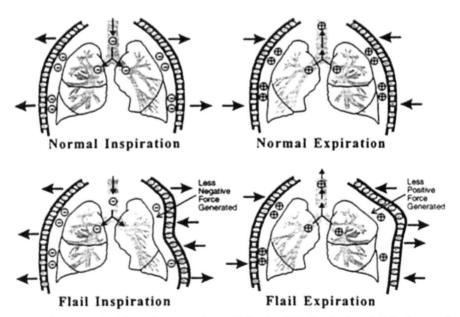

Normal Inspiration   **Normal Expiration**

Flail Inspiration   **Flail Expiration**

Fig. 1. Flail chest physiology. (*From* Mayberry JC, Trunkey DD. The fractured rib in chest wall trauma. Chest Surg Clin N Am 1997;7(2):253; with permission.)

multimodal analgesia over opioids alone in patients with blunt thoracic trauma.[11] This multimodal approach involving scheduled nonsteroidal antiinflammatory drugs, acetaminophen, and/or gabapentin and pregabalin with opioids as needed should be attempted for mild to moderate chest wall injury. Oral opioids are preferred to intravenous when possible. Additionally, when intravenous opioids are required, patient-controlled analgesia should be used if possible.[10] For patients requiring more aggressive pain control, lidocaine or ketamine infusions can be considered, although these modalities come with weaker recommendations.[10]

Regional anesthetic techniques should be considered to optimize pain control for patients with chest wall injury that are considered at higher risk of respiratory complications. This population includes more severe chest wall injury (>4 fractured ribs), over 45 years of age, insufficient respiratory effort (based on incentive spirometry or pulmonary function tests), and/or inadequate pain control with multimodal analgesia.[3–7,12–14] Regional anesthesia consists of intercostal nerve blocks, paravertebral blocks and thoracic epidural catheters (TEC).

The intercostal nerve block involves blocking the intercostal nerves individually with an injection of local anesthetic, typically bupivacaine. To ensure an adequate block and avoid missing overlapping innervating nerves, intercostal blocks require injection at the level of the fractured rib plus 1 rib above and below.[15] Identification of the appropriate location for injection involves manual palpation of the ribs, which can contribute to pain. Additionally, identification of landmarks becomes increasingly difficult above the seventh thoracic vertebral level. Local anesthetic toxicity and pneumothorax are risks with repeated injections.[15] A continuous infusion catheter with slow release of anesthetic has been developed to minimize these complications and increase the duration of pain relief. These catheters are placed in an extrathoracic, paraspinous location using manual palpation or ultrasound guidance. A long infusion catheter is placed and connected to an infusion pump that administers a continuous infusion of local anesthetic for up to 5 days. Truitt and colleagues[13,16] demonstrated in 2 studies that use of this technique significantly improved pain control at rest and after coughing, increased sustained maximal inspiratory lung volumes, and shortened duration of stay.

Paravertebral blocks offer broader, dermatomal, coverage, and avoid manual palpation of the fractured ribs. The technique involves blocking the nerve root in the paravertebral space as it exits the thoracic vertebrae. Although technically easier than TEC placement, there is a small pneumothorax risk.[17] Because it does not enter the epidural space, paravertebral blocks offer some distinct advantages compared with TEC, namely, no urinary retention, no systemic vasodilation, and accessibility to those with thoracic spine fractures or moderate coagulopathy.[17] In a small randomized trial, paravertebral block and TEC were found to be equally effective at relieving pain and improving respiratory function in patients with unilateral rib fractures with similar pulmonary complications and duration of ICU and hospital stay.[18]

TEC are the regional anesthetic modality of choice for patients with bilateral chest wall injury, and ideal for patients with more than 2 fractured ribs. The procedure is technically more challenging than the other regional approaches, however.[15,17] A catheter is inserted at the vertebral level that corresponds with the midpoint of the fractured ribs. The epidural space is entered and a local anesthetic and/or a narcotic (eg, bupivacaine and fentanyl) are infused.[17] This epidural location eliminates the risk of pneumothorax as well as local anesthetic toxicity. It does, however, carry certain unique risks, including dural puncture and spinal cord injury, hypotension, urinary retention, pruritus, and motor block limiting mobility.[15,17] Spinal epidural hematoma is a rare but significant complication of TEC insertion and removal. As such, coagulopathy, thrombocytopenia, anticoagulation, and antiplatelet therapy are contraindications to placement or removal. Deep sedation or severe head injury are also relative contraindications to placement of TEC. Outcomes for use in chest wall injury are somewhat mixed. Early studies demonstrated improved analgesia compared with other approaches.[12,19,20] Subsequent studies revealed that mortality and pulmonary complications were not significantly different with TEC use.[18,21] More recently, however, reductions in mortality have been seen with more widespread use of TEC.[22,23] These mixed data resulted in a conditional recommendation for epidural analgesia over opioids alone for patients with blunt chest trauma.[11] Rib fixation is also an option for managing pain in patients who are refractory to medical management, as will be discussed elsewhere in this article.

Respiratory therapy is arguably the most important component of the management of chest wall injury. Aggressive pulmonary hygiene is necessary to clear airway secretions and prevent atelectasis. Pneumonia and respiratory failure are the major complications of poor pulmonary hygiene in patients with chest wall injury. Lung expansion and secretion clearance are key interventions in preventing pneumonia and respiratory complications.[24–26] Respiratory therapists and bedside nurses are critical personnel in preventing these complications.[27,28] Therapies to aid lung expansion include incentive spirometry and positive expiratory pressure therapy devices. Secretion clearance is achieved with vibratory mechanisms, coughing, and airway suctioning (nasotracheal or tracheal). Protocolized application of these therapies as initiated by both physicians and respiratory therapists may reduce hospital duration of stay and unplanned ICU admissions.[24,25,29]

Mobility is a key component to the management of trauma patients with chest wall injury, allowing for optimal ventilation and perfusion matching. Additionally, upright positioning encourages better diaphragm excursion and subsequently higher tidal volumes compared with supine positioning. Progressive mobility has been associated with decreased rates of deep venous thrombosis and pulmonary embolism, and lower pneumonia rates, less ventilator days, and shorter durations of hospital and ICU stays.[24–26,30–32]

Multidisciplinary clinical pathways for rib fracture management are beneficial. In a study by Todd and associates,[14] all patients over 45 years of age with more than 4 fractured ribs were entered into a clinical rib fracture pathway (**Fig. 2**).

A preassessment–postassessment comparison of the pathway revealed significantly shortened ICU and hospital durations of stay (2.4 days vs 3.7 days, respectively). Logistic regression analysis showed an 88% reduction in pneumonia and a 63% reduction in mortality.[14]

A more controversial approach to chest wall injury is rib fixation. This has been a topic of increasing debate for many years now. Proponents of the rib fixation point to decreases in ICU duration of stay, duration of mechanical ventilation, pulmonary function tests, tracheostomy rates, and treatment costs.[33–42] Opponents have pointed to no improvements in mortality, mixed results in terms of pain control, few long-term outcome data, virtually no studies comparing rib fixation with multimodal analgesia, and questionable indications for operation.[34,40,43,44] Schuurmans and associates[40] recently performed a systematic review of operative versus nonoperative management of flail chest. Three small, randomized, controlled trials were identified, totaling 123 patients.[36,37,41] There was no difference in mortality between the operative and nonoperative groups, although the authors note that the sample size is underpowered to adequately determine this outcome. Of note, the relative risk of pneumonia was decreased by 55% in the operative management group. Duration of mechanical ventilation was reduced by an average of 6.5 days; ICU duration of stay and hospital

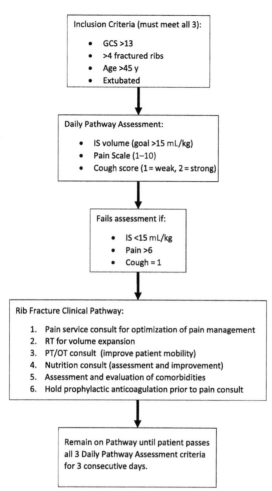

Fig. 2. Rib fracture management clinical pathway. Daily pathway assessment performed on morning rounds. Intubated patients may be included in clinical pathway if eye and motor components of GCS are intact and extubation is anticipated within next 7 days. GCS, Glasgow Coma Scale; IS, incentive spirometry; OT, occupational therapy; PT, physical therapy; RT, respiratory therapy. (*Adapted from* Todd SR, McNally MM, Holcomb JB, et al. A multidisciplinary clinical pathway decreases rib fracture-associated infectious morbidity and mortality in high-risk trauma patients. Am J Surg 2006;192(6):806–11; with permission.)

duration of stay were also shortened by 5.2 and 11.4 days, respectively.[40] A Cochrane review noted similar findings as well as a decrease in tracheostomy rates and improvement in chest wall deformity.[34]

Among the most common points of contention regarding operative fixation of chest wall injury are the indications for fixation.[44] Flail chest is considered among the most widely accepted indications for operative management.[33,34,37,41–43,45,46] A recent EAST practice management guidelines conditionally recommended rib fixation in patients with flail chest. A very low quality of evidence and risk of bias were reasons cited for only giving a conditional recommendation.[47] Other indications include significant chest wall deformity, inadequate pain control, and fracture nonunion.[45,48] **Table 1**

Table 1	
Relative indications and contraindications for rib fixation	
Relative Indications	**Contraindications**
Pain refractory to medical management	Respiratory failure not related to
Flail chest causing respiratory compromise	chest wall injury
Respiratory failure owing to chest wall instability	Significant pulmonary contusion
Rib fractures with fragments impinging on vital	Other injuries requiring prolonged
structures	intubation
Impaired pulmonary function tests owing to chest	Patients unable to tolerate surgery
wall deformity	
Symptomatic rib fracture nonunion or malunion	

shows the common indications and contraindications for rib fixation. The majority of the published outcomes involve ventilated patients. As a result, guidance for the management of nonintubated patients is greatly lacking.

Additionally, none of the published randomized studies compare operative fixation with current nonoperative multidisciplinary approaches. One study mentioned a comparison with TEC use.[41] In another study, nonoperative management included securing plaster over the fractured ribs, essentially splinting—a practice abandoned in the United States long ago.[36] Using modern multidisciplinary approach to chest wall trauma, patients managed nonoperatively were found to have better outcomes compared with surgical management. The duration of mechanical ventilation (3.1 days vs 6.1 days), ICU duration of stay (3.7 days vs 7.4 days), hospital duration of stay (16.0 days vs 21.9 days), and pneumonia rates (22% vs 63%) were all significantly less in the nonoperative group compared with the operative group.[43] Although a small, retrospective study, these findings may suggest that more modern approaches to critical care and rib fracture management have reopened the question of the role of surgery in chest wall injury.

Pieracci and coworkers[39] conducted a study that evaluated outcomes of early rib fixation (<72 hours after injury) as compared with a modern nonoperative, multidisciplinary approach. In this study, the authors noted a 76% reduction in odds of respiratory failure, 82% reduction in odds of tracheostomy, and a 5-day reduction in duration of mechanical ventilation.[39] This study is compelling, not in its results, which are similar to previous studies, but rather in its design. It is the first study to actually compare surgical fixation with the current best available multidisciplinary practices for nonoperative management of chest wall injury. Additionally, it describes outcomes for rib fixation for expanded indications beyond flail chest only. Other surgical indications in the study were 3 or more severely (bicortical) displacement, 30% or greater hemithorax volume loss, and failure of medical management.[39] It is unclear how, or if, these expanded indications or the earlier operative timing explain the differences in outcomes from the previous multidisciplinary study, but it certainly leaves open the question as to the best approach for managing patients with severe chest wall injury.

There are multiple different types of fixation systems in existence, including wire cerclage, clamping braces, external plate and screw fixation, and intramedullary fixation.[35] The most commonly used technique for rib fixation is the external plate and screw system.[35] Just as there are multiple commercially available fixation products, there are multiple surgical approaches to rib fixation. Traditionally, fixation has been performed through a single lateral thoracotomy-type incision. Modifications have been made to this technique based on unique fracture patterns (anterior, bilateral, flail, etc).[48–50] More recently, minimally invasive techniques have been reported, but no comparison of outcomes has been performed at this time.[51,52]

LUNG INJURY
Pulmonary Contusion

Pulmonary contusion often occurs in conjunction with chest wall injury. The contused lung is often damaged and unable to participate in the gas exchange of respiration.[53–55] If large enough in volume, this condition can result in significant respiratory distress. In flail chest, pulmonary contusions are frequently present and contribute to respiratory compromise. There are few clinical signs of pulmonary contusion. Concomitant injuries should raise a suspicion for the possible presence of pulmonary contusion and lead to further investigation. Chest radiographs and CT scanning are the 2 methods of diagnosing pulmonary contusions. The appearance of pulmonary contusion on chest radiographs is often delayed. CT scanning has proven to be a more accurate method for diagnosing pulmonary contusions. In a study by Miller and colleagues,[56] CT scans identified 100% of pulmonary contusions compared with just 38% identified by chest radiographs. Rodriguez and coworkers[57] noted in a study of more than 1000 patients with pulmonary contusion that more than 73% of contusions were seen only on CT imaging. In addition to early diagnosis, CT imaging can also determine the total contused lung volume. Pulmonary contusions have been identified as an independent risk factor for respiratory complications.[58,59] Miller and associates[56] found that patients with severe pulmonary contusions (contused lung ≥20% of total lung volume) developed acute respiratory distress syndrome at much higher rates (82% vs 22%; $P<.001$) than those with moderate contusions (<20% contused lung volume). The treatment of pulmonary contusion is supportive. Historically, judicious fluid administration was advocated to prevent "fluffing out" of contusions. As fluid management strategies have shifted away from aggressive crystalloid resuscitation, so has the concern of worsening pulmonary contusions. For severe contusions, intubation and mechanical ventilation may be necessary. For the most severe injuries, life-threatening hypoxia owing to pulmonary hemorrhage can result. Advanced ventilator modes, including extracorporeal membrane oxygenation, may be necessary.[60]

Pneumothorax

Pneumothorax is a common injury in both blunt and penetrating thoracic trauma. Typically, pneumothorax is not an immediately threatening condition, but there is potential for progression that can evolve to life threatening. Simple pneumothorax is characterized clinically in a variety of presentations. Although some patients may present asymptomatically, many present with ipsilateral chest pain, absent or diminished breath sounds, hyperresonance to percussion, shortness of breath, dyspnea, and subcutaneous emphysema of the chest wall. Hypoxia and tachypnea may also be present.

Tension pneumothorax presents in much more dramatic manner. The physical examination findings of simple pneumothorax are present, but with added physiologic derangements of obstructive shock. Tachycardia and hypotension are the result of increased intrathoracic pressure causing decreased venous return to the heart. Tracheal deviation away from the affected side, distended neck veins, and an elevated hemothorax also result from the building pressure from accumulating air within the hemothorax. Respiratory distress and cyanosis ultimately result if not identified and treated promptly.

A third, and much rarer, type of pneumothorax is the open pneumothorax. This diagnosis is the result of a penetrating wound that creates a direct connection between the pleural space and the outside world. This equilibrates the intrathoracic pressure with atmospheric pressure and disrupts the physiologic pressure gradient that drives respiration. Alternatively, the negative intrathoracic pressure generated during inspiration draws air into the chest via wound. The wound subsequently closes down creating a large pneumothorax. This so-called "sucking chest wound" can occur in a variety of traumatic mechanisms, including blast injuries, high-velocity gunshot wounds, slash injuries with large soft tissue defects, and impalement.

The diagnosis of a simple pneumothorax is confirmed by chest radiographs or CT scan. With the increasing prevalence of CT imaging in the evaluation of blunt trauma patients, some pneumothoraces are now identified that are not seen on radiographs. These 'occult' pneumothoraces are not altogether uncommon, occurring in 15% to 20% of blunt trauma patients and even up to 17% of penetrating trauma patients.[61–63] Ultrasound imaging has also emerged as a means to diagnose pneumothorax. On ultrasound examination, normal lung seems to slide along the thoracic wall. Ultrasonographic findings, such as comet tail artifacts or B-lines (**Fig. 3**), are created between the water and air interface of the visceral pleura in normal lung.[64] Pneumothorax is identified by the absence of lung sliding, loss of comet tail artifacts, the presence of A-lines, and the "lung point sign" all suggest pneumothorax. A-lines are artifacts reflecting off the parietal pleura that appear as equally spaced, hyperechoic horizontal lines (**Fig. 4**). These are present in pneumothoraces, but not visible when B-lines are present.[64,65] The so-called "lung point sign" is created by the intermittent contact between the lung and the chest wall in the setting of pneumothorax (**Fig. 5**). Although it lacks some sensitivity (66%), it is 100% specific for pneumothorax when present on ultrasonographic examination.[66] Negative predictive values for lung sliding and comet tail artifacts approach 100% for each finding.[64] Sensitivity and specificity of the combined finding of absent lung sliding with present A-lines is 95% and 94%, respectively.[65] Tension pneumothorax should be diagnosed based on clinical presentation and should not be confirmed with imaging studies. Rather, the diagnosis should be suspected and treatment rendered immediately. This is applicable to any patient in extremis with suspected pneumothorax.

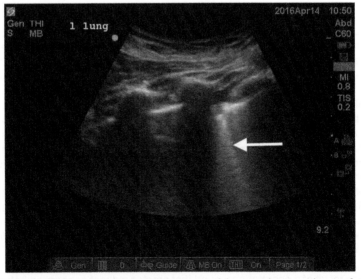

Fig. 3. Thoracic ultrasound imaging showing normal lung without evidence of pneumothorax. Comet tail artifacts, or B-lines (*arrow*), are created between the water and air interface of the visceral pleura in the absence of pneumothorax. (*Courtesy of* Jeremy Boyd, MD, RDMS, FACEP; Nashville, TN.)

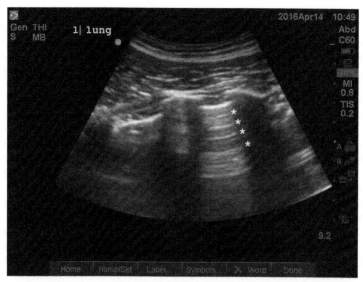

Fig. 4. Thoracic ultrasound examination suggestive of pneumothorax. A-lines (*asterisks*) are artifacts reflecting off the parietal pleura that appear as equally spaced, hyperechoic horizontal lines. These are present, but most often not visible when B-lines are present. (*Courtesy of* Jeremy Boyd, MD, RDMS, FACEP; Nashville, TN.)

The treatment of pneumothorax depends on patient stability. Unstable patients with pneumothorax require immediate decompression. Needle decompression or tube thoracostomy are the procedures of choice. Needle decompression occurs in the second intercostal space at the midclavicular line. Alternatively, needle decompression

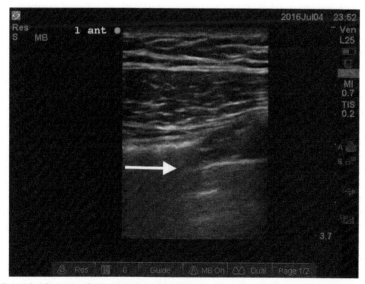

Fig. 5. Thoracic ultrasound examination showing the "lung point sign." This ultrasonographic finding is created by the intermittent contact between the lung and the chest wall in the setting of pneumothorax. (*Courtesy of* Jeremy Boyd, MD, RDMS, FACEP; Nashville, TN.)

can be effectively performed in the fourth or fifth intercostal space at the anterior axillary line.[67,68] A metaanalysis by Laan and associates[69] demonstrated a lower failure rate ($P = .01$) for needle thoracostomy performed at anterior axillary location (13%) compared with midclavicular (38%) and midaxillary (31%). Questions regarding the effectiveness and durability of needle decompression have led others to advocate for tube thoracostomy as the primary treatment for tension pneumothorax.[70]

In stable patients, consideration should be given to the need for any pneumothorax evacuation. EAST practice management guidelines support observation without chest tube for occult pneumothoraces.[71] Even simple pneumothoraces that are small on chest radiographs can likely be managed with a 12- to 24-hour clinical observation period. Kong and coworkers[72] reported on the outcomes of 125 patients with pneumothoraces from stab wounds that measured less than 2 cm on chest radiographs. Only 4 (3%) required chest tube placement.

Larger, enlarging, or symptomatic pneumothoraces should be managed with tube thoracostomy. Size of the chest tube is an area of ongoing research. Inaba showed that smaller chest tubes (28-F or 32-F) were just as effective as larger tubes (36-F or 40-F) in evacuating pneumothoraces.[73] A recent, small, randomized clinical trial demonstrated that 14-F chest tubes were equivalent to 28-F chest tubes in terms of success evacuating pneumothorax and insertion-related complications.[74]

Open pneumothorax requires immediate treatment in the prehospital setting. An occlusive dressing secured on 3 sides is the preferred initial treatment for this injury.[75] In the prehospital setting, this may require the addition of needle decompression if tension physiology develops after the dressing is applied. In the emergency department, a chest tube should be placed away from the soft tissue defect. Operative repair of the soft tissue defect is required to reestablish the intrathoracic pressure gradients necessary for ventilation.

Hemothorax

Hemothorax can result from both blunt and penetrating mechanisms. Simple hemothorax is not directly fatal, but can be associated with significant morbidity. Failure to completely evacuate blood can result in retained hemothorax. This is associated with an empyema rate between 27% and 33%.[76,77] Additionally, fibrothorax can result and cause significant respiratory complications owing to entrapped lung. Massive hemothorax is a life-threatening condition that is associated with a high mortality rate and requires prompt intervention. Rib fractures with or without intercostal vessel laceration and lung laceration most commonly result in mild to moderate hemorrhage, but on rare occasion can cause massive hemothorax. Massive hemothorax is typically the result of more significant injuries, such as those involving the pulmonary vasculature, great vessels, or heart.

The initial treatment of hemothorax is the same whether simple or massive. EAST practice management guidelines suggest all hemothoraces should be considered for drainage regardless of size.[71] When considering drainage of a hemothorax, its effect on respiratory function should be the primary consideration. Although the optimal hemothorax size requiring drainage has not been demonstrated in the literature, consideration should be given to those with additional thoracic trauma. Multiple rib fractures, flail chest, and pneumothorax are concomitant injuries that warrant consideration for hemothorax drainage.[78]

After a chest tube is placed, the adequacy of the drainage should be assessed with daily chest radiographs. Patients with persistent opacities obscuring the costophrenic angle may be at risk of retained hemothorax. These patients should receive a contrasted chest CT scan to evaluate for retained hemothorax because chest radiographs alone are insufficient to determine the presence of retained hemothorax.[79] Chest CT scanning should be used for volumetric analysis of the retained blood within the hemithorax. A validated formula, $v = d^2l$, is used to calculate the fluid volume, where d represents the greatest depth (in cm) of the hemothorax on a single axial CT slice and l represents the greatest length (in cm) of the hemothorax in craniocaudal direction.[80] Dubose and colleagues[81] showed that retained hemothoraces of greater than 300 mL were unlikely to be resolve with observation and required intervention to drain. Patients with chest radiographs that showed clearing of the costophrenic angle or those with retained hemothorax volume 300 mL or less, observation and management of the initial chest alone is adequate treatment.[71,81] Chest tubes should remain in place until the air leak subsides and drainage is 200 mL or less per day.[82]

For those patients with retained hemothorax volumes of greater than 300 mL on volumetric analysis, surgical intervention is required to evacuate hematoma. Meyer and associates[83] demonstrated that video-assisted thoracoscopic surgery (VATS) drainage is more effective than placing a second chest tube for drainage of retained hemothorax. The goal of surgical intervention for retained hemothorax is 2-fold: (1) evacuate the retained blood and (2) free any entrapped lung to allow maximal expansion. Whether VATS or open approach is used, the same goals apply.

Although open thoracotomy would be considered the gold standard therapy for retained hemothorax, VATS is a much more common initial approach to operative drainage.[81] A prospective observational study by Dubose and colleagues[81] showed that 79% of patients undergoing open thoracotomy required no further intervention. The minimally invasive approach of VATS was shown to require no further intervention in 70% of cases.[81] The benefit of VATS lies in its minimally invasive, yet effective nature. The ability to remain minimally invasive is important in limiting postoperative pain, improving pulmonary function, reducing postoperative infectious complications, and shortening the recovery period, making it the recommended treatment of choice for retained hemothorax.[71] Timing correlates with the success of the minimally invasive approach. Early VATS has shown to be more effective in evacuating hemothorax and limiting conversion to open thoracotomy, considered to be before hospital day 7.[71,83–86] However, for interventions after day 7, it is still appropriate to first attempt a VATS and convert to open if ineffective.[71]

Other approaches to evacuation of retained hemothorax include image-guided catheters and intrapleural thrombolytics. In the study from Dubose and associates,[81] 41% of patients who received image-guided catheters for retained hemothorax failed this treatment and required an additional treatment. Intrapleural thrombolytics have shown promise as an alternative for patients not able to undergo VATS. In observational studies, thrombolytics were successful in clearing traumatic hemothoraces in 92% of cases.[87,88] Unfortunately, there are no prospective, randomized studies comparing thrombolytics to surgical intervention. The only retrospective study to compare these 2 approaches evaluated streptokinase as compared with VATS. The thrombolytic group had a failure rate of 29%, compared with 6% for the VATS group ($P<.02$). Hospital duration of stay was longer for the thrombolytic group also (mean 14.5 days vs 9.8 days; $P<.0001$).[89] In light of these data, thrombolytic therapy and image-guided catheters are considered to be a second-line therapies for retained hemothorax and reserved for patients who are not considered surgical candidates.[90]

Tracheobronchial Injury

Injury to the tracheobronchial tree is a rare, but potentially life-threatening event. Penetrating mechanisms are more common than blunt, but still quite rare. The proposed mechanisms in blunt tracheobronchial injury include rapid deceleration in which the airway is lacerated near a fixed point, often the carina or cricoid cartilage; airway rupture from high airway pressures owing to compressive forces generated by the blunt trauma; and airway disruption owing to traction injuries created by the lateral displacement of intrathoracic organs during chest wall compression.[91] Stab wounds result in lacerations of the trachea that typically appear as a puncture wound or a linear slash-type wound. Gunshot wounds create larger wounds that frequently have some element of tracheal tissue loss, depending on the ballistic caliber, muzzle velocity, and associated cavitary effect.

In terms of anatomic location, 75% to 80% of penetrating airway injuries occur in the cervical trachea.[92] Blunt tracheobronchial injuries occur much more commonly in the thoracic trachea and proximal mainstem bronchi, with 75% of blunt airway injuries occurring within 2 cm of the carina, lending credence to the deceleration injury mechanism theory.[93,94]

Clinical symptoms vary somewhat based on the anatomic location and mechanism of injury. In general, though, subcutaneous emphysema, dyspnea, and respiratory distress are common findings.[95] Persistent air leak after chest tube placement for pneumothorax should raise suspicion for a tracheobronchial injury. For patients with penetrating cervical injuries, air escaping from the wound is common and is considered pathognomonic for tracheal injury.[96]

Radiographic imaging studies can identify findings suggestive of possible tracheobronchial injury. Subcutaneous emphysema, pneumothorax, and pneumomediastinum are the most common findings in patients with intrathoracic airway injuries. Cervical tracheal injuries are less commonly associated with pneumothorax, but may show deep cervical emphysema.[95] CT imaging often shows similar findings and occasionally visualize defects in the tracheal wall suggesting disruption.

A definitive diagnosis is made by bronchoscopy. Fiberoptic bronchoscopy is an easy and fast method to determine the location and extent of the injury. A disruption of the tracheobronchial tree is often easily identified and may be associated with blood in the airway or an inability to assess the airway distal to the injury.[97] In a review by Symbas and associates,[94] nearly 75% of blunt injuries resulted in transverse tears; only 18% were longitudinal.

Treatment consists of 2 components: securing the airway and injury management. Endotracheal intubation should be performed on all patients with suspected tracheobronchial injury. Fiberoptic intubation is an extremely useful method for intubating these patients.[95] The patient's neck remains in a neutral position, which prevents traction or stretching of the injured airway and addresses some of the technical challenges of intubating an 'uncleared' cervical spine. Without the need for direct laryngoscopy, fiberoptic intubation can be performed relatively easily without paralysis or sedation. This is useful in spontaneously breathing patients who are at risk of airway loss with rapid sequence induction.[98] Additionally, bronchoscopic intubation potentially allows for direct visualization of the injury. This can allow for both diagnostic and therapeutic interventions. Guiding the endotracheal tube beyond the injury can be safely accomplished with the aid of the bronchoscope. In patients with other significant injuries, this may potentially serve as a temporary, or occasionally a definitive, treatment until more concerning issues can be addressed. For injuries of the distal trachea, carina, or mainstem bronchi, single lung ventilation of the uninjured side is recommended, preferably under bronchoscopic guidance.[95,97] Distal airway injuries may require bronchial blockers to prevent ventilating injured segments.

Surgical repair is associated with a 10-fold improvement in survival odds and should be considered the management option of choice.[93] Definitive surgical management varies depending on the location and extent of the injury, as well as individual patient factors. Injuries to the proximal two-thirds of the trachea are most easily approached through the neck. Slash or stab wounds involving the cervical trachea often leave the injured segment of trachea exposed and provide a direct path to the injury, simple extension of the wound is usually adequate. For injuries without a large open wound, a collar incision is often the best approach for injuries in this area.[99] Occasionally, extending the collar incision inferiorly and splitting the manubrium may allow further exposure of the trachea to the aortic arch.[95] Injuries to the distal trachea, carina, right mainstem bronchus, and even the proximal left mainstem bronchus are best approached through a right thoracotomy.[94] Distal left mainstem bronchus injuries are best approached via a left thoracotomy incision. Sternotomy offers no advantages in exposure owing to overlying cardiac and vascular structures.

Suture repair should be performed whenever possible. For penetrating wounds or large tears, the wound edges may require debridement before suture closure. Some injuries may be too large for primary closure. For these wounds, the damaged area should be circumferentially resected and primary end-to-end anastomosis should be performed. Careful dissection is required to prevent devascularization of the anastomosis. In particular, excessive circumferential dissection beyond area of injury can result in damage to the blood supply to the tracheobronchial tree, which can threaten the healing and lead to stenosis or leak. If resection of a small portion of the trachea is required, the neck should be flexed during repair and maintained postoperatively by using a chin-to-chest stitch. If more mobility is needed, blunt dissection of the pretracheal plane anteriorly may provide additional tracheal mobility in this avascular space.[100] Almost any area of the tracheobronchial tree can be resected; the carina, however, is the exception to this rule. Resection of the carina should not be performed. To protect the repair, buttressing using pleural flaps has been described.[99] Flaps can also be used as tissue interposition in cases of combined tracheal and esophageal injuries.

Tracheostomy is seldom required for these injuries if successful endotracheal intubation is performed. For patients unable to be intubated orally, a tracheostomy may be necessary for airway control. Tracheostomy is also indicated for proximal airway injuries near the vocal cords, where airway obstruction owing to edema can occur. For relatively small anterior penetrating cervical tracheal injuries, tracheostomy via the tracheal injury defect may be an alternative to primary repair.[101]

REFERENCES

1. Ziegler DW, Agarwal NN. The morbidity and mortality of rib fractures. J Trauma 1994;37(6):975–9.
2. Lee RB, Bass SM, Morris JA Jr, et al. Three or more rib fractures as an indicator for transfer to a Level I trauma center: a population-based study. J Trauma 1990; 30(6):689–94.
3. Flagel BT, Luchette FA, Reed RL, et al. Half-a-dozen ribs: the breakpoint for mortality. Surgery 2005;138(4):717–23 [discussion: 723–5].
4. Bulger EM, Arneson MA, Mock CN, et al. Rib fractures in the elderly. J Trauma 2000;48(6):1040–6 [discussion: 1046–7].
5. Brasel KJ, Guse CE, Layde P, et al. Rib fractures: relationship with pneumonia and mortality. Crit Care Med 2006;34(6):1642–6.
6. Bergeron E, Lavoie A, Clas D, et al. Elderly trauma patients with rib fractures are at greater risk of death and pneumonia. J Trauma 2003;54(3):478–85.
7. Holcomb JB, McMullin NR, Kozar RA, et al. Morbidity from rib fractures increases after age 45. J Am Coll Surg 2003;196(4):549–55.

8. Mayberry JC, Trunkey DD. The fractured rib in chest wall trauma. Chest Surg Clin N Am 1997;7(2):239–61.

9. Dehghan N, de Mestral C, McKee MD, et al. Flail chest injuries: a review of outcomes and treatment practices from the National Trauma Data Bank. J Trauma Acute Care Surg 2014;76(2):462–8.

10. Chou R, Gordon DB, de Leon-Casasola OA, et al. Management of Postoperative Pain: a Clinical Practice Guideline from the American Pain Society, the American Society of Regional Anesthesia and Pain Medicine, and the American Society of Anesthesiologists' Committee on Regional Anesthesia, Executive Committee, and Administrative Council. J Pain 2016;17(2):131–57.

11. Galvagno SM Jr, Smith CE, Varon AJ, et al. Pain management for blunt thoracic trauma: a joint practice management guideline from the Eastern Association for the Surgery of Trauma and Trauma Anesthesiology Society. J Trauma Acute Care Surg 2016;81(5):936–51.

12. Moon MR, Luchette FA, Gibson SW, et al. Prospective, randomized comparison of epidural versus parenteral opioid analgesia in thoracic trauma. Ann Surg 1999;229(5):684–91 [discussion: 691–2].

13. Truitt MS, Murry J, Amos J, et al. Continuous intercostal nerve blockade for rib fractures: ready for primetime? J Trauma 2011;71(6):1548–52 [discussion: 1552].

14. Todd SR, McNally MM, Holcomb JB, et al. A multidisciplinary clinical pathway decreases rib fracture-associated infectious morbidity and mortality in high-risk trauma patients. Am J Surg 2006;192(6):806–11.

15. Karmakar MK, Ho AM. Acute pain management of patients with multiple fractured ribs. J Trauma 2003;54(3):615–25.

16. Truitt MS, Mooty RC, Amos J, et al. Out with the old, in with the new: a novel approach to treating pain associated with rib fractures. World J Surg 2010; 34(10):2359–62.

17. Ho AM, Karmakar MK, Critchley LA. Acute pain management of patients with multiple fractured ribs: a focus on regional techniques. Curr Opin Crit Care 2011;17(4):323–7.

18. Mohta M, Verma P, Saxena AK, et al. Prospective, randomized comparison of continuous thoracic epidural and thoracic paravertebral infusion in patients with unilateral multiple fractured ribs–a pilot study. J Trauma 2009;66(4):1096–101.

19. Luchette FA, Radafshar SM, Kaiser R, et al. Prospective evaluation of epidural versus intrapleural catheters for analgesia in chest wall trauma. J Trauma 1994;36(6):865–9 [discussion: 869–70].

20. Wu CL, Jani ND, Perkins FM, et al. Thoracic epidural analgesia versus intravenous patient-controlled analgesia for the treatment of rib fracture pain after motor vehicle crash. J Trauma 1999;47(3):564–7.

21. Carrier FM, Turgeon AF, Nicole PC, et al. Effect of epidural analgesia in patients with traumatic rib fractures: a systematic review and meta-analysis of randomized controlled trials. Can J Anaesth 2009;56(3):230–42.

22. Gage A, Rivara F, Wang J, et al. The effect of epidural placement in patients after blunt thoracic trauma. J Trauma Acute Care Surg 2014;76(1):39–45 [discussion: 45–6].

23. Jensen CD, Stark JT, Jacobson LL, et al. Improved Outcomes Associated with the Liberal Use of Thoracic Epidural Analgesia in Patients with Rib Fractures. Pain Med 2016. [Epub ahead of print].

24. Cassidy MR, Rosenkranz P, McCabe K, et al. I COUGH: reducing postoperative pulmonary complications with a multidisciplinary patient care program. JAMA Surg 2013;148(8):740-5.

25. Wren SM, Martin M, Yoon JK, et al. Postoperative pneumonia-prevention program for the inpatient surgical ward. J Am Coll Surg 2010;210(4):491-5.

26. Strickland SL, Rubin BK, Drescher GS, et al. AARC clinical practice guideline: effectiveness of nonpharmacologic airway clearance therapies in hospitalized patients. Respir Care 2013;58(12):2187-93.

27. Hanlon VD, White F, Hustosky AE, et al. Benefits of standardizing additional airway clearance in the trauma patient population. J Trauma Nurs 2014;21(3): 127-32.

28. Brown SD, Walters MR. Patients with rib fractures: use of incentive spirometry volumes to guide care. J Trauma Nurs 2012;19(2):89-91 [quiz: 92-3].

29. Nyland BA, Spilman SK, Halub ME, et al. A Preventative Respiratory Protocol to Identify Trauma Subjects at Risk for Respiratory Compromise on a General In-Patient Ward. Respir Care 2016;61(12):1580-7.

30. Booth K, Rivet J, Flici R, et al. Progressive mobility protocol reduces venous thromboembolism rate in trauma intensive care patients: a quality improvement project. J Trauma Nurs 2016;23(5):284-9.

31. Haines KJ, Skinner EH, Berney S. Association of postoperative pulmonary complications with delayed mobilisation following major abdominal surgery: an observational cohort study. Physiotherapy 2013;99(2):119-25.

32. Morris PE, Goad A, Thompson C, et al. Early intensive care unit mobility therapy in the treatment of acute respiratory failure. Crit Care Med 2008;36(8):2238-43.

33. Bhatnagar A, Mayberry J, Nirula R. Rib fracture fixation for flail chest: what is the benefit? J Am Coll Surg 2012;215(2):201-5.

34. Cataneo AJ, Cataneo DC, de Oliveira FH, et al. Surgical versus nonsurgical interventions for flail chest. Cochrane Database Syst Rev 2015;(7):CD009919.

35. Fitzpatrick DC, Denard PJ, Phelan D, et al. Operative stabilization of flail chest injuries: review of literature and fixation options. Eur J Trauma Emerg Surg 2010; 36(5):427-33.

36. Granetzny A, Abd El-Aal M, Emam E, et al. Surgical versus conservative treatment of flail chest. Evaluation of the pulmonary status. Interact Cardiovasc Thorac Surg 2005;4(6):583-7.

37. Marasco SF, Davies AR, Cooper J, et al. Prospective randomized controlled trial of operative rib fixation in traumatic flail chest. J Am Coll Surg 2013;216(5): 924-32.

38. Nirula R, Allen B, Layman R, et al. Rib fracture stabilization in patients sustaining blunt chest injury. Am Surg 2006;72(4):307-9.

39. Pieracci FM, Lin Y, Rodil M, et al. A prospective, controlled clinical evaluation of surgical stabilization of severe rib fractures. J Trauma Acute Care Surg 2016; 80(2):187-94.

40. Schuurmans J, Goslings JC, Schepers T. Operative management versus nonoperative management of rib fractures in flail chest injuries: a systematic review. Eur J Trauma Emerg Surg 2016;43(2):163-8.

41. Tanaka H, Yukioka T, Yamaguti Y, et al. Surgical stabilization of internal pneumatic stabilization? A prospective randomized study of management of severe flail chest patients. J Trauma 2002;52(4):727-32 [discussion: 732].

42. Leinicke JA, Elmore L, Freeman BD, et al. Operative management of rib fractures in the setting of flail chest: a systematic review and meta-analysis. Ann Surg 2013;258(6):914-21.

43. Farquhar J, Almahrabi Y, Slobogean G, et al. No benefit to surgical fixation of flail chest injuries compared with modern comprehensive management: results of a retrospective cohort study. Can J Surg 2016;59(5):299–303.

44. Mayberry J. Surgical stabilization of severe rib fractures: several caveats. J Trauma Acute Care Surg 2015;79(3):515.

45. Nirula R, Diaz JJ Jr, Trunkey DD, et al. Rib fracture repair: indications, technical issues, and future directions. World J Surg 2009;33(1):14–22.

46. Lafferty PM, Anavian J, Will RE, et al. Operative treatment of chest wall injuries: indications, technique, and outcomes. J Bone Joint Surg Am 2011;93(1):97–110.

47. Kasotakis G, Hasenboehler EA, Streib EW, et al. Operative fixation of rib fractures after blunt trauma: a practice management guideline from the Eastern Association for the Surgery of Trauma. J Trauma Acute Care Surg 2017;82(3):618–26.

48. Sarani B, Schulte L, Diaz JJ. Pitfalls associated with open reduction and internal fixation of fractured ribs. Injury 2015;46(12):2335–40.

49. Pieracci FM, Rodil M, Stovall RT, et al. Surgical stabilization of severe rib fractures. J Trauma Acute Care Surg 2015;78(4):883–7.

50. Bonne SL, Turnbull IR, Southard RE. Technique for repair of fractures and separations involving the cartilaginous portions of the anterior chest wall. Chest 2015;147(6):e199–204.

51. Sales JR, Ellis TJ, Gillard J, et al. Biomechanical testing of a novel, minimally invasive rib fracture plating system. J Trauma 2008;64(5):1270–4.

52. Bemelman M, van Baal M, Yuan JZ, et al. The role of minimally invasive plate osteosynthesis in rib fixation: a review. Korean J Thorac Cardiovasc Surg 2016;49(1):1–8.

53. Cohn SM, Zieg PM. Experimental pulmonary contusion: review of the literature and description of a new porcine model. J Trauma 1996;41(3):565–71.

54. Leone M, Albanese J, Rousseau S, et al. Pulmonary contusion in severe head trauma patients: impact on gas exchange and outcome. Chest 2003;124(6):2261–6.

55. Oppenheimer L, Craven KD, Forkert L, et al. Pathophysiology of pulmonary contusion in dogs. J Appl Physiol Respir Environ Exerc Physiol 1979;47(4):718–28.

56. Miller PR, Croce MA, Bee TK, et al. ARDS after pulmonary contusion: accurate measurement of contusion volume identifies high-risk patients. J Trauma 2001;51(2):223–8 [discussion: 229–30].

57. Rodriguez RM, Friedman B, Langdorf MI, et al. Pulmonary contusion in the pan-scan era. Injury 2016;47(5):1031–4.

58. Miller PR, Croce MA, Kilgo PD, et al. Acute respiratory distress syndrome in blunt trauma: identification of independent risk factors. Am Surg 2002;68(10):845–50 [discussion: 850–1].

59. Cohn SM, Dubose JJ. Pulmonary contusion: an update on recent advances in clinical management. World J Surg 2010;34(8):1959–70.

60. Simon B, Ebert J, Bokhari F, et al. Management of pulmonary contusion and flail chest: an Eastern Association for the Surgery of Trauma practice management guideline. J Trauma Acute Care Surg 2012;73(5 Suppl 4):S351–61.

61. Wilson H, Ellsmere J, Tallon J, et al. Occult pneumothorax in the blunt trauma patient: tube thoracostomy or observation? Injury 2009;40(9):928–31.

62. Ball CG, Dente CJ, Kirkpatrick AW, et al. Occult pneumothoraces in patients with penetrating trauma: does mechanism matter? Can J Surg 2010;53(4):251–5.

63. Ball CG, Kirkpatrick AW, Laupland KB, et al. Incidence, risk factors, and outcomes for occult pneumothoraces in victims of major trauma. J Trauma 2005; 59(4):917–24 [discussion: 924–5].

64. Husain LF, Hagopian L, Wayman D, et al. Sonographic diagnosis of pneumothorax. J Emerg Trauma Shock 2012;5(1):76–81.

65. Lichtenstein DA, Meziere G, Lascols N, et al. Ultrasound diagnosis of occult pneumothorax. Crit Care Med 2005;33(6):1231–8.

66. Lichtenstein D, Meziere G, Biderman P, et al. The "lung point": an ultrasound sign specific to pneumothorax. Intensive Care Med 2000;26(10):1434–40.

67. Inaba K, Ives C, McClure K, et al. Radiologic evaluation of alternative sites for needle decompression of tension pneumothorax. Arch Surg 2012;147(9):813–8.

68. Chang SJ, Ross SW, Kiefer DJ, et al. Evaluation of 8.0-cm needle at the fourth anterior axillary line for needle chest decompression of tension pneumothorax. J Trauma Acute Care Surg 2014;76(4):1029–34.

69. Laan DV, Vu TD, Thiels CA, et al. Chest wall thickness and decompression failure: a systematic review and meta-analysis comparing anatomic locations in needle thoracostomy. Injury 2016;47(4):797–804.

70. Martin M, Satterly S, Inaba K, et al. Does needle thoracostomy provide adequate and effective decompression of tension pneumothorax? J Trauma Acute Care Surg 2012;73(6):1412–7.

71. Mowery NT, Gunter OL, Collier BR, et al. Practice management guidelines for management of hemothorax and occult pneumothorax. J Trauma 2011;70(2):510–8.

72. Kong VY, Oosthuizen GV, Clarke DL. The selective conservative management of small traumatic pneumothoraces following stab injuries is safe: experience from a high-volume trauma service in South Africa. Eur J Trauma Emerg Surg 2015; 41(1):75–9.

73. Inaba K, Lustenberger T, Recinos G, et al. Does size matter? A prospective analysis of 28-32 versus 36-40 French chest tube size in trauma. J Trauma 2012;72(2):422–7.

74. Kulvatunyou N, Erickson L, Vijayasekaran A, et al. Randomized clinical trial of pigtail catheter versus chest tube in injured patients with uncomplicated traumatic pneumothorax. Br J Surg 2014;101(2):17–22.

75. ATLS Subcommittee; American College of Surgeons' Committee on Trauma, International ATLS working group. Advanced trauma life support (ATLS(R)): the ninth edition. J Trauma Acute Care Surg 2013;74(5):1363–6.

76. Karmy-Jones R, Holevar M, Sullivan RJ, et al. Residual hemothorax after chest tube placement correlates with increased risk of empyema following traumatic injury. Can Respir J 2008;15(5):255–8.

77. DuBose J, Inaba K, Okoye O, et al. Development of posttraumatic empyema in patients with retained hemothorax: results of a prospective, observational AAST study. J Trauma Acute Care Surg 2012;73(3):752–7.

78. Boersma WG, Stigt JA, Smit HJ. Treatment of haemothorax. Respir Med 2010; 104(11):1583–7.

79. Velmahos GC, Demetriades D, Chan L, et al. Predicting the need for thoracoscopic evacuation of residual traumatic hemothorax: chest radiograph is insufficient. J Trauma 1999;46(1):65–70.

80. Mergo PJ, Helmberger T, Didovic J, et al. New formula for quantification of pleural effusions from computed tomography. J Thorac Imaging 1999;14(2):122–5.

81. Dubose J, Inaba K, Demetriades D, et al. Management of post-traumatic retained hemothorax: a prospective, observational, multicenter AAST study. J Trauma 2012;72(1):11–24.

82. Younes RN, Gross JL, Aguiar S, et al. When to remove a chest tube? A randomized study with subsequent prospective consecutive validation. J Am Coll Surg 2002;195(5):658–62.

83. Meyer DM, Jessen ME, Wait MA, et al. Early evacuation of traumatic retained hemothoraces using thoracoscopy: a prospective, randomized trial. Ann Thorac Surg 1997;64(5):1396–400 [discussion: 1400–1].

84. Heniford BT, Carrillo EH, Spain DA, et al. The role of thoracoscopy in the management of retained thoracic collections after trauma. Ann Thorac Surg 1997; 63(4):940–3.

85. Morales Uribe CH, Villegas Lanau MI, Petro Sanchez RD. Best timing for thoracoscopic evacuation of retained post-traumatic hemothorax. Surg Endosc 2008; 22(1):91–5.

86. Vassiliu P, Velmahos GC, Toutouzas KG. Timing, safety, and efficacy of thoracoscopic evacuation of undrained post-traumatic hemothorax. Am Surg 2001; 67(12):1165–9.

87. Inci I, Ozcelik C, Ulku R, et al. Intrapleural fibrinolytic treatment of traumatic clotted hemothorax. Chest 1998;114(1):160–5.

88. Kimbrell BJ, Yamzon J, Petrone P, et al. Intrapleural thrombolysis for the management of undrained traumatic hemothorax: a prospective observational study. J Trauma 2007;62(5):1175–8 [discussion: 1178–9].

89. Oguzkaya F, Akcali Y, Bilgin M. Videothoracoscopy versus intrapleural streptokinase for management of post traumatic retained haemothorax: a retrospective study of 65 cases. Injury 2005;36(4):526–9.

90. Dennis BM, Gondek SP, Guyer RA, et al. Use of an evidence-based algorithm for patients with traumatic hemothorax reduces need for additional interventions. J Trauma Acute Care Surg 2017;82(4):728–32.

91. Kirsh MM, Orringer MB, Behrendt DM, et al. Management of tracheobronchial disruption secondary to nonpenetrating trauma. Ann Thorac Surg 1976;22(1): 93–101.

92. Lee RB. Traumatic injury of the cervicothoracic trachea and major bronchi. Chest Surg Clin N Am 1997;7(2):285–304.

93. Kiser AC, O'Brien SM, Detterbeck FC. Blunt tracheobronchial injuries: treatment and outcomes. Ann Thorac Surg 2001;71(6):2059–65.

94. Symbas PN, Justicz AG, Ricketts RR. Rupture of the airways from blunt trauma: treatment of complex injuries. Ann Thorac Surg 1992;54(1):177–83.

95. Karmy-Jones R, Wood DE. Traumatic injury to the trachea and bronchus. Thorac Surg Clin 2007;17(1):35–46.

96. Symbas PN, Hatcher CR Jr, Vlasis SE. Bullet wounds of the trachea. J Thorac Cardiovasc Surg 1982;83(2):235–8.

97. Prokakis C, Koletsis EN, Dedeilias P, et al. Airway trauma: a review on epidemiology, mechanisms of injury, diagnosis and treatment. J Cardiothorac Surg 2014;9:117.

98. Abernathy JH 3rd, Reeves ST. Airway catastrophes. Curr Opin Anaesthesiol 2010;23(1):41–6.

99. Rossbach MM, Johnson SB, Gomez MA, et al. Management of major tracheobronchial injuries: a 28-year experience. Ann Thorac Surg 1998;65(1):182–6.

100. Heitmiller RF. Tracheal release maneuvers. Chest Surg Clin N Am 1996;6(4): 675–82.

101. Pate JW. Tracheobronchial and esophageal injuries. Surg Clin North Am 1989; 69(1):111–23.

Blunt and Penetrating Cardiac Trauma

Seth A. Bellister, MD, Bradley M. Dennis, MD*, Oscar D. Guillamondegui, MD, MPH

KEYWORDS

- Cardiac trauma • Blunt cardiac injury • Penetrating cardiac injury • Cardiac box

KEY POINTS

- Blunt cardiac injury diagnosis requires a high index of suspicion. Treatment is supportive care in almost all instances.
- Penetrating cardiac injuries are highly lethal. The 3-dimensional cardiac box defines anatomic areas that are at highest risk of underlying cardiac wounds.
- Treatment of penetrating cardiac injuries requires emergent surgical intervention. Cardiac surgical support, including cardiopulmonary bypass, may be required.

BLUNT CARDIAC INJURY

The earliest reports of nonpenetrating cardiac injury date back to the seventeenth century; however, the first successful repair would not take place until 4 centuries later.[1] Blunt cardiac injury (BCI) is a challenging clinical entity to fully understand. This challenge is due to a lack of clear diagnostic criteria and further complicated by a lack of a uniform grading system. The American Association for the Surgery of Trauma (AAST) has created an injury scale to define BCI.[2] By the admission of the AAST, this grading is limited by the spectrum of injuries and lack of diagnostic test. Although this grading scale provides some language to discuss these injuries, there is no large-scale validation of this system against mortality.

The best evidence within the body of literature cites an incidence of BCI between 3% and 76% of trauma patients.[3] It may cause as many as 20% of motor vehicle collision–related deaths.[2] Minor injuries may be asymptomatic. Severe injury can manifest as a highly morbid constellation of symptoms making the true incidence impossible to quantify. Autopsy reports suggest that severe cardiac injury may carry a prehospital mortality as high as 95%.[4] The population of patients that survive to hospitalization

Disclosure Statement: The authors have nothing to disclose.
Division of Trauma and Surgical Critical Care, Emergency General Surgery, Department of Surgery, Vanderbilt University Medical Center, 1211 21st Avenue South, 404 Medical Arts Building, Nashville, TN 37212, USA
* Corresponding author.
E-mail address: Bradley.m.dennis@vanderbilt.edu

can be divided into 3 groups: (1) hemodynamically stable patients with conduction abnormalities, (2) hemodynamically unstable patients with isolated conduction abnormalities, or (3) those with conduction abnormalities and structural defects.[5,6]

EVALUATION

During the initial evaluation of the injured patient, recognition of a pattern of injuries or symptoms at high risk for BCI is critical but challenging, and the clinician must maintain a high index of suspicion in any patient sustaining chest trauma. Physical examination may demonstrate a "seat-belt sign," subcutaneous emphysema, or obvious deformity of the chest wall.[7] It should not be interpreted that these findings necessarily mandate workup, but rather should be part of the astute clinician's overall gestalt in deciding which patients need further evaluation (**Fig. 1**). Unfortunately, significant physical examination findings may be absent in a patient with severe BCI, and the clinician must remain vigilant in monitoring their patient's physiologic progression. The difficulty with studying BCI is that there is no clear diagnostic test. This creates significant heterogeneity within the literature.

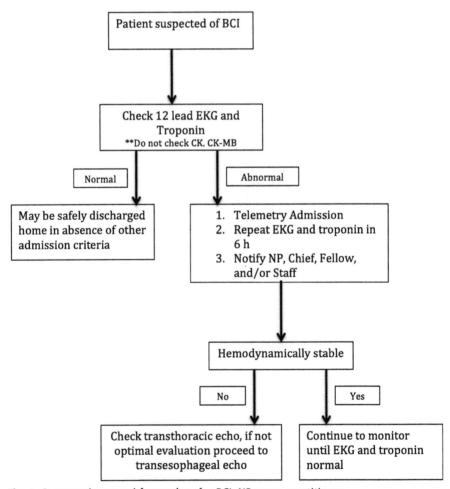

Fig. 1. Suggested protocol for workup for BCI. NP, nurse practitioner.

The most essential screening component in the workup of the patient with suspected BCI is an electrocardiogram (EKG). When performed serially, the sensitivity is reported as high as 89%. The negative predictive value (NPV) of EKG in identifying BCI approaches 98%.[8,9] Discussion remains within the literature that an NPV of 98% may preclude the use of further testing. Nevertheless, with the wide availability of troponin I testing (discussed later), the recommendation remains that EKG should not be used as the sole screening modality.[10]

There is a wide spectrum of electrical disturbances identified on screening EKG. Most studies eliminate sinus bradycardia and tachycardia as being abnormal because of the wide spectrum of causes that may lead to their development in the multiply injured patient.[8] The most common abnormalities identified on EKG are right bundle branch blocks.[11] This abnormality is presumably due to the anterior position of the right heart and its subsequent susceptibility to injury. Of note, it cannot be assumed that all EKG abnormalities will not require treatment. Approximately one-quarter to one-third of all patients with BCI require some intervention, whether chemical or otherwise, for arrhythmia.[9,12]

With the identification of assays for cardiac troponin I (cTnI), the specificity of biochemical assays has improved over creatine kinase (CK), although the sensitivity remains poor.[3,13] The sensitivity of cTnI for significant BCI is 23%. In concert with findings on the EKG, the use of cTnI is synergistic. The sensitivity decreases as the threshold defining "elevated" increases. When defined as greater than 0.1 ng/mL, cTnI only identifies an injury in approximately 8% of cases at presentation and 24% at 24 hours.[14] The troponin T is only slightly better at 10% at presentation and 24% at 24 hours. These data were later confirmed, suggesting that sensitivities of cTnI and T were 23% and 12%, respectively.[9] Regardless, significant cardiac injury can be ruled out within 8 hours of presentation in the setting of normal EKG and cTnI, because this combination has a 100% NPV for significant cardiac injury.[9] These data would suggest that in the setting of significant blunt chest trauma after the initial EKG and serial cTnI need only be checked for 8 hours. If normal, the patient can be safely discharged in the absence of other indications for admission. Although cTnI may be elevated more than 36 hours after injury, there appears to be no benefit in checking serially if the overall trend is downward. After multiple sources demonstrated very little predictive value in terms of actual cardiac injury, the use of CK in BCI has fallen out of favor.[3,13,14] In addition, CK-MB was noted to be elevated in patients with only isolated extremity injuries, bringing into question its utility in polytrauma at all.[14] The current body of literature does not support the use of CK in the evaluation of BCI.

Hemodynamically stable patients with normal EKG and cTnI need no further workup. Those with ongoing arrhythmia or hemodynamic instability after resuscitation or those with elevated troponin require further workup. The use of transthoracic echocardiography is useful in determining structural abnormalities or wall motion defects. The difficulty with transthoracic echocardiography is that it may prove technically difficult or impossible to obtain optimal images in the setting of significant blunt trauma. If so, the use of transesophageal echocardiography can be used successfully, when available.

The use of multidetector computed tomographic (CT) scanners has revolutionized the decision making in the acute trauma setting. Although highly accurate for identification of most osseous and nonosseous injuries, the cardiac motion limits the ability to identify BCI on the initial "traumagram." It may be useful in revealing pericardial effusions, or even pericardial rupture. Traditional dogma is that sternal fractures may necessitate workup for BCI. However, there currently is no indication for workup of

BCI after sternal fracture in the absence of other clinical indicators.[12,15] In fact, there are no radiographic findings that should prompt workup for BCI.

The EKG-gated CT scan, timed by concurrent use of EKG to capture images of the heart without motion artifact, is useful in identifying structural injuries to the heart or differentiating between myocardial infarction and BCI.[16,17] MRI of the heart in a gated fashion is also described and may provide valuable insight regarding diagnostic challenges of acute myocardial infarction or BCI. There is no clear literature to suggest superiority of CT over MRI; however, the speed and accessibility of CT make it likely the favored choice.

TREATMENT

The mainstay of BCI management is supportive care. Vasopressors and inotropes are needed on occasion to support patients through the initial period of myocardial stunning resulting from the injury itself. Surgical intervention is extremely rare. The role of surgery in BCI should be restricted to patients with structural abnormalities, that is, ruptured papillary muscle, valvular abnormalities, cardiac rupture or, more commonly, diagnosis and treatment of pericardial effusions. Patients with pericardial effusions identified on a FAST (focused abdominal with sonogram For trauma) examination in the trauma bay should proceed expeditiously to the operative theater for a subxiphoid pericardial window. The patient should be prepared for the possibility of extending the incision into a formal median sternotomy should the pericardial fluid return sanguineous. It is incumbent on the trauma surgeon to maintain open communication with anesthesia team, such that induction of anesthesia does not occur before the arrival of the surgical team and completion of the standard preoperative preparation and draping. A pericardial window is favored over traditional pericardiocentesis because the latter has a false negative rate as high as 80%.[2] Surgeons proceeding to operative intervention on a presumed BCI should be clear that cardiopulmonary bypass might be necessary in the setting of significant intracardiac injury. Early consultation with cardiac surgery and mobilization of a perfusion team should be initiated in these circumstances. Should a hemodynamically significant lesion be identified, surgical intervention is associated with poor outcomes for atrial or ventricular injuries with mortality between 40% and 70%.[18–21] Mitral, tricuspid, and aortic valve abnormalities may have better outcomes than chamber injuries.[22–24] Pulmonary valve injury is the least commonly reported in the literature, but appears to present late and overall has good outcomes. Valve replacement is more common and generally has better outcomes than repair, although large randomized series are lacking.[25–27] It should also be noted that hemodynamically stable patients with valve injuries may be repaired in a delayed fashion, days or up to years later.

PENETRATING CARDIAC INJURY
History

Of the myriad injuries confronting the trauma surgeon, none may be more daunting than the patient presenting with a penetrating cardiac injury. Battlefield descriptions of injuries to the heart punctuate the Homerian epics as a novel graphic way into the pantheon of Mount Olympus.[28] As early as the first century BC anatomists and surgeons recognized the imminent and nearly universal fatality associated with these injuries.[29] By the nineteenth century, a few rogue surgeons began to experiment with suture repair of the heart in both human and experimental models. Although the early descriptions of these injuries demonstrate technically successful operations, in-hospital mortality was extremely high. The earliest series of penetrating cardiac injuries corroborated the expected intraoperative and postoperative lethality of these injuries.[30]

Incidence

Contemporary series have shown a tremendous improvement in outcomes over the past centuries. A recent series from a high-volume center demonstrated that current mortality for penetrating cardiac injuries is approximately 40%,[31] mirroring the current body of literature with survival being reported between 19% and 73%.[32–37] Outcomes within individual centers may vary depending on available institutional resources, including cardiopulmonary bypass capabilities, massive transfusion protocols, and immediate availability of surgical staff.[38]

Secondarily, outcomes from penetrating cardiac injuries are related to the mechanism of injury. Over the last 2 decades, there has been a shift in frequency from knife-based "stab" injuries to gunshot wounds.[31,39] During the 1980s and 1990s, the number of stab wounds nearly doubled the number of gunshot wounds. This gap has closed in many urban centers in the new millennium. The prognostic difference between these injury types is not wholly unpredictable.

Between both mechanisms, the most frequently injured chamber of the heart is the right ventricle (RV).[31,40] This injury pattern has been consistent through history.[30] When combined with left ventricle injuries, ventricle injuries may represent up to 87% of all penetrating cardiac injuries.[31] The location of individual injuries may affect prognosis. RV injuries appear to have the best "to discharge" survival, at nearly 60%, whereas injuries to the right atrium are reportedly half.[34] These data are potentially biased by the difference in frequency of the 2 injuries, with some series demonstrating no difference in mortality.[32] Injury to more than one chamber is increasing with the increase in contemporary gun violence. Some series identify multichamber injury as both an independent predictor of mortality and a unique product of gunshot wounds.[31] Ballistic injuries, overall, are more lethal than stab wounds, and this may be due to the increase in multichamber injury.[31,34,36]

Diagnosis

Diagnosis should begin with physical examination. Penetrating wounds in the anatomic area known as the "cardiac box" should elicit highest levels of concern for penetrating cardiac injury. The "cardiac box" is an area of the anterior thorax bordered superiorly by the clavicles, inferiorly by the xiphoid, and the nipples laterally.[41] Recent literature has identified that corresponding lateral and posterior areas of the thorax are also associated with high rates of cardiac injury.[42] These data, along with the classic anatomic areas of concern, have led to the development of a more inclusive area defining possible injury. This "three-dimensional cardiac box" (**Fig. 2**) represents a modern structure for penetrating wounds that should be of highest concern for cardiac injury. Other clinical findings can suggest cardiac injury as well. Beck Triad of hypotension, jugular venous distention, and muffled heart sounds constitutes the classic clinical presentation of pericardial tamponade. The findings of Beck's Triad should be considered within the context of a complete workup, as Demetriades[43] demonstrated that these findings may not be present in up to 25% of patients with cardiac injuries.

The increased use of ultrasonography has made early recognition of penetrating cardiac injuries obtainable, even in the prehospital setting. Pericardial tamponade identified preoperatively may be an independent risk factor for survivability of penetrating cardiac injuries.[44] In the trauma bay, the increased use of surgeon-led ultrasonography has led to a decrease in time to operating room for patients with pericardial

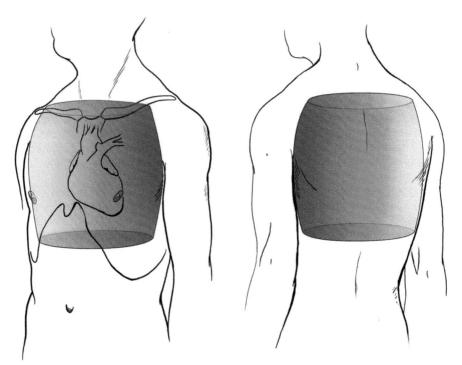

Fig. 2. The 3-dimensional cardiac box. Red gradient indicates likelihood of cardiac injury with brighter red being of higher degree of likelihood.

blood identified on ultrasound.[45] The use of ultrasound may have up to 100% sensitivity in experienced hands.[46] Ultrasound has use beyond identifying hemopericardium. It may also rule out risky operative procedures with narrow therapeutic benefit, like resuscitative thoracotomies.[36] The surgeon-ultrasonographer must always remain vigilant in the setting of penetrating cardiac injury because violation of the pericardium may allow necessitation of blood into the left or right hemithorax, leading to false negative results.[47] Historically, blind pericardiocentesis was performed to identify hemopericardium; however, this practice has largely been supplanted by ultrasound. Ultrasound has many advantages, including reproducibility, minimal false positive rate, and speed.

Chest radiography as part of a ballistic survey may allow some prognostic information of 2-compartment or transmediastinal injury and identify massive thoracic cage hemorrhage. In hemodynamically stable patients, proceeding to the CT scanner is also safe to identify trajectory and characterize potential injured structures.[48] The caveats of CT use in the evaluation of thoracoabdominal ballistic injury are the following: (1) there is no role for CT evaluation of patients that do not respond to resuscitation, (2) CT should not preclude transport of stable patients to a center that is better equipped to deal with cardiac injuries, (3) in the setting of an ultrasound positive pericardial effusion, the surgeon should not delay operative intervention to perform a CT scan. CT findings that correlate strongly with penetrating cardiac injury include primarily hemopericardium and pneumopericardium. Other more subtle findings that suggest cardiac injury include hemothorax with trajectory in close proximity to heart, retained ballistic fragments, hemomediastinum, or pneumomediastinum.[49]

Preoperative Care

As the identification of hemopericardium can be performed rapidly and reliably with minimal equipment, it is a logical conclusion that the envelope would be pushed further in the hope that early relief of tamponade may allow increased survival. This has led to the idea of early implementation of resuscitative thoracotomy in the prehospital setting in some areas of the world.[50,51] Vital signs on arrival to an emergency center are a strong predictor of outcomes in the penetrating cardiac injury. Presumably the restoration of vital signs as early as possible is the rationale for roadside operative intervention; however, this idea is largely disregarded in the America trauma literature, where the trauma system does not allow for a trauma surgeon in the prehospital setting.[40] In fact, patients that suffer cardiac arrest in the field have a survival of 0% in some studies, and even patients who arrest in the ambulance have dismal predicted survival. The window for potential salvage of patients undergoing resuscitative thoracotomy in the setting of penetrating thoracic trauma is approximately 15 minutes. Beyond that timeframe, the yield of performing resuscitative thoracotomy is less than 1.5%.[34,52,53] This is not to say that the performance of a resuscitative thoracotomy is a hopeless procedure. In fact, of all patients undergoing resuscitative thoracotomy, penetrating cardiac injuries portend the most favorable outcomes, with stab victims surviving neurologically intact between 15% and 50% of the time, and gunshot victims about half that.[52,54] These data have remained remarkably consistent over time.[53]

Intraoperative Care

What has not remained consistent is the management of exsanguinating hemorrhage. The advent of damage control surgery revolutionized the approach to the patient arriving in hemorrhagic shock due to injury.[55] However, techniques for damage control surgery to the chest may not be as familiar to the surgeon covering the trauma bay. In principle, the concept of damage control thoracic surgery is the same: abbreviated hemorrhage control followed by resuscitation and planned reoperation. In fact, the use of this technique in thoracic surgery is well accepted and safe.[56] Temporary packing of a thoracotomy or sternotomy wound as a temporizing measure should be performed when the injured patient enters into the triad of death: acidosis, coagulopathy, hypothermia.[56,57] Additional temporizing maneuvers for damage control cardiac surgery include the use of Foley balloon tamponade.[58] This technique however has fallen out of favor according to a contemporary panel of expert opinion.[57] Stapled cardiorrhaphy is another technique that permeates the surgical lore. This technique has proven safe and expeditious in both the preclinical setting and clinical setting for damage control of an exsanguinating cardiac laceration.[59–61] This technique may not be as useful in gunshot wounds with significant tissue loss. When faced with a lacerated coronary artery, suture ligation is a possible maneuver. The heart muscle must be subsequently observed for ischemia. If a focal area of muscle appears to be suffering compromise, the suture should be removed and finger occlusion applied until the necessary technical expertise can arrive. Although distal ligation is usually well tolerated, proximal narrowing or ligation will ultimately require revascularization.

In the setting of hemodynamic stability or after the successful completion of a damage control procedure, the next conundrum facing the trauma surgeon is definitive repair of penetrating cardiac injury. Most lacerations to the muscle of the heart can be repaired with simple interrupted monofilament suture with or without pledgets. When the injury is through or near a coronary vessel in a hemodynamically stable patient, the artery should be spared by placing mattress sutures underneath the bed of the artery using a polypropylene monofilament suture on a tapered needle. Complex injuries involving valves, multiple chambers, or the great vessels require cardiac surgery involvement.

Postoperative Care

In the postoperative period, management of penetrating cardiac injury should focus on the normal sequelae of cardiac operations. These sequelae may warrant echocardiography postoperatively to evaluate function.[31] The exact incidence of postoperative complications is unknown. Improved resuscitation practices, critical care, and trauma systems may have changed the patterns of postoperative complications after penetrating cardiac injuries. In the 1960s and 1970s, the University of Pennsylvania published a series of complications after cardiac repair.[62] The frequency of complication was nearly 50%, with ventricular septal defect (VSD) being the most common. In this series, the secondary lesion was picked up using a combination of EKG, echocardiography, and catheterization for patients with symptoms. The incidence of postoperative complications in a series out of Houston was nearly 30%. Again, patients with symptoms were worked up with echocardiogram and catheterization. The reoperative rate in this series was 20% of symptomatic patients and ~6% of patients surviving their injury.[63]

Because the nature of postoperative complications can likely be predicted based on the location of the injury, the recovery of patients in the intensive care unit should be focused on symptom management. Transient (~72 hour) symptomatic bradycardia and hypotension due to complete heart block are described and may necessitate temporary pacemaker placement.[64] This series also noted the relatively high incidence of VSD in survivors. Extrapolations of these data are difficult given the small number of cases in the series. Reports of complete heart block permeate the literature, however.[65–67] Thrombus formation, well described in BCI, is less frequent in penetrating cardiac injury, although possible.[63,68]

FUTURE DIRECTIONS

Penetrating cardiac injuries continue to be highly lethal. As technology has raced to keep up with cardiac surgery, the availability of adjuncts to support the injured heart has also appeared. Older technology such as extracorporeal membrane oxygenation (ECMO) is finding more and more places to fit in the care of the trauma patient.[69–75] These reports document successful management of many different injury patterns using both venovenous and venoarterial ECMO. Included in these data is a report of the successful use of venoarterial ECMO for a penetrating cardiac injury. All centers may not maintain expertise or interest in an expensive and labor-intensive technology like ECMO, but there is a developing role for this technology in the care of trauma patients. In addition to ECMO, ventricular assist devices may be safe to include in rare well-considered situations of penetrating cardiac injury complicated by acute heart failure.[76]

REFERENCES

1. Warburg E. Myocardial and pericardial lesions due to non-penetrating injury. Br Heart J 1940;2(4):271–80.
2. Ottosen J, Guo A. Blunt cardiac injury. 2012. Accessed January 1, 2017.
3. Bertinchant JP, Polge A, Mohty D, et al. Evaluation of incidence, clinical significance, and prognostic value of circulating cardiac troponin I and T elevation in

hemodynamically stable patients with suspected myocardial contusion after blunt chest trauma. J Trauma 2000;48(5):924–31.

4. Fedakar R, Turkmen N, Durak D, et al. Fatal traumatic heart wounds: review of 160 autopsy cases. Isr Med Assoc J 2005;7(8):498–501.

5. Yousef R, Carr JA. Blunt cardiac trauma: a review of the current knowledge and management. Ann Thorac Surg 2014;98(3):1134–40.

6. Brewer B, Zarzaur B. Cardiac contusions. Curr Trauma Rep 2015;1:5.

7. Velmahos GC, Tatevossian R, Demetriades D. The "seat belt mark" sign: a call for increased vigilance among physicians treating victims of motor vehicle accidents. Am Surg 1999;65(2):181–5.

8. Velmahos GC, Karaiskakis M, Salim A, et al. Normal electrocardiography and serum troponin I levels preclude the presence of clinically significant blunt cardiac injury. J Trauma 2003;54(1):45–50 [discussion: 50–1].

9. Salim A, Velmahos GC, Jindal A, et al. Clinically significant blunt cardiac trauma: role of serum troponin levels combined with electrocardiographic findings. J Trauma 2001;50(2):237–43.

10. Clancy K, Velopulos C, Bilaniuk JW, et al. Screening for blunt cardiac injury: an Eastern Association for the Surgery of Trauma practice management guideline. J Trauma Acute Care Surg 2012;73(5 Suppl 4):S301–6.

11. Berk WA. ECG findings in nonpenetrating chest trauma: a review. J Emerg Med 1987;5(3):209–15.

12. Joseph B, Jokar TO, Khalil M, et al. Identifying the broken heart: predictors of mortality and morbidity in suspected blunt cardiac injury. Am J Surg 2016; 211(6):982–8.

13. Biffl WL, Moore FA, Moore EE, et al. Cardiac enzymes are irrelevant in the patient with suspected myocardial contusion. Am J Surg 1994;168(6):523–7 [discussion: 527–8].

14. Swaanenburg JC, Klaase JM, DeJongste MJ, et al. Troponin I, troponin T, CKMB-activity and CKMB-mass as markers for the detection of myocardial contusion in patients who experienced blunt trauma. Clin Chim Acta 1998;272(2):171–81.

15. Oyetunji TA, Jackson HT, Obirieze AC, et al. Associated injuries in traumatic sternal fractures: a review of the National Trauma Data Bank. Am Surg 2013;79(7): 702–5.

16. Sade R, Kantarci M, Ogul H, et al. The feasibility of dual-energy computed tomography in cardiac contusion imaging for mildest blunt cardiac injury. J Comput Assist Tomogr 2016;41(3):354–9.

17. Baxi AJ, Restrepo C, Mumbower A, et al. Cardiac injuries: a review of multidetector computed tomography findings. Trauma Mon 2015;20(4):e19086.

18. Marcolini EG, Keegan J. Blunt cardiac injury. Emerg Med Clin North Am 2015; 33(3):519–27.

19. Teixeira PG, Inaba K, Oncel D, et al. Blunt cardiac rupture: a 5-year NTDB analysis. J Trauma 2009;67(4):788–91.

20. Namai A, Sakurai M, Fujiwara H. Five cases of blunt traumatic cardiac rupture: success and failure in surgical management. Gen Thorac Cardiovasc Surg 2007;55(5):200–4.

21. Nan YY, Lu MS, Liu KS, et al. Blunt traumatic cardiac rupture: therapeutic options and outcomes. Injury 2009;40(9):938–45.

22. Pasquier M, Sierro C, Yersin B, et al. Traumatic mitral valve injury after blunt chest trauma: a case report and review of the literature. J Trauma 2010;68(1):243–6.

23. Tsugu T, Murata M, Mahara K, et al. Long-term survival on medical therapy alone after blunt-trauma aortic regurgitation: report of a new case with summary of 95 others. Tex Heart Inst J 2016;43(5):446–52.

24. van Son JA, Danielson GK, Schaff HV, et al. Traumatic tricuspid valve insufficiency. Experience in thirteen patients. J Thorac Cardiovasc Surg 1994;108(5): 893–8.

25. Fuglsang S, Heiberg J, Hjortdal VE. Severe pulmonary valve regurgitation 40 years after blunt chest trauma. Ann Thorac Surg 2015;100(4):1458–9.

26. Yousaf H, Ammar KA, Tajik AJ. Traumatic pulmonary valve injury following blunt chest trauma. Eur Heart J Cardiovasc Imaging 2015;16(11):1206.

27. Parmley LF, Manion WC, Mattingly TW. Nonpenetrating traumatic injury of the heart. Circulation 1958;18(3):371–96.

28. Murray AT, Wyatt WF. Homer Iliad translated. 2nd edition. Cambridge (MA): Harvard University Press; 1999.

29. Beck CS. Wounds of the heart. The technique of suture. Arch Surg 1926;(13): 205–27.

30. Peck CH. XI. The operative treatment of heart wounds: report of a case of wound of the right auricle; suture; recovery. Tabulation of 158 cases of sutured heart wounds. Ann Surg 1909;50(1):100–34.

31. Morse BC, Mina MJ, Carr JS, et al. Penetrating cardiac injuries: a 36-year perspective at an urban, level I trauma center. J Trauma Acute Care Surg 2016;81(4):623–31.

32. Asensio JA, Murray J, Demetriades D, et al. Penetrating cardiac injuries: a prospective study of variables predicting outcomes. J Am Coll Surg 1998;186(1): 24–34.

33. Feliciano DV, Bitondo CG, Mattox KL, et al. Civilian trauma in the 1980s. A 1-year experience with 456 vascular and cardiac injuries. Ann Surg 1984;199(6):717–24.

34. Tyburski JG, Astra L, Wilson RF, et al. Factors affecting prognosis with penetrating wounds of the heart. J Trauma 2000;48(4):587–90 [discussion: 590–1].

35. Rhee PM, Foy H, Kaufmann C, et al. Penetrating cardiac injuries: a population-based study. J Trauma 1998;45(2):366–70.

36. Mina MJ, Jhunjhunwala R, Gelbard RB, et al. Factors affecting mortality after penetrating cardiac injuries: 10-year experience at urban level I trauma center. Am J Surg 2017;213(6):1109–15.

37. Bowley DM, Saeed M, Somwe D, et al. Off-pump cardiac revascularization after a complex stab wound. Ann Thorac Surg 2002;74(6):2192–3.

38. Demetriades D, Martin M, Salim A, et al. The effect of trauma center designation and trauma volume on outcome in specific severe injuries. Ann Surg 2005;242(4): 512–7 [discussion: 517–9].

39. Campbell NC, Thomson SR, Muckart DJ, et al. Review of 1198 cases of penetrating cardiac trauma. Br J Surg 1997;84(12):1737–40.

40. Topal AE, Celik Y, Eren MN. Predictors of outcome in penetrating cardiac injuries. J Trauma 2010;69(3):574–8.

41. Asensio JA, Stewart BM, Murray J, et al. Penetrating cardiac injuries. Surg Clin North Am 1996;76(4):685–724.

42. Jhunjhunwala R, Mina MJ, Roger EI, et al. Reassessing the cardiac box: a comprehensive evaluation of the relationship between thoracic gunshot wounds and cardiac injury. J Trauma Acute Care Surg 2017. [Epub ahead of print].

43. Demetriades D. Cardiac wounds. Experience with 70 patients. Ann Surg 1986; 203(3):315–7.

44. Moreno C, Moore EE, Majure JA, et al. Pericardial tamponade: a critical determinant for survival following penetrating cardiac wounds. J Trauma 1986;26(9): 821–5.

45. Rozycki GS, Feliciano DV, Schmidt JA, et al. The role of surgeon-performed ultrasound in patients with possible cardiac wounds. Ann Surg 1996;223(6):737–44 [discussion: 744–6].

46. Rozycki GS, Feliciano DV, Ochsner MG, et al. The role of ultrasound in patients with possible penetrating cardiac wounds: a prospective multicenter study. J Trauma 1999;46(4):543–51 [discussion: 551–2].

47. Ball CG, Williams BH, Wyrzykowski AD, et al. A caveat to the performance of pericardial ultrasound in patients with penetrating cardiac wounds. J Trauma 2009; 67(5):1123–4.

48. Stassen NA, Lukan JK, Spain DA, et al. Reevaluation of diagnostic procedures for transmediastinal gunshot wounds. J Trauma 2002;53(4):635–8 [discussion: 638].

49. Plurad DS, Bricker S, Van Natta TL, et al. Penetrating cardiac injury and the significance of chest computed tomography findings. Emerg Radiol 2013;20(4): 279–84.

50. Coats TJ, Keogh S, Clark H, et al. Prehospital resuscitative thoracotomy for cardiac arrest after penetrating trauma: rationale and case series. J Trauma 2001; 50(4):670–3.

51. Davies GE, Lockey DJ. Thirteen survivors of prehospital thoracotomy for penetrating trauma: a prehospital physician-performed resuscitation procedure that can yield good results. J Trauma 2011;70(5):E75–8.

52. Seamon MJ, Shiroff AM, Franco M, et al. Emergency department thoracotomy for penetrating injuries of the heart and great vessels: an appraisal of 283 consecutive cases from two urban trauma centers. J Trauma 2009;67(6):1250–7 [discussion: 1257–8].

53. Rhee PM, Acosta J, Bridgeman A, et al. Survival after emergency department thoracotomy: review of published data from the past 25 years. J Am Coll Surg 2000;190(3):288–98.

54. Seamon MJ, Haut ER, Van Arendonk K, et al. An evidence-based approach to patient selection for emergency department thoracotomy: a practice management guideline from the Eastern Association for the Surgery of Trauma. J Trauma Acute Care Surg 2015;79(1):159–73.

55. Rotondo MF, Schwab CW, McGonigal MD, et al. 'Damage control': an approach for improved survival in exsanguinating penetrating abdominal injury. J Trauma 1993;35(3):375–82 [discussion: 382–3].

56. Mackowski MJ, Barnett RE, Harbrecht BG, et al. Damage control for thoracic trauma. Am Surg 2014;80(9):910–3.

57. Roberts DJ, Bobrovitz N, Zygun DA, et al. Indications for use of thoracic, abdominal, pelvic, and vascular damage control interventions in trauma patients: a content analysis and expert appropriateness rating study. J Trauma Acute Care Surg 2015;79(4):568–79.

58. Cowling K, Eidah A. In: Atlas of surgical techniques in trauma. Demetriades D, Inaba K, Velmahos G, editors vol. 23. New York: Cambridge University Press; 2015. p. 336, e6–7.

59. Mayrose J, Jehle DV, Moscati R, et al. Comparison of staples versus sutures in the repair of penetrating cardiac wounds. J Trauma 1999;46(3):441–3 [discussion: 443–4].

60. Macho JR, Markison RE, Schecter WP. Cardiac stapling in the management of penetrating injuries of the heart: rapid control of hemorrhage and decreased risk of personal contamination. J Trauma 1993;34(5):711–5 [discussion: 715–6].
61. Bowman MR, King RM. Comparison of staples and sutures for cardiorrhaphy in traumatic puncture wounds of the heart. J Emerg Med 1996;14(5):615–8.
62. Fallahnejad M, Kutty AC, Wallace HW. Secondary lesions of penetrating cardiac injuries: a frequent complication. Ann Surg 1980;191(2):228–33.
63. Mattox KL, Limacher MC, Feliciano DV, et al. Cardiac evaluation following heart injury. J Trauma 1985;25(8):758–65.
64. Jhunjhunwala R, Dente CJ, Keeling WB, et al. Injury to the conduction system: management of life-threatening arrhythmias after penetrating cardiac trauma. Am J Surg 2016;212(2):352–3.
65. O'Byrne GT, Nalos PC, Gang ES, et al. Progression of complete heart block to isolated infra-Hisian block following penetrating cardiac trauma. Am Heart J 1987;113(3):839–42.
66. Eckart RE, Falta EM, Stewart RW. Complete heart block following penetrating chest trauma in Operation Iraqi Freedom. Pacing Clin Electrophysiol 2008; 31(5):635–8.
67. Kennedy F, Duffy B, Stiles G, et al. Gunshot wound traversing the ventricular septum with peripheral embolization presenting as complete heart block. J Trauma 1998;45(3):620–2.
68. Neidlinger NA, Puzziferri N, Victorino GP, et al. Cardiac thromboemboli complicating a stab wound to the heart. Cardiovasc Pathol 2004;13(1):56–8.
69. Ahmad SB, Menaker J, Kufera J, et al. Extracorporeal membrane oxygenation after traumatic injury. J Trauma Acute Care Surg 2017;82(3):587–91.
70. Biscotti M, Agerstrand C, Abrams D, et al. Extracorporeal membrane oxygenation transport after traumatic aortic valve injury. ASAIO J 2014;60(3):353–4.
71. Gatti G, Forti G, Bologna A, et al. Rescue extracorporeal membrane oxygenation in a young man with a stab wound in the chest. Injury 2014;45(9):1509–11.
72. Ried M, Bein T, Philipp A, et al. Extracorporeal lung support in trauma patients with severe chest injury and acute lung failure: a 10-year institutional experience. Crit Care 2013;17(3):R110.
73. Schmoekel NH, O'Connor JV, Scalea TM. Nonoperative damage control: the use of extracorporeal membrane oxygenation in traumatic bronchial avulsion as a bridge to definitive operation. Ann Thorac Surg 2016;101(6):2384–6.
74. Tseng YH, Wu TI, Liu YC, et al. Venoarterial extracorporeal life support in post-traumatic shock and cardiac arrest: lessons learned. Scand J Trauma Resusc Emerg Med 2014;22:12.
75. Jacobs JV, Hooft NM, Robinson BR, et al. The use of extracorporeal membrane oxygenation in blunt thoracic trauma: a study of the Extracorporeal Life Support Organization database. J Trauma Acute Care Surg 2015;79(6):1049–53 [discussion: 1053–4].
76. Chavanon O, Dutheil V, Hacini R, et al. Treatment of severe cardiac contusion with a left ventricular assist device in a patient with multiple trauma. J Thorac Cardiovasc Surg 1999;118(1):189–90.

Surgical Management of Solid Organ Injuries

Niels V. Johnsen, MD[a], Richard D. Betzold, MD[b],
Oscar D. Guillamondegui, MD, MPH[b], Bradley M. Dennis, MD[b,*],
Nicole A. Stassen, MD[c], Indermeet Bhullar, MD[d],
Joseph A. Ibrahim, MD[d]

KEYWORDS

- Spleen trauma • Liver trauma • Pancreas trauma • Kidney trauma • Hepatic injury
- Renal injury • Angioembolization

KEY POINTS

- The management of solid organ injuries has become progressively less operative over the past 20 years. The need for initial operative management of solid organ injuries is determined by the patient's clinical status, not the extent of the solid organ injury.
- Patients presenting with hemodynamic instability and peritonitis still warrant emergent operative intervention. Intravenous contrast-enhanced computed tomographic scan is the diagnostic modality of choice for evaluating solid organ injuries in the stable patient.
- Major liver trauma with extensive parenchymal injury and uncontrollable bleeding in hemodynamically unstable patients is challenging and the adoption of a combination of effective damage control resuscitation and damage control surgery strategies have been demonstrated to be associated with improved outcomes.
- Adjunctive therapies like angiography, percutaneous drainage, endoscopy/endoscopic retrograde cholangiopancreatography, and laparoscopy remain important adjuncts to solid organ injury management.
- The status of the pancreatic duct and the location of the injury guide surgical management of pancreatic trauma whether it is diagnosed during a laparotomy or with preoperative imaging. Pancreatic head injuries typically are treated with wide drainage, whereas injuries to the pancreatic tail are most often treated with surgical resection.

Disclosure: No commercial or financial conflicts of interest related to this article.
[a] Urological Surgery, Department of Urological Surgery, Vanderbilt University Medical Center, A-1302 Medical Center North, Nashville, TN 37232, USA; [b] Division of Trauma, Surgical Critical Care, Emergency General Surgery, Department of Surgery, Vanderbilt University Medical Center, 1211 21st Avenue South, 404 Medical Arts Building, Nashville, TN 37212, USA; [c] Surgical Critical Care Fellowship and Surgical Sub-Internship, University of Rochester, Kessler Family Burn Trauma Intensive Care Unit, 601 Elmwood Avenue, Box Surg, Rochester, NY 14642, USA; [d] Orlando Health Physicians Surgical Group, Orlando Regional Medical Center, 86 West Underwood, Suite 201, Orlando, FL 32806, USA
* Corresponding author.
E-mail address: Bradley.m.dennis@vanderbilt.edu

INTRODUCTION: THE EVOLUTION OF SOLID ORGAN INJURY MANAGEMENT

Surgery used to be the treatment of choice in patients with solid organ injuries. This approach has gradually changed over the past 2 decades as nonoperative management (NOM) has become the primary management strategy used for solid organ injuries. The improvement in critical care monitoring and computed tomographic (CT) scanning, as well as the more frequent use of interventional radiology techniques, has helped to bring about this change to NOM. Additionally, the availability of less invasive procedures has dramatically expanded the treatment options for these patients, optimizing the outcomes of initial NOM.[1–4] Even though NOM has become the standard of care in patients with solid organ in most trauma center, surgeons should not hesitate to operate on a patient to control life-threatening hemorrhage.

LIVER

Management of liver trauma is challenging and may vary widely given the heterogeneity of liver injuries' anatomic configuration, the hemodynamic status of the patient, and the settings and resources available. Hepatic injury ranges from a small capsular tear, without parenchymal laceration, to massive parenchymal injury with major hepatic vein/retrohepatic vena cava lesions[5] (**Table 1**). Expeditious initial diagnosis is paramount to the management of hepatic injury, as most Grade I-III hepatic injuries are successfully treated with NOM, whereas two-thirds of grade IV or V injuries necessitate intervention.[6] In the hemodynamically stable trauma patient without peritonitis, an abdominal CT scan with intravenous contrast should be performed to identify and assess the severity of injury to the liver. The greatest advantages of CT lie in its ability to determine the extent of the hepatic injury, document the presence of active hemorrhage, and assess for associated injuries.[7] The severity of hepatic injury (as suggested by CT grade or degree of hemoperitoneum), neurologic status, presence of a "blush" on CT scan, age older than 55 years, and/or the presence of associated injuries are no longer considered absolute contraindications to a trial of nonoperative management in the hemodynamically stable patient.[8–11] Improvements in intensive care monitoring and multidisciplinary treatment options have changed the philosophy of NOM even in those patients who in the recent past were consistently managed in a surgical manner. Adjunctive interventions, as well as application of endovascular,

Table 1
Routine angiogram strategy with angiograms performed on all hemodynamically stable patients with BST on admission CT

Institution	Journal	Year	Total, n	NOM, n (%)	Angiograms	AE, %	FNOM, %
State University of New York[20]	Radiology	1991	44	44 (100)	44 (100%)	17 (39%)	3
State University of New York[21]	J Trauma	1995	172	150 (87)	150 (100%)	56 (37%)	3
Kyorin University Japan[27]	AJR	1996	31	28 (90)	28 (100%)	15 (53%)	7
University of Maryland[18]	J Trauma	2001	352	136 (39)	29%	8%	8

Angioembolization was performed for those with active extravasation on angiogram and bed rest without embolization those without extravasation.

Abbreviations: AE, angioembolization; BST, blunt splenic trauma; CT, computed tomography; FNOM, failure of nonoperative management; NOM, nonoperative management.

percutaneous, and endoscopic methods, have decreased the morbidity that was once commonly associated with high-grade liver injuries.[12–14]

The hemodynamically unstable patient or the patient with peritonitis should proceed emergently to the operating room for exploration. In this instance, the grade of hepatic injury and most effective management strategy is determined intraoperatively.

Management of Hepatic Injury

Operative management of hepatic injury as a primary intervention

Primary surgical intervention for hepatic injury is an option that is now reserved for patients who remain hemodynamically abnormal despite aggressive resuscitation. Such patients are extremely challenging for the trauma team, as they may rapidly evolve toward the development of the lethal triad of hypothermia, acidosis, and coagulopathy. The advent of the use of damage control laparotomy has revolutionized the operative management of patients with high-grade liver injury resulting in improved survival in multiple series.[2,14–16] The main goals of the initial damage control operation in this setting are to control hemorrhage and control visible bile leak.

Damage control surgery must proceed in tandem with damage control resuscitation in the management of these patients to achieve the best clinical outcome. Damage control resuscitation combines 2 strategies: permissive hypotension and hemostatic resuscitation. Permissive hypotension is a strategy of restricting crystalloid administration until the bleeding is controlled, while accepting a limited period of suboptimal end-organ perfusion. This strategy derives from the assumption that hypotension facilitates coagulation, whereas a more elevated blood pressure may contribute to "pop the clot" and subsequently more bleeding. Permissive hypotension is not without risks, as prolonged hypotension can lead to aggravated postinjury coagulopathy and ischemic damage secondary to poor tissue perfusion and lactic acidosis.[17–19] Hemostatic resuscitation instead applies to massively bleeding patients and derives from the attempt of approximating whole blood, providing patients transfusions with plasma and platelets in addition to packed red blood cells (PRBCs).[18] The massive transfusion protocol should be activated to ensure the blood bank is always ahead of the patient's needs for PRBCs, fresh frozen plasma, platelets, and cryoprecipitate. Adequate vascular access and arterial blood pressure monitoring are essential.

The surgical approach to control of liver bleeding follows a stepwise progression. The patient should be widely prepped, neck to knees and table to table. The initial operative incision will be a xiphoid to pubis midline laparotomy. A right subcostal extension can be added if needed for exposure and hemorrhage control. The first step in hepatic hemorrhage control is manual compression of the liver.[20,21] The hepatic compression serves 2 main functions: to control hemorrhage and to further diagnose the potential etiology of the hemorrhage. The hurried tendency is to pack laparotomy pads anteriorly only. This can exacerbate the hepatic hemorrhage rather than diminish it by splaying open the hepatic defect. Proper compression of the liver grossly closes the defect, compressing the liver into its natural configuration. The liver should be mobilized by taking down the falciform, coronary, and triangular ligaments. Laparotomy pads are packed around the liver in a "sandwich" fashion to both compress the injury and to assist in hemostasis. Inappropriate or inadequate packing has been shown to lead to worsened patient outcomes.[22] For parenchymal bleeding, large liver sutures may be an adequate treatment. Liver sutures are typically large chromic sutures on a blunt or tapered needle to allow passage through a large swath of liver parenchyma without causing additional bleeding.[23] Placing large liver sutures can often reapproximate injured and oozing liver parenchymal surfaces enough to allow tamponade and cessation of bleeding. Another option for parenchymal bleeding is omental packing. In addition to the tamponade effect, omental tissue has extremely high levels of tissue factor, which allows it to augment hemostasis.[24] Although most applicable for penetrating trauma with deep tracts into the liver parenchyma, balloon tamponade using a Penrose or Foley catheter can be a useful adjunct to control exsanguinating hemorrhage in patients not responding to packing alone.[25] If the hemorrhage is controlled with suture or packing, the laparotomy should be abbreviated and the patient taken to the intensive care unit (ICU) for further resuscitation. Perihepatic packing will control profuse hemorrhaging in up to 80% of patients undergoing laparotomy, allowing intraoperative resuscitation.[26]

If the hemorrhage is not controlled by packing alone, it raises concern for a more complex hepatic injury. The next move is to perform a Pringle maneuver. The porta hepatis should be identified and either an atraumatic vascular clamp or a Rummel tourniquet should be placed and tightened. If the bleeding is controlled with the Pringle, the source of hemorrhage is likely a hepatic artery or portal vein branch. These can be identified and repaired or selectively ligated. Hepatotomy and selective vascular ligation is one technique for management of portal venous and arterial injuries. With Pringle control, the injured portion of the liver is further fractured with the surgeon's finger to allow direct ligation of the bleeding vessels. Intermittent release of the Pringle clamp may allow identification of deep bleeding sites and control by direct suture.[27,28] For hepatic parenchymal devascularization or destruction, resectional debridement along nonsegmental planes should be performed. Angiography with selective arterial embolization can be a useful adjunct in these cases.

If the Pringle maneuver fails to control bleeding from within a liver injury or dark venous bleeding persists from behind a hepatic lobe, a juxtahepatic venous injury is likely. Injuries to the juxtahepatic veins, that is, the retrohepatic vena cava or major hepatic veins, although representing only a small proportion of all liver injuries, constitute the most difficult and most deadly form of liver trauma.[29–31] The mortality for such injuries has ranged between 50% and 80%.[27,32–34] The extreme lethality of juxtahepatic venous injuries has generally been attributed to the surgically inaccessible location of the major hepatic veins and retrohepatic vena cava, which lie within and behind the thickest and least mobile portion of the liver.[35] Any attempt to rotate the liver for exposure of the veins tends to increase hemorrhage and presents an additional risk of fatal air embolization. Major juxtahepatic venous injuries fall into 1 of 2 general wounding patterns: intraparenchymal hepatic venous injury (bleeding emanates through the liver tissue) and extraparenchymal hepatic venous injury (bleeding emanates around the liver tissue).[36] Intraparenchymal hepatic venous injuries are often controlled by reinforcement and restoration of torn containment around the injury either by packing or suturing. Extraparenchymal hepatic venous injuries require direct exposure and control. Total vascular isolation of the liver is often needed for repair of these injuries. This can be done in several ways, by placing an atriocaval shunt, utilization of venovenous bypass, or by clamping the suprahepatic inferior vena cava (IVC), the suprarenal IVC, and the porta hepatis.[37–39] The liver can then be further mobilized and the injury repaired. Assistance from a transplant surgeon in these cases is quite beneficial. It is critical that "audible" surgical bleeding is controlled before truncating any operation on the liver.

Once operative hemorrhage control is obtained, further resuscitation may require ICU management and possible adjunctive angiography with selective embolization if there is evidence of ongoing hemorrhage. With adequate resuscitation, to include correction of hypothermia, acidosis, and coagulopathy, the patient should return to the operating room. The packs should be removed for assessment of hemorrhage. Devitalized tissues should be debrided and bile leaks controlled. Closed suction drains should be placed if there is a high concern for bile leak. Secondary procedures may be necessary, as potential complications such as persistent bile leak, biloma, bile peritonitis, hepatic abscess/necrosis, and hemobilia arise.

Operative management of hepatic injury as a secondary intervention

As the success of NOM of liver injuries has increased, so has the need to treat different complications related to its use.[40] Although uncommon, these complications usually require accurate diagnosis and multimodal interventions.[13,14] By far, delayed hemorrhage is the most common complication.[41] In those patients with delayed hemorrhage, selective arterial transcatheter embolization is vital to determine the precise location of the source of hemorrhage and also can be extremely useful as an adjunct to operative packing.[42] Bile leaks or bile peritonitis may also occur after severe parenchymal disruption or injuries to the extrahepatic biliary ducts. Diagnosis and treatment can be performed with endoscopic retrograde cholangiopancreatography.[43] Bile peritonitis associated with a systemic inflammatory response has been described in the days after extensive liver injuries. Patients may present with leukocytosis, right upper quadrant pain, fever, and worsening multiple system organ dysfunction. Laparoscopic evaluation and wash-out is a technique described to remove bile and old blood as an alternative to laparotomy after stabilization of the injury.[44,45] Early use of these adjunctive techniques has been shown to improve outcomes after NOM by avoiding surgical laparotomy and decreasing mortality.[42,46] Retained blood or bile may lead to hepatic abscess, perihepatic infection, or abdominal compartment syndrome. Delayed development of liver abscess or intra-abdominal fluid collections resulting from liver injuries are best treated with percutaneous drainage by the interventional radiology team. More significant hepatic necrosis can be treated with nonanatomic hepatic resection.

After massive resuscitation, abdominal compartment syndrome has also been reported in association with liver injuries.[47] Percutaneous drainage in lieu of laparotomy has been described as a technique to decrease intra-abdominal pressure.[13]

SPLEEN

Management of blunt splenic trauma (BST) has substantially evolved over the past century. More than 100 years ago, evaluation of postmortem findings led Bilroth to suggest that the injured spleen has the ability of self-healing, and may be observed with NOM.[48–59] The landmark Eastern Association for the Surgery of Trauma (EAST) trial in 2000 established the failure rates based on grade of injury for BST with little to no intervention.[60] Prohibitive failure rates of 33% to 75% for high-grade (IV-V) injuries led to the recommendation of operative management for this group.[60] Since its introduction in 1981 by Sclafani,[61] angioembolization (AE) has increasingly been used as an adjunct to NOM of hemodynamically stable patients with BST. Although many centers have reported significant reductions in failure rates of NOM (FNOM) using AE, its benefit and indications remain unclear.[61–75] There have been no randomized trials of its role, and some retrospective studies have concluded that AE does not improve success of NOM.[76–80]

Management

Operative management

All hemodynamically unstable patients with BST should undergo immediate operative intervention with splenectomy; attempt at NOM both with and without AE results in high failure rates and increased mortality. Bhullar and colleagues[63,80] demonstrated an FNOM rate of 100% and spleen-related mortality of 13% in hemodynamically unstable patients in whom NOM was attempted. Peitzman and colleagues[81] also demonstrated the dangers of attempting NOM in hemodynamically unstable patients by reporting a spleen-related mortality of 37% in this group. An undue delay in laparotomy was responsible for 60% of the deaths, and 3 patients exsanguinated without laparotomy.[81] Blood transfusion in an effort to stabilize hemodynamically unstable patients has been shown to be an independent risk factor for failure of NOM.[63,82] A study of the role of blood transfusion in BST by Velmahos and colleagues[82] identified, among other variables, that transfusion of more than 1 unit of blood was an independent risk factor for FNOM. In their study, patients with grade III-IV BST injuries who received more than 1 unit of blood transfusion during NOM had a 100% FNOM rate.[82] With the introduction of the new resuscitative endovascular balloon occlusion of the aorta (REBOA) system, the Japanese have reported successful salvage of the spleen in hemodynamically unstable patients using REBOA deployment as a bridge to AE.[83] However, further study regarding safety of this approach is needed before further recommendations, because a mortality of 14% (1 of 7 patients) was reported with this technique.[83]

Nonoperative management

Extreme scrutiny must to be exercised to select patients for NOM to limit overall failure rates. As discussed previously, all hemodynamically unstable patients need immediate operative intervention. This group comprises approximately 20% to 40% of all BST admissions (**Fig. 1**).[60–63] Patients with acute abdomen or peritonitis or concerns for other intra-abdominal injuries also should undergo immediate operative intervention. Patients requiring ongoing resuscitation with fluids and blood transfusions also should be excluded from consideration of NOM, as discussed previously. Of the remaining hemodynamically stable patients, success of NOM is determined by 2 factors: grade of injury (I-V) and presence of contrast blush (CB) on admission CT.[60,84] The EAST trial in 2000 established the failure rates based on grade of injury for BST with little to no intervention.[60] Of the total population studied, 39% went immediately to the operating room. The overall FNOM rate was reported as 11%. FNOM increased significantly by grade of splenic injury: grade I, 5%; grade II, 10%; grade III, 20%; grade IV, 33%; and grade V, 75%. Prohibitive failure rates of 33% to 75% for high-grade (IV-V) injuries led to the recommendation of operative management for this group.[60] In 1995, the Memphis group also identified CB on admission CT as a strong indicator for active bleeding resulting in high failure rates (67%) with observation alone,[62] predicting 25 times the likelihood of FNOM. Similarly, Bhullar and colleagues[63] found that 71% of patients with CB who were observed FNOM and the likelihood of failure was 22 times higher for those with CB on initial CT. Based on these findings, NOM was considered a contraindication and operative intervention was recommended for 2 groups of patients with BST: (1) CB on CT, and (2) high-grade (IV-V) injuries without CB. However, with the evolution of AE as an adjunct to NOM these contraindications have moved from absolute to controversial.

Grade I-II

For hemodynamically stable grade I-II patients who lack other indications for laparotomy, NOM should be used because the FNOM is very low. The presence of CB still carries a high failure rate (70%) even for low-grade I-II injuries.[63,69,85] The failure rate reported by the EAST trial for grade I and grade II with observation alone was 5% and 10%, respectively.[60] A recent study reported significant reduction in FNOM compared with the EAST trial for grade I-II injuries with the addition of AE for CB: grade

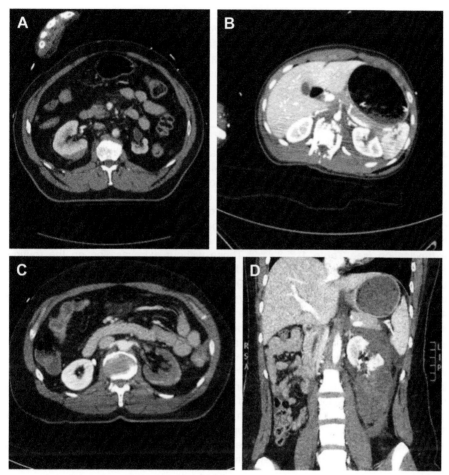

Fig. 1. CT imaging of traumatic renal injuries. (*A*) Small right perinephric hematoma (grade I). (*B*) Left renal laceration >1.0 cm without urinary extravasation (grade III). (*C*) Left renal artery thrombosis with devascularized left kidney (grade IV). (*D*) Shattered left kidney with large surrounding hematoma and devascularized lower pole (grade V).

I, 5% vs 1%, *P* = .01; grade II, 10% vs 2%, *P* = .01.[63] Based on limited data, AE of grade I-II with CB should be strongly considered.

Grade III

Grade III remains a controversial group. The FNOM with observation alone for grade III injuries in the EAST trial was 20%. Although some have advocated selective AE for grade III with CB, others have recommended routine AE of all grade III injuries. However, the FNOM rate reported for grade III injuries using routine AE (7.5%)[86] is similar to the FNOM for selective AE for CB (5%–6%).[63,87–89] Therefore, currently a selective AE approach to limit unnecessary angiograms is recommended.

Grade IV-V

High-grade (IV-V) injuries behave distinctly differently from the other grades, and are a unique group given their consistently high failure rates with observation alone

(40%–64%).[60,63,64,85,88,90] Grade IV-V injuries with CB have nearly a 100% FNOM with observation.[90] Protocols using selective AE for CB still reported failure rates as high as 18%.[63] However, 2 institutions using routine AE of all grade IV-V injuries with or without CB have reported FNOM rates as low as 3% to 8%.[80,86] Further studies are needed to determine if these new routine AE strategies will allow for safe NOM of high-grade injuries.

Angioembolization

Since its introduction in 1981 by Sclafani,[61] AE has increasingly been used as an adjunct to NOM of hemodynamically stable patients with BST. Although many centers have reported significant reductions in FNOM rates using AE, its benefits and indications remain unclear.[62–75] There have been no randomized trials of its role, and some retrospective studies have concluded that AE does not improve success of NOM.[76–78] For hemodynamically stable patients, 2 divergent angiogram strategies have evolved over the past 2 decades. The first strategy performed mandatory angiograms on all hemodynamically stable patients with BST and only embolized those with active extravasation (see **Table 1**).[65,67,68,73] Those without extravasation on the routine angiogram were admitted and observed with bedrest. A series of studies published using this strategy over the decade of 1990 to 2001 reported encouraging overall failure rates of 1.5% to 7.9%; however, they also noted an unnecessary angiogram rate of 46% to 68%.[65,67,68,72] These unnecessary angiograms were primarily in the low-grade injuries (I-II) resulting in additional cost and risk to the patients with little benefit to overall success.[65,67,68,72] In an effort to eliminate these unnecessary angiograms, a second more selective strategy evolved with angiograms being performed only on patients with BST who demonstrated a CB on admission CT (**Table 2**). This was based primarily on the fact that CB had a strong correlation with active bleeding during angiography.[62] Using this selective angiogram strategy, a series of studies was published over the next decade (1998–2012) with FNOM rates ranging from 2% to 9% (see **Table 2**).[63,66,69,73,74,91–93] Although a drop was noted in the overall FNOM with the selective AE for CB in comparison with the EAST trial that had no intervention (11% vs 2%–9%), conclusions regarding effectiveness of AE were limited by confounding

Table 2
Selective angiogram strategy with angiograms performed on all hemodynamically stable patients with BST and CB on admission CT

Institution	Journal	Year	Total, n	NOM, n (%)	AE, %	FNOM, %
University of Tennessee Memphis[69]	*J Trauma*	1998	524	322 (61)	7	6
University of Texas San Antonio[66]	*J Trauma*	2004	168	139 (83)	10	2
University of Michigan[91]	*Surgery*	2004	164	131 (80)	18	5
University of Maryland[74]	*J Trauma*	2005	648	368 (57)	81	8
Case Western[92]	*Surgery*	2005	403	344 (85)	25	2
University of Tennessee Memphis[93]	*J Trauma*	2007	426	341 (80)	12	4
University of Pittsburgh[77]	*J Trauma*	2007	570	349 (61)	13	9
University of Florida Jacksonville[63]	*J Trauma*	2012	1039	539 (64)	19	4

Angioembolization was performed for those with active extravasation on angiogram and bed rest without embolization those without extravasation.

Abbreviations: AE, angioembolization; BST, blunt splenic trauma; CB, contrast blush; CT, computed tomography; FNOM, failure of nonoperative management; NOM, nonoperative management.

factors such as improved patient selection, evolution of CT technology, and varying definitions of FNOM. Although unnecessary angiograms of low-grade injuries (grade I-II) were limited using this approach, high-grade (IV-V) injuries without CB had a 26% failure rate with observation alone; operative intervention was again recommended for this group given the high failures.[63,90] Further analysis revealed that high failure rates in grade (IV-V) injuries without CB may be due to failure of CT scans to identify active bleeding. Bhullar and colleagues[80,90] reported that 85% (20 of 51) of patients with high-grade (IV-V) injury and no CB who were sent for angiograms in noncompliance to the protocol had active extravasation that was missed by the admission CT. All 20 were AE and 0% failed. There was a significant decrease in the failure rate with routine AE of high-grade (IV-V) injuries without CB compared with observation alone (NO-AE vs AE, 26% [8 of 31] vs 0% [0 of 20], $P = .04$).[80,90]

Based on these findings, 2 groups have combined Selective and Routine strategies to form a hybrid protocol that attempts to compensate for the high false-negative rate of CT scans as well as preventing unnecessary angiograms of low-grade injuries (**Table 3**). These protocols perform routine embolization on all high-grade injuries grade III-IV or IV-V and selective embolization of all low-grade injuries with CB. Using this hybrid protocol, Miller and colleagues[86] performed routine embolization of all grade III-V injuries and reported an FNOM rate of 6%, whereas Bhullar and colleagues[80] performed routine embolization of grade IV-V injuries and reported an FNOM rate of 1%. In the latter study, 68 patients had high-grade IV-V injuries (36 with no CB and 32 with CB). All 68 were embolized. FNOM for high-grade (IV-V) injuries was 3% (2 of 68) with 0 failures among the 36 without the CB and 2 failures for the 32 with CB.[80] Although a significant drop was noted with both protocols for high-grade injuries (40%–67% vs 1%–6%), further multicenter studies are necessary to better define the safety of NOM of high-grade IV-V injuries before conclusions regarding operative versus embolization intervention.[80,86]

Advances in Embolization Techniques

Advancements in the embolization techniques also may be contributing to the lower failure rates reported recently. Previous protocol used gel foam, steel wool, or Tornado

Table 3
Selective angiogram strategy with angiograms performed on all hemodynamically stable patients with BST and CB on admission CT

Institution	Journal (Year)	Total, n	NOM, n (%)	Routine AE Grade	Overall FNOM, %	Successful Management of High-Grade III-V or IV-V with NOM, %
State University of New York[86]	J Trauma (2005)	648	368 (57)	III-IV	6	80
University of Florida Jacksonville[80]	J Trauma (2017)	712	190 (85)	IV-V	1	97

Angioembolization was performed for those with active extravasation on angiogram and bed rest without embolization those without extravasation. In addition, routine embolization was performed on all high-grade injuries III-IV or IV-V regardless of CB or not.

Abbreviations: AE, angioembolization; BST, blunt splenic trauma; CB, contrast blush; CT, computed tomography; FNOM, failure of nonoperative management; NOM, nonoperative management.

coils (https://www.cookmedical.com/products/di_mwcet_webds/, Bloomington, IN) and primarily embolized distal vessels in the splenic parenchyma close to the point of bleeding. This technique had a theoretic risk of limiting collateral blood flow to distal embolized regions and may have increased spleen necrosis and abscess formation. In response, newer techniques use primarily proximal main splenic artery embolization with selective distal embolization. Proximal main splenic artery embolization does not completely stop blood flow to the spleen parenchyma but decreases the pressure head, resulting in lower possible complications of infarction and abscess. Human studies of proximal main splenic artery embolization have demonstrated a decrease in splenic blood pressure of 47% to 58%.[75] However, given limited studies with low statistical power and lack of randomized data, conclusions regarding distal versus proximal embolization and subsequent complications are limited.

Immune Function

Immunologic function of the spleen after angiographic embolization remains questionable, although existing studies seem to suggest that splenic function is preserved.[94–96] To date, no specific marker of splenic immune function has been identified, and immune function is assessed by means of indirect tests of the spleen's viability, spleen size and perfusion, hemofiltrate, and immunologic markers (memory B-lymphocytes; total immunoglobulin (Ig)A, IgM, and IgG levels; Howell-Jolly [HJ] bodies, platelets, white blood cells, and T-cell levels).[97,98] A recent review of 11 studies with adult patients evaluated immunologic function after embolization and reported no overwhelming postsplenectomy infections and preserved immunologic function.[99] Patients treated with splenic artery ligation have been reported to have normal immunologic outcome.[100] Bessoud and colleagues[97] reported that after proximal AE, the spleens remained well perfused with HJ bodies and a sufficient immunoglobulin response to *Haemophilus influenzae* and pneumococci. Nakae and colleagues[98] compared AE patients with those who had a splenectomy; significantly higher lymphocytes, total B-cell and T-cell counts, and serum IgG levels were noted in the AE group. Malhotra and colleagues[101] reported that T-cell subgroups after AE were similar to those in healthy controls. Existing studies on immune function after AE are not sufficient for any firm conclusions to be drawn about preservation of splenic immunocompetence, but current knowledge seems to support the view that vaccination is unnecessary after embolization in most patients.[94–104]

Complications After Angioembolization

Reported complications of AE include splenic infarction, abscess, subcapsular hematoma, left pleural effusion and atelectasis, and complications due to angiography.[65,68,73,74,105–108] Aiolfi and colleagues[109] recently compared the infectious complications and mortality for patients undergoing AE versus splenectomy for high-grade IV-V injuries. The early infectious complications (11.7% vs 23.1%, $P<.001$) and mortality (5.4% vs 12.7%, $P<.001$) were significantly lower for the AE group as compared with the splenectomy group, respectively.[109]

Complications After Splenectomy

One of the driving forces for NOM was the 1952 description of overwhelming postsplenectomy infection (OPSI) and sepsis that led surgeons to look for alternative management strategies for splenic preservation.[110] Although rare in adults (estimated incidence of 0.05%), OPSI is a potentially lethal complication that can occur after splenectomy.[111] A prospective multicenter study by Demetraides and colleagues[112] recently reported that splenectomy was an independent risk factor for postinjury infectious complications, such as intra-abdominal abscesses, wound infections, pneumonia, and septicemia. A 2017 follow-up study by the same group compared splenectomy with AE for high-grade IV-V injuries and again reported significantly higher infectious complications and mortality.[109] Others have reported an increased rate of type II diabetes, thrombocytosis, and persistent hypercoagulable state, as well as venous thromboembolism after splenectomy.[113–116] Splenectomy also has been reported to be associated with a longer hospital length of stay and higher overall cost as compared to NOM.[117]

Role of Age

There remains controversy as to whether older patients (older than 55 years) with BST should undergo NOM. Several investigators have recommended routine operative management of hemodynamically stable patients with BST and age older than 55 years due to high failure rates (60%–100%) with NOM strategies.[118–122] The EAST study found a significantly higher FNOM rate in those 55 years or older than those younger than 55 years (19% vs 10%, $P<.05$).[60] More recent data have refuted age older than 55 as a contraindication to NOM. Three large retrospective studies have reported no difference in FNOM rate between age younger than 55 and age 55 or older.[123–126]

PANCREAS

The incidence of pancreatic trauma is less than 10% overall, but it varies based on mechanism of injury. Despite the low incidence, significant morbidity exists in this population, and there are times when traditional dogma must be ignored in favor of maneuvers that require a gloved hand on the human pancreas.[127,128] This section will characterize the current trends in the diagnosis and treatment of traumatic pancreatic injuries.

Diagnosis

The American Association for the Surgery of Trauma (AAST) organ injury scale for pancreatic injury is based on anatomic severity of injury, and it is displayed in **Table 4**.[128] Despite the lack of quality prospective data on the treatment of pancreatic trauma, the AAST organ injury grade for pancreatic trauma allows individualized treatment of this population.[129] Surrogates for gross anatomic description require further diagnostic testing with varying success, as summarized in the following sections (**Table 5**).

Table 4		
American Association for the Surgery of Trauma pancreas organ injury scale		
Grade[a]		**Injury Description**
I	Hematoma	Major contusion without duct injury or tissue loss
	Laceration	Major laceration without duct injury or tissue loss
II	Hematoma	Involving more than 1 portion
	Laceration	Disruption <50% of circumference
III	Laceration	Distal transection or parenchymal injury with duct injury
IV	Laceration	Proximal (to right of superior mesenteric vein) transection or parenchymal injury
V	Laceration	Massive disruption of pancreatic head

[a] Advance 1 grade for multiple injuries to the same organ.

From Moore EE, Cogbill TH, Malangoni MA, et al. Organ injury scaling, II: pancreas, duodenum, small bowel, colon, and rectum. J Trauma 1990;30(11):1427; with permission.

Table 5
Sensitivity and specificity of diagnostic tests for pancreatic trauma

Diagnostic Modality	Utility
Amylase/lipase	85% Sensitive, 100% Specific
Computed tomography	>36% sensitive, >90% specific
MRI/MRCP	Accuracy approaches 100%
ERCP	Accuracy approaches 100%

Abbreviations: ERCP, endoscopic retrograde cholangiopancreatography; MRCP, magnetic resonance cholangiopancreatography.

Laboratory tests

Serum pancreatic enzyme levels for the diagnosis of pancreatic trauma are limited in their usefulness. Studies that detail the utility of both serum amylase and lipase in the diagnosis of abdominal injury were shown to be 85% sensitive for the diagnosis of pancreatic injury when obtained in concert.[130] Serum amylase and lipase levels also increase with hollow viscus injury, so true organ injury localization is difficult without imaging.[131] Because the treatment of pancreatic injury hinges on the grade of pancreatic injury,[132] the true application of laboratory analysis for the diagnosis of pancreatic injury in trauma is limited to countries where access to advanced imaging is not possible or in the pediatric population in which reduction in the quantity of radiation exposure is standard of care.[130,131] In this way, laboratory values also may be used as a screening tool in settings in which CT imaging of the abdomen and pelvis is not routinely performed.

Computed tomography

CT is the diagnostic imaging modality in trauma, and the utilization of cross-sectional imaging has even been validated in the postoperative setting after laparotomy for penetrating trauma.[133] Unfortunately, the yield of CT in the diagnosis of pancreatic injury, especially in the setting of blunt trauma, remains low.[134–137] In a multicenter AAST study, patients who underwent laparotomy after preoperative CT were evaluated for pancreatic parenchymal and ductal injury. The sensitivity of CT for diagnosis of pancreatic injury was between 47% and 60%, and the specificity for the diagnosis of pancreatic duct injury was between 90% and 94%.[136] In an updated study in which only modern CT technology was used, the sensitivity for identification of pancreatic injury was 36%.[137] When focusing on pancreatic ductal injury, there is a greater than 90% sensitivity and specificity for injury diagnosis.[137] The distinction between the diagnosis of pancreatic parenchymal injury and ductal injury is critical because of the difference in operative management between these 2 entities.[129]

MRI

The lengthy examination time of MRI makes it prohibitive in the acute trauma setting, but it does correlate well with the capabilities of CT in the diagnosis of both pancreatic injury and pancreatic duct injury in the setting of blunt force trauma.[138] Magnetic resonance cholangiopancreatography (MRCP) also has been used with and without secretin stimulation to image the pancreas after trauma. In a small series, MRCP identified both parenchymal and ductal injuries with 100% accuracy, rivaling endoscopic retrograde cholangiopancreatography (ERCP) without adding procedural risk.[139]

Endoscopic retrograde cholangiopancreatography

A technique that can be both diagnostic and therapeutic, ERCP has proven to be valuable in the management of pancreatic trauma.[140–143] In a recent study, Kim and colleagues[141] found that in a population of patients with known pancreatic trauma, ERCP identified pancreatic ductal injuries with a greater efficacy than that of CT imaging. In fact, 41% of patients who had pancreatic ductal injuries were missed by initial cross-sectional imaging, but were appropriately identified with ERCP.

Nonoperative Management

NOM of pancreatic trauma can, in general, be guided by the same continuum that guides NOM of all traumatic injuries. It should be considered only in the absence of peritonitis and hemodynamic instability. An additional consideration in pancreatic trauma is the status of the pancreatic duct. Follow-up of pancreatic injury managed nonoperatively should include serial physical and laboratory examinations, with deteriorations in either necessitating early action with cross-sectional imaging.[131,132,144]

External drainage

Studies that describe NOM of pancreatic ductal injury are few, but with careful follow-up, the combination of bowel rest, serial imaging, and percutaneous image-directed drainage can be effective. In a recent analysis, there was no difference in complication rate between groups managed operatively and those managed nonoperatively. The nonsurgical group did have a longer length of stay and some went home with percutaneous drains in place, but the utilization of this approach maybe valuable in patients with prohibitive surgical risk.[145]

Internal drainage

ERCP was described previously in the diagnosis of pancreatic ductal injuries. Ductal imaging using real-time intraluminal contrast allows for superior visualization of the pancreatic ductal system, along with the additional benefit of therapeutic intervention at the time of diagnosis. In a series of 43 pancreatic ductal injuries, there were no differences in mortality or pancreas-related complications in either the ERCP stent or operative resection groups. Thus, ERCP provides a less invasive way of controlling pancreatic drainage in the setting of ductal injury.[141] In a smaller study with long-term follow-up, the incidence of pancreatic stricture after stenting for pancreatic ductal injury approached 100%.[146] Additionally, ERCP carries procedural risks of pancreatitis (3%) and bleeding (<1%).[147] Although ERCP has a role in the diagnosis of pancreatic ductal injury, its role in the pancreatic duct injury management algorithm remains unsettled due to its long-term complication risks.

Octreotide

There is a paucity of data to promote octreotide use after pancreatic trauma. Amirata and colleagues[148] showed elimination of all pancreatic complications in a small sample size with use of prophylactic octreotide after pancreatic trauma. A larger study by Nwariaku and colleagues[149] showed directly oppositional results with the use of octreotide after pancreatic trauma, and these results support the largest meta-analysis showing no influence on pancreatic fistula rate with octreotide use after pancreaticoduodenectomy.[150] Importantly, the cost of octreotide often makes its use prohibitive.

Operative Management

The status of the pancreatic duct and the location of the injury guide surgical management of pancreatic trauma whether it is diagnosed during a laparotomy or with preoperative imaging (**Table 6**). In general, the "crawfish approach" (suck the head and eat

Table 6		
Operative management of pancreatic trauma by AAST organ injury scale		
AAST Grade	**Preferred Treatment**	
I-II	Observation/Drainage	
III	Distal pancreatectomy	
IV-V	Drainage, endoscopic stenting, pancreaticoduodenectomy, enteral drainage options	

Abbreviation: AAST, American Association for the Surgery of Trauma.

From Moore EE, Cogbill TH, Malangoni MA, et al. Organ injury scaling, II: pancreas, duodenum, small bowel, colon, and rectum. J Trauma 1990;30(11):1427–9; with permission.

the tail) to pancreatic trauma treatment continues to hold true, with drainage being appropriate for most injuries to the pancreatic head and resection being appropriate for ductal injuries to the pancreatic tail. The presence of pancreatic ductal injury advances AAST grade into the III-V categories, which are generally managed with resection or stenting.[132,151] Injuries discovered at the time of laparotomy that do not have duct involvement can be managed with surgical drainage alone.[128]

Surgical drainage

In the absence of main duct injury, drainage of the pancreas is the recommended operative treatment. The continuum of pancreatic drainage has evolved from open drainage, to sump drainage, and finally closed suction drainage. The use of closed suction drainage was validated in a randomized trial that showed a reduction in septic complications of pancreatic trauma in the patients with closed suction drainage.[152]

Resection

Pancreatic resection is recommended when the pancreatic duct is injured. The resection plan is determined by 2 factors: the proximity of the injury to the superior mesenteric vasculature and status of the duodenum.

For those injuries to the left of the mesenteric vasculature, distal pancreatectomy is the preferred operation.[153–155] When choosing the modality of pancreatic closure, there is likely no superior method, and this trend was observed in a multicenter retrospective study of outcomes after distal pancreatectomy.[155] The value of splenic preservation during distal pancreatectomy is another option, and it may be considered in the hemodynamically stable pediatric trauma patient. There are certainly studies that support splenic preservation,[156,157] but in the adult trauma population, an expeditious operation is preferred.

For complex injuries that are anatomically located adjacent to or to the right of the mesenteric vessels, there is no unanimous treatment algorithm. Options range from duodenal and pancreatic drainage procedures to the pancreaticoduodenectomy,[132] and the current prevailing methodology is that "less is more," particularly in the acute trauma setting. The most aggressive surgical option is the pancreaticoduodenectomy, which is sometimes the only surgical option in combined pancreatic and duodenal injuries. In an assessment from the National Trauma Data Bank, increasing injury severity score was associated with worse outcomes after pancreaticoduodenectomy. In this analysis, the patients who were treated with operative intervention short of pancreaticoduodenectomy had equivalent outcomes despite worse initial physiologic parameters.[158] There are data to support the use of pancreaticoduodenectomy, and in a large single-center study, there was 28% mortality for patients who underwent said operation even in the era of the damage control laparotomy. In this study, combined vascular and pancreaticoduodenal injury was associated with worsened mortality.[159]

Outcomes

Trauma to the pancreas is associated with significant morbidity. In a large, single-center study, Kao and colleagues[160] reported 50% morbidity for patients with pancreatic trauma, and 22% of these patients had pancreas-related complications. Additionally, higher grades of pancreatic injury were associated with increased rates of both morbidity and mortality. With regard to pancreatic function after pancreatic trauma, insulin requirements are rare even after pancreatic resection for trauma. However, there was an association with insulin requirements in those patients who had a proximal pancreatic resection.[161] Delayed complications of pancreatic trauma include pseudocyst formation, pancreatic fistulas, and pancreatic strictures, with the incidence of complications reported to be less than 10%, pseudocyst formation being the most common of the three.[162]

Although prospective data for the diagnosis and treatment of pancreatic trauma is sparse, the following can summarize the management of this entity:

1. Identify the status of the pancreatic duct
2. Perform an anatomically guided resection if the duct is injured
3. Drain the peripancreatic space

Pancreatic trauma continues to be problematic, but choosing simple treatment options seems to be the best way to prevent major complications.

KIDNEY

Although traumatic renal injuries are relatively uncommon and are present in only 1% of patients hospitalized following a traumatic injury, the kidney remains the most commonly injured genitourinary organ.[163–165] Present in approximately one-quarter of patients with blunt abdominal trauma and affecting men 3 times more frequently than women, traumatic renal injuries represent a significant disease burden in both the developed and developing worlds.[166,167] Blunt trauma is the causative mechanism in the vast majority of renal injuries, comprising approximately 80% to 90% of injuries in most contemporary series.[163,165–169] This is largely due to the particular vulnerability of the kidney to deceleration injuries following high-velocity impact trauma, as it is essentially tethered in place by just the vascular pedicle and renal pelvis.[170,171] However, in more urban areas with higher rates of gun and knife violence, or regions with high levels of civil unrest, rates of penetrating renal trauma are much higher.[163,172–174]

Renal injuries occur along a spectrum, with most injuries being on the milder side of this range.[164] However, for those with more severe traumas, these injuries can cause significant hemorrhage and be life-threatening. As such, appropriate evaluation and grading is essential to risk-stratify patients for the potential need for intervention and to prevent potentially devastating complications. It has become the general consensus of most experts in the field of genitourinary trauma that the vast majority of renal injuries can be managed conservatively; however, there are still a number of indicators for intervention. Recognition of these indicators requires appropriate patient evaluation and injury grading, as well as close collaboration among trauma surgeons, urologists, and interventional radiologists.

Evaluation and Grading

The American Urological Association (AUA), European Association of Urology (EAU), and the Société Internationale d'Urologie (SIU) all have guideline statements regarding the recommended evaluation and management of renal trauma.[175–177] In all 3 guidelines, the initial step in evaluation of patients with potential renal injury is assessment of hemodynamic stability. Hemodynamically unstable patients should be considered for immediate intervention, the modality of which depends on associated injury patterns and institutional expertise. Patients undergoing exploratory laparotomy should undergo retroperitoneal exploration to manage life-threatening retroperitoneal bleeds, although this often results in nephrectomy. Otherwise, patients at high-volume, experienced trauma centers who do not require open operative intervention for other indications should be considered for AE with interventional radiology, as this has been shown to increase rates of renal salvage and decrease need for nephrectomy.[165,178] However, this should be undertaken only at centers in which patients can be actively resuscitated and monitored during preparation for and transport to the interventional radiology suite, and where quick access to the operating room is readily available in cases of AE failure.

All hemodynamically stable patients presenting with a history of blunt abdominal trauma and gross hematuria warrant intravenous contrast-enhanced spiral CT imaging with 10-minute delayed excretory images to rule out renal injury at presentation. Similarly, the AUA guidelines recommend performing dedicated imaging for patients with microscopic hematuria (>5 RBCs per high power field) and initial systolic blood pressures lower than than 90 mm Hg, or in cases in which the mechanism of injury or physical examination findings raise significant suspicion for potential renal injury.[175] Such findings include significant flank ecchymosis, rib fractures, history of targeted flank or rib injury, or rapid deceleration injury. Similarly, patients presenting with penetrating trauma to the flank or upper back, regardless of the presence or absence of hematuria, should have dedicated renal imaging, given the high incidence of associated renal injury.[177]

The AAST proposed a standardized grading system for renal trauma in 1989, which remains to this day the gold standard tool for assessment of traumatic renal injuries.[179] This scoring system is based on imaging findings seen on initial presenting CT scans (see **Fig. 1**) and has been shown in numerous studies to significantly correlate with prognosis, need for intervention, and mortality.[180–182] An additional substratification scheme was published in 2009 that further classified grade IV injuries into low-risk and high-risk categories.[183] These investigators found that patients presenting with grade IV injuries with 2 to 3 high-risk radiographic findings (medial renal laceration, large perirenal hematoma >3.5 cm, or evidence of intravascular contrast extravasation) were significantly more likely to require intervention for renal bleeding and, thus, these investigators concluded, should be considered for earlier intervention. Taken together, the AAST grading of renal injuries serves as an important diagnostic and prognostic marker, as management decisions are significantly influenced by injury grade, as are risks of long-term complications.

Indications for Intervention

There has been a significant shift over time as to the preferred management strategies for both blunt and penetrating renal traumas, and the AUA guidelines, in accordance, recommend a trial period of conservative management in all stable patients before intervention for injuries of any grade.[175] Although higher-grade injuries have been shown to be associated with higher rates of operative intervention, appropriately staged grade IV and V injuries can potentially be managed conservatively if carefully selected and monitored.[177,183–185] Recent data show that fewer than 5% of blunt injuries and 36% of penetrating renal injuries undergo operative intervention, suggesting that even in cases of penetrating trauma, conservative management appears to serve an appropriate role.[165] Renal artery thrombosis can similarly be expectantly managed, presuming there is a functional and uninvolved contralateral kidney.[177,186,187]

Patients with grade IV injuries with urinary extravasation may similarly be managed expectantly, as 75% to 85% of these injuries will resolve without intervention.[176,188,189] However, reimaging of all patients with grade IV or V injuries remains vital and an important component of the AUA guidelines, as patients with these injuries in particular are at risk for developing significant complications.[175] Patients with grade III or lower do not require routine follow-up imaging.[183] Follow-up imaging has been recommended at 48 to 72 hours following presentation to determine the size of the perirenal hematoma and degree of urinary extravasation in all grade IV or V patients. Patients who show evidence of stable or worsening urinary extravasation likely require intervention in the form of cystoscopy and ureteral stenting, and possible percutaneous urinoma drainage, as well as bladder decompression with a Foley to optimize urinary drainage.[172,188]

The only absolute indication for intervention, either surgical or percutaneous, remains life-threatening hemorrhage in an unstable patient.[176] Similarly, unstable patients brought to the operating room for laparotomy who are noted to have a pulsatile, expanding retroperitoneal hematoma should undergo retroperitoneal exploration. Relative indications that remain a point of discussion in the literature include patients whose injuries are incompletely staged radiographically and who are undergoing operations for other indications, as well as patients who display a significant volume of devitalized parenchymal tissue on cross-sectional imaging. Historically, penetrating injuries were absolute indications for intervention; however, more contemporary series have shown that these patients can similarly be managed conservatively in most settings.[190,191] NOM in stable patients following penetrating trauma has previously been shown to be successful in 50% of stab injuries and up to 40% of gunshot wounds, although data are beginning to show even higher success rates.[192] Last, stable patients with persistent blood loss should be considered for intervention, although these patients can often forego open surgical procedures and proceed directly to interventional radiology for AE.

Angioembolization

Although many patients are able to avoid any sort of intervention for traumatic renal injuries, a subset of patients will ultimately require intervention for persistent renal bleeding. This bleeding can be due to the injury itself, as well as to subsequent arteriovenous fistulas or pseudoaneurysms that develop following the initial insult. Angiography and AE represent the primary management option in patients requiring intervention who are not undergoing laparotomy for other indications and should be the first therapy offered to most patients.[177] One recent institutional series showed that 94.4% of grade IV and V renal traumas were successfully managed with a combination of observation and AE.[193] In general, patients are best served by AE if bleeding is limited to segmental vessels rather than the main renal vasculature, as studies have shown poor success in attempts to embolize these larger vessels.[194–196]

Grade V renal injuries represent a unique controversy in management. Although some studies have shown 100% failure of embolization of grade V injuries, others have noted 100% success.[194,197] As such, there remains a significant need for more data to better evaluate angiographic management for high-grade injuries. It should be noted that embolization has been shown to be 3 times more likely to fail following penetrating trauma, and, thus, options after failed conservative management of these injuries must be carefully considered.[177,198]

Open Surgical Intervention

Open surgical exploration is indicated in cases of initial hemodynamic instability on presentation and where an expanding, pulsatile retroperitoneal hematoma is encountered in the operating room, as well as in cases in which patients show evidence of persistent intravascular contrast extravasation and ongoing blood loss. Similarly, patients with persistent bleeding in the setting of grade V renal injuries should be considered for open surgical intervention, although some centers may advocate for AE, as previously discussed. Last, patients with significantly devascularized segments of the affected kidney should be considered for debridement and renal reconstruction in attempts for renal salvage, although this is generally performed only at high-volume centers with significant experience with urologic trauma. Even in patients undergoing laparotomy for other indications, conservative management of renal trauma often can be used as long as the patient is hemodynamically stable and there is no evidence of a pulsatile or expanding retroperitoneal hematoma.[199] This is because most retroperitoneal bleeding can usually be contained within the Gerota fascia, leading to a tamponade effect.

Patients with higher-grade renal injuries are much more likely to undergo nephrectomy once operative intervention is undertaken and even patients who undergo operations in which renorrhaphy or partial nephrectomy of devitalized tissues are intended, nephrectomy is often the end result.[165,177,200] As such, operative intervention should be limited to extreme cases, as preservation of functioning renal parenchyma should be prioritized whenever reasonably possible. Attempts at renal salvage in patients with significant vascular injuries involving the main renal arteries have been attempted; however, even in the most experienced of hands, salvage rates are low, ranging from just 6% to 40%.[201-204] As such, these types of procedures should be reserved for patients with either a solitary kidney or bilateral renal injury.

Follow-up and Complications

Patients who are managed conservatively, as well as those who undergo intervention for renal trauma are at risk for complications in the postacute and chronic settings. In general, following repeat imaging 48 to 72 hours after injury, routing imaging is not a requirement in the absence of clinical concern. The SIU and EAU recommend routine nuclear renal scans in follow-up as an outpatient to evaluate differential renal function return, whereas the AUA recommends against routine imaging due to inadequate benefit, as this information would be useful only in the presence of a compelling clinical indication for further intervention.[175-177] However, all 3 guidelines recommend that patients undergo routine blood pressure monitoring due to the small risk of postinjury hypertension.

As previously discussed, worsening urinary extravasation with conservative management puts patients at risk for subsequent infection and persistence of a urine leak. As such, if enlargement of the urinoma is encountered on follow-up imaging 48 to 72 hours after instituting conservative management, endoscopic placement of a ureteral stent should be performed with Foley catheter placement.[188] In the absence of confirmatory imaging, clinical signs, such as worsening renal function, worsening flank pain, decreased urine output, fever, and leukocytosis, may be evidence of an accumulating urinoma.[199] Percutaneous drainage of urinoma collections may in addition to stent placement, specifically if clinical signs of infection are present. As advocated by Alsikafi and colleagues,[188] ureteral stents are usually left in place for approximately 6 weeks, after which time the stent can be removed with or without repeat retrograde pyelography to confirm cessation of extravasation. The recommended duration of Foley catheterization in this setting is not uniform, although in the previously referenced report catheters remained indwelling for an average of 7 days after stent placement.

Delayed hemorrhage is a particularly devastating potential complication after renal trauma. Seen in up to 25% of patients with grade III or higher injuries managed conservatively, providers must have a high suspicion for either arteriovenous fistulization or pseudoaneurysm formation in patients who present with either recurrent gross hematuria or a drifting hematocrit days to weeks after trauma.[176,205] This is particularly true for patients after penetrating traumas, as they are at significantly higher risk for delayed bleeding relative to patients with blunt trauma.[176,177] Initial management is generally conservative with bed rest and hydration, although for patients with persistent bleeding, AE is often required.

Hypertension is often noted as a potential complication after renal trauma, although the true rate of occurrence is likely less than 5% and is directly related to the severity of injury experienced.[199,206] The etiology of hypertension can be due to 1 or more factors directly resulting from injury, including injury to and compression of the renal artery leading elevated renin release (Goldblatt kidney), direct compression of the renal parenchyma from a surrounding hematoma (Page kidney), or from an arteriovenous fistula formation. Medical management is generally used as first-line therapy; however, some patients ultimately require decortication of subcapsular hematomas (in the case of Page kidneys) or nephrectomy to control refractory renovascular hypertension.

The kidney remains the most commonly injured genitourinary organ, as well as one of the most commonly injured solid organs of the abdomen. Although historical practice was to operatively intervene on most patients with significant renal trauma, current guidelines recommend attempts at conservative management to preserve as many functioning nephrons as possible, even in cases of high-grade injury. For those patients who do require intervention, percutaneous approaches by interventional radiology have grown in favor and success and represent the preferred initial management strategy. Formal operative intervention is now reserved for those who require emergent laparotomy or in centers in which AE is not available.

SUMMARY

In summary, the management of solid organ injuries has greatly evolved over the past 20 years. NOM has become the initial management strategy used for most solid organ injuries. Even though NOM has become the standard of care in patients with solid organ injuries in most trauma centers, surgeons should not hesitate to operate on a patient to control life-threatening hemorrhage. A safe and effective surgical hemostasis and a carefully planned multidisciplinary approach can improve the outcome of severe liver trauma.

REFERENCES

1. Malhotra AK, Fabian TC, Croce MA, et al. Blunt hepatic injury: a paradigm shift from operative to nonoperative management in the 1990s. Ann Surg 2000;231: 804–13.
2. Richardson JD, Franklin GA, Lukan JK, et al. Evolution in the management of hepatic trauma: a 25-years perspective. Ann Surg 2000;232:324–30.
3. Stassen NA, Bhullar I, Cheng JD, et al, Eastern Association for the Surgery of Trauma. Nonoperative management of blunt hepatic injury: an Eastern Association for the Surgery of Trauma practice management guideline. J Trauma Acute Care Surg 2012;73(5 Suppl 4):S288–93.
4. Richardson JD. Changes in the management of injuries to the liver and spleen. J Am Coll Surg 2005;200(5):648–69.

5. Moore EE, Shackford SR, Pachter HL. Organ injury scaling: spleen, liver and kidney. J Trauma 1995;38:323–4.
6. Piper GL, Peitzman AB. Current management of hepatic trauma. Surg Clin North Am 2010;90:775–85.
7. Carrillo EH, Richardson JD. The current management of hepatic trauma. Adv Surg 2001;35:39–59.
8. Christmas AB, Wilson AK, Manning B, et al. Selective management of blunt hepatic injuries including non-operative management is a safe and effective strategy. Surgery 2005;138:606–11.
9. Poletti PA, Mirvis SE, Shanmuganathan K, et al. CT criteria for management of blunt liver trauma: correlation with angiography and surgical findings. Radiology 2000;216:418–27.
10. Gaarder C, Naess PA, Eken T, et al. Liver injuries—improved results with a formal protocol including angiography. Injury 2007;38:1075–83.
11. Hagiwara AT, Yukioka T, Ohta S, et al. Nonsurgical management of patients with blunt hepatic injury: efficacy of transcatheter arterial embolization. AJR Am J Roentgenol 1997;169:1151–6.
12. Croce MA, Fabian TC, Menke PG, et al. Nonoperative management of blunt hepatic trauma is the treatment of choice for hemodynamically stable patients. Results of a prospective trial. Ann Surg 1995;221:744–53.
13. Yang EY, Marder SR, Hastings G, et al. The abdominal compartment syndrome complicating nonoperative management of major blunt liver injuries: recognition and treatment using multimodality therapy. J Trauma 2002;52:982–6.
14. Asensio JA, Demetriades D, Chahwan S, et al. Approach to the management of complex hepatic injuries. J Trauma 2000;48:66–9.
15. Shapiro M, Jenkins D, Schwab CW, et al. Damage control: collective review. J Trauma 2000;49:969–78.
16. Sriussadaporn S, Pak-art R, Tharavej C, et al. A multidisciplinary approach in the management of hepatic injuries. Injury 2002;33:309–15.
17. Jansen JO, Thomas R, Loudon MA, Brooks A. Damage control resuscitation for patients with major trauma. BMJ 2009;338:b1778.
18. Jansen JO, Thomas R, Loudon MA, et al. Damage control resuscitation for patients with major trauma. BMJ 2009;338:b1778.
19. Duchesne JC, Barbeau JM, Islam TM, et al. Damage control resuscitation: from emergency department to the operating room. Am Surg 2011;77:201–6.
20. Biffl WL, Barnett CC Jr. Surgical treatment of liver and biliary tree trauma. Chapter 8. In: Di Saverio S, Tugnoli G, Catena F, et al, editors. Trauma surgery. Milan (Italy): Springer-Verlag; 2014. p. 99–115.
21. Kozar RA, Feliciano DV, Moore EE, et al. Western Trauma Association critical decisions in trauma: operative management of adult blunt hepatic trauma. J Trauma 2011;71:1–5.
22. Aydin U, Yazici P, Zeytunlu M, et al. Is it more dangerous to perform inadequate packing? World J Emerg Surg 2008;14(3):1.
23. Brasfield RD. New liver suture. JAMA 1960;173(2):162.
24. Logmans A, Schoenmakers CH, Haensel SM, et al. High tissue factor concentration in the omentum, a possible cause of its hemostatic properties. Eur J Clin Invest 1996;26(1):82–3.
25. Demetriades D. Balloon tamponade for bleeding control in penetrating liver injuries. J Trauma 1998;44:538–9.
26. Badger SA, Barclay R, Campbell P, et al. Management of liver trauma. World J Surg 2009;33:2522–37.

27. Pachter HL, Spencer FC, Hofstetter SR, et al. Significant trends in the treatment of hepatic injuries. Experience with 411 injuries. Ann Surg 1992;215:492–500.

28. Beal SL. Fatal hepatic hemorrhage: an unresolved problem in the management of complex liver injuries. J Trauma 1990;30:163–9.

29. Moore FA, Moore EE, Seagraves A. Non-resectional management of major hepatic trauma: an evolving concept. Am J Surg 1985;150:725–9.

30. Cogbill TH, Moore EE, Jurkovich GJ, et al. Severe hepatic trauma: a multicenter experience with 1335 liver injuries. J Trauma 1988;28:1433–8.

31. Fabian TC, Croce MA, Stanford GG, et al. Factors affecting morbidity following hepatic trauma: a prospective analysis of 482 injuries. Ann Surg 1991;213: 540–8.

32. Rovito PF. Atrial caval shunting in blunt hepatic vascular injury. Ann Surg 1987; 205:318–21.

33. Burch JM, Feliciano DV, Mattox KL. The atriocaval shunt: facts and fiction. Ann Surg 1988;207:555–68.

34. Buechter KJ, Sereda D, Gomez G, et al. Retrohepatic vein injuries: experience with 20 cases. J Trauma 1989;29:1698–704.

35. Walt AJ, Levison MA. Hepatic trauma: juxta-hepatic vena cava injury. In: Champion HE, Robbs JV, Trunkey DD, editors. Rob and Smith's operative surgery. Trauma surgery. Boston: Butterworths; 1992. p. 374–84.

36. Buckman RF, Miraliakbari R, Badellino MM. Juxtahepatic venous injuries: a critical review of reported management strategies. J Trauma 2000;48:978–84.

37. Schrock T, Blaisdell W, Mathewson C Jr. Management of blunt trauma to the liver and hepatic veins. Arch Surg 1968;96:698–704.

38. Baumgartner F, Scudamore C, Nair C, et al. Venovenous bypass for major hepatic and caval trauma. J Trauma 1995;39:671–3.

39. Abdalla EK, Noun R, Belghiti J. Hepatic vascular occlusion: which technique? Surg Clin North Am 2004;84:563–85.

40. Carrillo EH, Wohltmann C, Richardson JD, et al. Evolution in the treatment of complex blunt liver injuries. Curr Probl Surg 2001;38:1–60.

41. Kozar RA, Moore JB, Niles SE, et al. Complications of nonoperative management of high-grade blunt hepatic injuries. J Trauma 2005;59:1066–71.

42. Ciraulo DL, Luk S, Palter M, et al. Selective hepatic arterial embolization of grade IV and V blunt hepatic injuries: an extension of resuscitation in the nonoperative management of traumatic hepatic injuries. J Trauma 1998;45:353–8.

43. Wahl WL, Brandt MM, Hemmila MR, et al. Diagnosis and management of bile leaks after blunt liver injury. Surgery 2005;138:742–7.

44. Carrillo EH, Spain DA, Wohltmann CD, et al. Interventional techniques are useful adjuncts in nonoperative management of hepatic injuries. J Trauma 1999;46: 619–22.

45. Carrillo EH, Reed DN Jr, Gordon L, et al. Delayed laparoscopy facilitates the management of biliary peritonitis in patients with complex liver injuries. Surg Endosc 2001;15:319–22.

46. Carrillo EH, Richardson JD. Delayed surgery and interventional procedures in complex liver injuries. J Trauma 1999;46:978.

47. MacKenzie S, Kortbeek JB, Mulloy R, et al. Recent experiences with a multidisciplinary approach to complex hepatic trauma. Injury 2004;35:869–77.

48. Billroth T. Clinical Surgery. London: New Sydenham Society; 1881.p. 229.

49. Sherman R. Perspectives in management of trauma to the spleen: 1979 presidential address, American Association for the Surgery of Trauma. J Trauma 1980 Jan;20(1):1–13.

50. Gross SD. System of surgery. Philadelphia: H.C. Lea; 1866. Available at: https://archive.org/details/systemofsurgeryp001gros. Accessed July 24, 2017.
51. Upadhyaya P, Simpson JS. Splenic trauma in children. Surg Gynecol Obstet 1968;126(4):781–90.
52. Upadhyaya P, Nayak NC, Moitra S. Experimental study of splenic trauma in monkeys. J Pediatr Surg 1971;6(6):767–73.
53. Malangoni MA, Levine AW, Droege EA, et al. Management of injury to the spleen in adults. Ann Surg 1994;200:702–5.
54. Mahon PA, Sutton JE. Nonoperative management of adult splenic injury due to blunt trauma: a warning. Am J Surg 1985;149:716–21.
55. Pachter HL, Hofstetter SR, Spencer FC. Evolving concepts in splenic surgery. Ann Surg 1981;194:262–9.
56. Millikan JS, Moore EE, Moore GE, et al. Alternatives to splenectomy in adults after trauma. Am J Surg 1982;144:711–6.
57. Wesson DE, Filler RM, Ein SH, et al. Ruptured spleen—when to operate? J Pediatr Surg 1981;16:324–6.
58. Cogbill TH, Moore EE, Jurkovich GJ, et al. Nonoperative management of blunt splenic trauma: a multicenter experience. J Trauma 1989;29:1312–7.
59. Pachter HL, Guth AA, Hofstetter SR, et al. Changing patterns in the management of splenic trauma. Ann Surg 1998;227:708–19.
60. Peitzman AB, Heil B, Rivera L, et al. Blunt splenic injury in adults: multi-institutional study of the Eastern Association for the Surgery of Trauma. J Trauma 2000;49:187–9.
61. Sclafani SJ. The role of angiographic hemostasis in salvage of injured spleen. Radiology 1981;141:645–50.
62. Schurr MJ, Fabian TC, Gavant M, et al. Management of blunt splenic trauma: computed tomographic contrast blush predicts failure of nonoperative management. J Trauma 1995;39:507–13.
63. Bhullar IS, Frykberg ER, Siragusa D, et al. Selective angiographic embolization of blunt splenic traumatic injuries in adults decreases failure rate of nonoperative management. J Trauma 2012;72:1127–34.
64. Requarth JA, D'Agostino RB, Miller PR. Nonoperative management of adult blunt splenic injury with and without splenic artery embolotherapy: a meta-analysis. J Trauma 2011;71:898–903.
65. Haan J, Scott J, Boyd-Kranis RL, et al. Admission angiography for blunt splenic injury: advantages and pitfalls. J Trauma 2001;51:1161–5.
66. Dent D, Alsabrook G, Erickson BA, et al. Blunt splenic injuries: high nonoperative management rate can be achieved with selective embolization. J Trauma 2004;56:1063–7.
67. Sclafani SJ, Weisberg A, Scalea TM, et al. Blunt splenic injuries: nonsurgical treatment with CT, arteriography, and transcatheter arterial embolization of the splenic artery. Radiology 1991;18:189–96.
68. Sclafani SJ, Shaftan GW, Scalea TM, et al. Nonoperative salvage of computer tomography–diagnosed splenic injuries: utilization of angiography for triage and embolization for hemostasis. J Trauma 1995;39:818–25.
69. Davis KA, Fabian TC, Croce MA, et al. Improved success in the nonoperative management of blunt splenic injuries: embolization of splenic artery pseudoaneurysms. J Trauma 1998;44:1008–13.
70. Haan J, Ilahi ON, Kramer M, et al. Protocol-driven nonoperative management in patients with blunt splenic trauma and minimal associated injury decreases length of stay. J Trauma 2003;55:317–21.

71. Liu PP, Lee WC, Cheng YF, et al. Use of splenic artery embolization as an adjunct to nonsurgical management of blunt splenic injury. J Trauma 2004;56: 768–72.

72. Hagiwara A, Yukioka T, Ohta S, et al. Nonsurgical management of patients with blunt splenic injury: efficacy of transcatheter arterial embolization. AJR Am J Roentgenol 1996;167:159–66.

73. Haan JM, Biffl W, Knudson M, et al. Splenic embolization revisited: a multicenter review for the Western Trauma Association multi-institutional trials committee. J Trauma 2004;56:542–7.

74. Haan JM, Bochicchio GV, Kramer N, et al. Nonoperative management of blunt splenic injury: a 5-year experience. J Trauma 2005;58:492–8.

75. Bessoud B, Denys A. Main splenic artery embolization using coils in blunt splenic injuries: effects on the intrasplenic blood pressure. Eur Radiol 2004; 14:1718–9.

76. Duchesne JC, Simmons JD, McSwain NE, et al. Proximal splenic angioembolization does not improve outcomes in treating blunt splenic injuries compared with splenectomy: a cohort analysis. J Trauma 2008;65:1346–53.

77. Harbrecht BG, Ko SH, Watson GA, et al. Angiography for blunt splenic trauma does not improve the success rate of nonoperative management. J Trauma 2007;63:44–9.

78. Smith HE, Biffl WL, Majercik SD, et al. Splenic artery embolization: have we gone too far? J Trauma 2006;61:541–6.

79. Wu SC, Chen RJ, Yang AD, et al. Complications associated with embolization in the treatment of blunt splenic injury. World J Surg 2008;32:476–82.

80. Bhullar IS, Tepas JT, Siragusa D, et al. To nearly come full circle: Nonoperative management of high grade IV-V blunt splenic trauma is safe using a protocol with routine angioembolization. J Trauma Acute Care Surg 2017;82(4):657–64.

81. Peitzman AB, Harbrecht BG, Rivera L, et al. Failure of observation of blunt splenic injury in adults: variability in practice and adverse consequences. J Am Coll Surg 2005;201(2):179–87.

82. Velmahos GC, Chan LS, Kamel E, et al. Nonoperative management of splenic injuries: have we gone too far? Arch Surg 2000;201:179–87.

83. Ogura T, Lefor AT, Nakano M, et al. Nonoperative management of hemodynamically unstable abdominal trauma patients with angioembolization and resuscitative endovascular balloon occlusion of the aorta. J Trauma Acute Care Surg 2015;78:132–5.

84. Moore EE, Cogbill TH, Juskovich GJ, et al. Organ injury scaling: spleen and liver (1994 revision). J Trauma 1995;38:323–4.

85. Velmahos GC, Zacharias N, Emhoff TA, et al. Management of the most severely injured spleen: a multicenter study of the Research Consortium of New England Centers for Trauma (ReCONECT). Arch Surg 2010;145:456–60.

86. Miller PR, Chang MC, Hoth JJ, et al. Prospective trial of angiography and embolization for all grade III to V blunt splenic injuries: nonoperative management success rate is significantly improved. J Am Coll Surg 2014;218:644–8.

87. Sabe AA, Claridge JA, Rosenblum DI, et al. The effects of splenic artery embolization on nonoperative management of blunt splenic injury: a 16-year experience. J Trauma 2009;67:565–72.

88. Skattum J, Naess PA, Eken T, et al. Refining the role of splenic angiographic embolization in high-grade splenic injuries. J Trauma Acute Care Surg 2013; 74:100–3.

89. McCray VW, Davis JW, Lemaster D, et al. Observation for nonoperative management of the spleen: how long is long enough? J Trauma 2008;65:1354–8.

90. Bhullar IS, Frykberg ER, Tepas JJ, et al. At first blush: absence of computed tomography contrast extravasation in grade IV or V adult blunt splenic trauma should not preclude angioembolization. J Trauma Acute Care Surg 2013;74: 105–11.

91. Wahl WL, Ahrns KS, Chen S, et al. Blunt splenic injury: operation versus angiographic embolization. Surgery 2004;136:891–9.

92. Rajani RR, Claridge JA, Yowler CH, et al. Improved outcome of adult splenic injury: a cohort analysis. Surgery 2006;140:625–32.

93. Weinberg JA, Magnotti LJ, Croce MA, et al. The utility of serial computed tomography imaging of blunt splenic injury: still worth a second look? J Trauma 2007; 62:1143–8.

94. Skattum J, Naess PA, Gaarder C. Non-operative management and immune function after splenic injury. Br J Surg 2012;99(Suppl 1):59–65.

95. Miller PR, Croce MA, Bee TK, et al. Associated injuries in blunt solid organ trauma: implications of missed injury in nonoperative management. J Trauma 2001;53:238–42.

96. Stylianos S. Evidence-based guidelines for resource utilization in children with isolated spleen or liver injury. The APSA trauma committee. J Pediatr Surg 2000;35:164–7.

97. Bessoud B, Duchosal MA, Siegrist CA, et al. Proximal splenic artery embolization for blunt splenic injury: clinical, immunologic, and ultrasound-Doppler follow-up. J Trauma 2007;62:1481–6.

98. Nakae H, Shimazu T, Miyauchi H, et al. Does splenic preservation treatment (embolization, splenorrhaphy, and partial splenectomy) improve immunologic function and long-term prognosis after splenic injury? J Trauma 2009;67: 557–63.

99. Schimmer JA, van der Steeg AF, Zudema WP. Splenic function after angioembolization for splenic trauma in children and adults: a systematic review. Injury 2016;47(3):525–30.

100. Dormagen JB, Gaarder C, Sandvik L, et al. Doppler ultrasound after proximal embolization of the splenic artery in trauma patients. Eur Radiol 2008;18: 1224–31.

101. Malhotra AK, Carter RF, Lebman DA, et al. Preservation of splenic immunocompetence after splenic artery angioembolization for blunt splenic injury. J Trauma 2010;69:1126–31.

102. Tominaga GT, Simon FJ, Dandan IS, et al. Immunologic function after splenic embolization, is there a difference? J Trauma 2009;67:289–95.

103. Shih HC, Wang CY, Wen YS, et al. Spleen artery embolization aggravates endotoxin hyporesponse of peripheral blood mononuclear cells in patients with spleen injury. J Trauma 2010;68:532–7.

104. Skattum J, Titze TL, Dormagen JB, et al. Preserved splenic function after angioembolization of high grade injury. Injury 2012;43(1):62–6.

105. Killeen KL, Shanmuganathan K, Boyd-Kranis R, et al. CT findings after embolization for blunt splenic trauma. J Vasc Interv Radiol 2001;12:209–14.

106. Marincek B, Dondelinger RF. Emergency radiology. Berlin: Springer; 2007. ISBN:3540689087.

107. Bilbao JI, Martínez-Cuesta A, Urtasun F, et al. Complications of embolization. Semin Intervent Radiol 2006;23(2):126–42.

108. Ekeh AP, McCarthy MC, Woods RJ, et al. Complications arising from splenic embolization after blunt splenic trauma. Am J Surg 2005;189(3):335–9.
109. Aiolfi A, Inaba K, Strumwasser A, et al. Splenic artery embolization versus splenectomy: analysis for early in-hospital infectious complications and outcomes. J Trauma Acute Care Surg 2017. [Epub ahead of print].
110. King H, Schumacher HB. Splenic studies I: susceptibility to infection after splenectomy performed in infancy. Ann Surg 1952;136:239–42.
111. Cullingford GL, Watkins DN, Watts AD, et al. Severe late post-splenectomy infection. Br J Surg 1991;78:716–21.
112. Demetraides D, Scalea TM, Degiannis E, et al. Blunt splenic trauma: splenectomy increases early infectious complications: a prospective multicenter study. J Trauma Acute Care Surg 2012;72:229–34.
113. Ley EJ, Singer MB, Clond MA, et al. Long-term effect of trauma splenectomy on blood glucose. J Surg Res 2012;177:152–6.
114. Wu SC, Fu CY, Muo CH, et al. Splenectomy in trauma patients is associated with an increased risk of postoperative type II diabetes: a nationwide population-based study. Am J Surg 2014;208:811–6.
115. Watters JM, Sambasivan CN, Zink K, et al. Splenectomy leads to a persistent hypercoagulable state after trauma. Am J Surg 2010;199:646–51.
116. Pimpl W, Dapunt O, Kaindl H, et al. Incidence of septic shock and thromboembolic-related deaths after splenectomy in adults. Br J Surg 1989; 76:517–21.
117. Hafiz S, Desale S, Sava J, et al. The impact of solid organ injury management on the US health care system. J Trauma Acute Care Surg 2014;77:310–4.
118. Esposito TJ, Gamelli RL. Injury to the spleen. In: Feliciano DV, Moore EE, Mattox KL, editors. Trauma. Stamford (CT): Appleton and Lange; 1996. p. 538–9.
119. Godley CD, Warren RL, Sheridan RL, et al. Nonoperative management of blunt splenic injury in adults: age over 55 years as a powerful indicator for failure. J Am Coll Surg 1996;183:133–9.
120. Smith JS Jr, Wengrovitz MA, DeLong BS. Prospective validation of criteria, including age, for safe, nonsurgical management of the ruptured spleen. J Trauma 1992;33:363–9.
121. Smith JS Jr, Cooney RN, Mucha P Jr. Nonoperative management of the ruptured spleen: a revalidation of criteria. Surgery 1996;120:745–51.
122. Longo WE, Baker CC, McMillen MA, et al. Nonoperative management of adult blunt splenic trauma. Ann Surg 1989;210:626–9.
123. Clancy TV, Ramshaw DG, Maxwell JG, et al. Management outcomes in splenic injury. Ann Surg 1997;226:17–24.
124. Cocanour CS, Moore FA, Ware DN, et al. Age should not be a consideration for nonoperative management of blunt splenic injury. J Trauma 2000;48:606–12.
125. Bhullar IS, Frykberg ER, Siragusa D, et al. Age does not affect outcomes of nonoperative management of blunt splenic trauma. J Am Coll Surg 2012; 214(6):958–64.
126. Kwok AM, Davis JW, Kirks RC, et al. Time is now: venous thromboembolism prophylaxis in blunt splenic injury. Am J Surg 2016;12(6):1231–6.
127. Lin BC, Chen RJ, Fang JF, et al. Management of blunt major pancreatic injury. J Trauma 2004;56(4):774–8.
128. Vasquez JC, Coimbra R, Hoyt DB, et al. Management of penetrating pancreatic trauma: an 11-year experience of a level-1 trauma center. Injury 2001;32(10): 753–9.

129. Ho VP, Patel NJ, Bokhari F, et al. Management of adult pancreatic injuries: a practice management guideline from the Eastern Association for the Surgery of Trauma. J Trauma Acute Care Surg 2017;82(1):185–99.

130. Mahajan A, Kadavigere R, Sripathi S, et al. Utility of serum pancreatic enzyme levels in diagnosing blunt trauma to the pancreas: a prospective study with systematic review. Injury 2014;45(9):1384–93.

131. Singh RP, Garg N, Nar AS, et al. Role of amylase and lipase levels in diagnosis of blunt trauma abdomen. J Clin Diagn Res 2016;10(2):PC20–3.

132. Subramanian A, Dente CJ, Feliciano DV. The management of pancreatic trauma in the modern era. Surg Clin North Am 2007;87(6):1515–32, x.

133. Mendoza AE, Wybourn CA, Charles AG, et al. Routine computed tomography after recent operative exploration for penetrating trauma: what injuries do we miss? J Trauma Acute Care Surg 2017. [Epub ahead of print].

134. Ilahi O, Bochicchio GV, Scalea TM. Efficacy of computed tomography in the diagnosis of pancreatic injury in adult blunt trauma patients: a single-institutional study. Am Surg 2002;68(8):704–7 [discussion: 707–8].

135. Teh SH, Sheppard BC, Mullins RJ, et al. Diagnosis and management of blunt pancreatic ductal injury in the era of high-resolution computed axial tomography. Am J Surg 2007;193(5):641–3 [discussion: 643].

136. Phelan HA, Velmahos GC, Jurkovich GJ, et al. An evaluation of multidetector computed tomography in detecting pancreatic injury: results of a multicenter AAST study. J Trauma 2009;66(3):641–6 [discussion: 646–7].

137. Vasquez M, Cardarelli C, Glaser J, et al. The ABC's of pancreatic trauma: airway, breathing, and computerized tomography scan? Mil Med 2017;182(S1):66–71.

138. Panda A, Kumar A, Gamanagatti S, et al. Evaluation of diagnostic utility of multi-detector computed tomography and magnetic resonance imaging in blunt pancreatic trauma: a prospective study. Acta Radiol 2015;56(4):387–96.

139. Ragozzino A, Manfredi R, Scaglione M, et al. The use of MRCP in the detection of pancreatic injuries after blunt trauma. Emerg Radiol 2003;10(1):14–8.

140. Bhasin DK, Rana SS, Rawal P. Endoscopic retrograde pancreatography in pancreatic trauma: need to break the mental barrier. J Gastroenterol Hepatol 2009;24(5):720–8.

141. Kim S, Kim JW, Jung PY, et al. Diagnostic and therapeutic role of endoscopic retrograde pancreatography in the management of traumatic pancreatic duct injury patients: single center experience for 34 years. Int J Surg 2017;42:152–7.

142. Wind P, Tiret E, Cunningham C, et al. Contribution of endoscopic retrograde pancreatography in management of complications following distal pancreatic trauma. Am Surg 1999;65(8):777–83.

143. Wolf A, Bernhardt J, Patrzyk M, et al. The value of endoscopic diagnosis and the treatment of pancreas injuries following blunt abdominal trauma. Surg Endosc 2005;19(5):665–9.

144. Mahajan A. Current status of role of serum amylase and lipase to triage blunt pancreatic trauma? J Clin Diagn Res 2016;10(11):PL02.

145. Hamidian Jahromi A, D'Agostino HR, Zibari GB, et al. Surgical versus nonsurgical management of traumatic major pancreatic duct transection: institutional experience and review of the literature. Pancreas 2013;42(1):76–87.

146. Lin BC, Liu NJ, Fang JF, et al. Long-term results of endoscopic stent in the management of blunt major pancreatic duct injury. Surg Endosc 2006;20(10):1551–5.

147. Cotton PB, Garrow DA, Gallagher J, et al. Risk factors for complications after ERCP: a multivariate analysis of 11,497 procedures over 12 years. Gastrointest Endosc 2009;70(1):80–8.

148. Amirata E, Livingston DH, Elcavage J. Octreotide acetate decreases pancreatic complications after pancreatic trauma. Am J Surg 1994;168(4):345–7.

149. Nwariaku FE, Terracina A, Mileski WJ, et al. Is octreotide beneficial following pancreatic injury? Am J Surg 1995;170(6):582–5.

150. Jin K, Zhou H, Zhang J, et al. Systematic review and meta-analysis of somatostatin analogues in the prevention of postoperative complication after pancreaticoduodenectomy. Dig Surg 2015;32(3):196–207.

151. Moore EE, Cogbill TH, Malangoni MA, et al. Organ injury scaling, II: pancreas, duodenum, small bowel, colon, and rectum. J Trauma 1990;30(11):1427–9.

152. Fabian TC, Kudsk KA, Croce MA, et al. Superiority of closed suction drainage for pancreatic trauma. A randomized, prospective study. Ann Surg 1990; 211(6):724–8 [discussion: 728–30].

153. Buccimazza I, Thomson SR, Anderson F, et al. Isolated main pancreatic duct injuries: spectrum and management. Am J Surg 2006;191(4):448–52.

154. Malgras B, Douard R, Siauve N, et al. Management of left pancreatic trauma. Am Surg 2011;77(1):1–9.

155. Cogbill TH, Moore EE, Morris JA, et al. Distal pancreatectomy for trauma: a multicenter experience. J Trauma 1991;31(12):1600–6.

156. Moore EE. Blunt transection of the pancreas treated by distal pancreatectomy, splenic salvage, and hyperalimentation. Ann Surg 1983;198(1):117.

157. Pachter HL, Hofstetter SR, Liang HG, et al. Traumatic injuries to the pancreas: the role of distal pancreatectomy with splenic preservation. J Trauma 1989; 29(10):1352–5.

158. van der Wilden GM, Yeh D, Hwabejire JO, et al. Trauma whipple: do or don't after severe pancreaticoduodenal injuries? An analysis of the National Trauma Data Bank (NTDB). World J Surg 2014;38(2):335–40.

159. Krige JE, Kotze UK, Setshedi M, et al. Surgical management and outcomes of combined pancreaticoduodenal injuries: analysis of 75 consecutive cases. J Am Coll Surg 2016;222(5):737–49.

160. Kao LS, Bulger EM, Parks DL, et al. Predictors of morbidity after traumatic pancreatic injury. J Trauma 2003;55(5):898–905.

161. Mansfield N, Inaba K, Berg R, et al. Early pancreatic dysfunction after resection in trauma: an 18-year report from a level I trauma center. J Trauma Acute Care Surg 2017;82(3):528–33.

162. Krige JE, Kotze UK, Navsaria PH, et al. Endoscopic and operative treatment of delayed complications after pancreatic trauma: an analysis of 27 civilians treated in an academic Level 1 trauma centre. Pancreatology 2015;15(5):563–9.

163. McAninch JW. Genitourinary trauma. World J Urol 1999;17:65.

164. Wessells H, Suh D, Porter JR, et al. Renal injury and operative management in the United States: results of a population-based study. J Trauma 2003;54:423.

165. Wright JL, Nathens AB, Rivara FP, et al. Renal and extrarenal predictors of nephrectomy from the national trauma data bank. J Urol 2006;175:970.

166. Smith J, Caldwell E, D'Amours S, et al. Abdominal trauma: a disease in evolution. ANZ J Surg 2005;75:790.

167. Paparel P, N'Diaye A, Laumon B, et al. The epidemiology of trauma of the genitourinary system after traffic accidents: analysis of a register of over 43,000 victims. BJU Int 2006;97:338.

168. Bariol SV, Stewart GD, Smith RD, et al. An analysis of urinary tract trauma in Scotland: impact on management and resource needs. Surgeon 2005;3:27.
169. Krieger JN, Algood CB, Mason JT, et al. Urological trauma in the Pacific Northwest: etiology, distribution, management and outcome. J Urol 1984;132:70.
170. Schmidlin F, Farshad M, Bidaut L, et al. Biomechanical analysis and clinical treatment of blunt renal trauma. Swiss Surg 1998;237:237–43.
171. Schmidlin FR, Iselin CE, Naimi A, et al. The higher injury risk of abnormal kidneys in blunt renal trauma. Scand J Urol Nephrol 1998;32:388.
172. Buckley JC, McAninch JW. Selective management of isolated and nonisolated grade IV renal injuries. J Urol 2006;176:2498.
173. Ersay A, Akgun Y. Experience with renal gunshot injuries in a rural setting. Urology 1999;54:972.
174. Madiba TE, Haffejee AA, John J. Renal trauma secondary to stab, blunt and firearm injuries–a 5-year study. S Afr J Surg 2002;40:5.
175. Morey AF, Brandes S, Dugi DD 3rd, et al. Urotrauma: AUA guideline. J Urol 2014;192:327.
176. Santucci RA, Wessells H, Bartsch G, et al. Evaluation and management of renal injuries: consensus statement of the renal trauma subcommittee. BJU Int 2004; 93:937.
177. Serafetinides E, Kitrey ND, Djakovic N, et al. Review of the current management of upper urinary tract injuries by the EAU trauma guidelines panel. Eur Urol 2015;67:930.
178. Myers JB, Brant WO, Broghammer JA. High-grade renal injuries: radiographic findings correlated with intervention for renal hemorrhage. Urol Clin North Am 2013;40:335.
179. Moore EE, Shackford SR, Pachter HL, et al. Organ injury scaling: spleen, liver, and kidney. J Trauma 1989;29:1664.
180. Kuan JK, Wright JL, Nathens AB, et al. American Association for the Surgery of Trauma Organ Injury Scale for kidney injuries predicts nephrectomy, dialysis, and death in patients with blunt injury and nephrectomy for penetrating injuries. J Trauma 2006;60:351.
181. Santucci RA, McAninch JW, Safir M, et al. Validation of the American Association for the Surgery of Trauma organ injury severity scale for the kidney. J Trauma 2001;50:195.
182. Shariat SF, Roehrborn CG, Karakiewicz PI, et al. Evidence-based validation of the predictive value of the American Association for the Surgery of Trauma kidney injury scale. J Trauma 2007;62:933.
183. Dugi DD 3rd, Morey AF, Gupta A, et al. American Association for the Surgery of Trauma grade 4 renal injury substratification into grades 4a (low risk) and 4b (high risk). J Urol 2010;183:592.
184. Simmons JD, Haraway AN, Schmieg RE Jr, et al. Blunt renal trauma and the predictors of failure of non-operative management. J Miss State Med Assoc 2010; 51:131.
185. Santucci RA, Fisher MB. The literature increasingly supports expectant (conservative) management of renal trauma–a systematic review. J Trauma 2005;59: 493.
186. Zinman LN, Vanni AJ. Surgical management of urologic trauma and iatrogenic injuries. Surg Clin North Am 2016;96:425.
187. Jawas A, Abu-Zidan FM. Management algorithm for complete blunt renal artery occlusion in multiple trauma patients: case series. Int J Surg 2008;6:317.

188. Alsikafi NF, McAninch JW, Elliott SP, et al. Nonoperative management outcomes of isolated urinary extravasation following renal lacerations due to external trauma. J Urol 2006;176:2494.
189. Matthews LA, Smith EM, Spirnak JP. Nonoperative treatment of major blunt renal lacerations with urinary extravasation. J Urol 1997;157:2056.
190. Voelzke BB, McAninch JW. Renal gunshot wounds: clinical management and outcome. J Trauma 2009;66:593.
191. Velmahos GC, Demetriades D, Cornwell EE 3rd, et al. Selective management of renal gunshot wounds. Br J Surg 1998;85:1121.
192. Hope WW, Smith ST, Medieros B, et al. Non-operative management in penetrating abdominal trauma: is it feasible at a Level II trauma center? J Emerg Med 2012;43:190.
193. Chow SJ, Thompson KJ, Hartman JF, et al. A 10-year review of blunt renal artery injuries at an urban level I trauma centre. Injury 2009;40:844.
194. Breyer BN, McAninch JW, Elliott SP, et al. Minimally invasive endovascular techniques to treat acute renal hemorrhage. J Urol 2008;179:2248.
195. Huber J, Pahernik S, Hallscheidt P, et al. Selective transarterial embolization for posttraumatic renal hemorrhage: a second try is worthwhile. J Urol 2011;185:1751.
196. Breyer BN, Master VA, Marder SR, et al. Endovascular management of trauma related renal artery thrombosis. J Trauma 2008;64:1123.
197. Brewer ME Jr, Strnad BT, Daley BJ, et al. Percutaneous embolization for the management of grade 5 renal trauma in hemodynamically unstable patients: initial experience. J Urol 2009;181:1737.
198. Armenakas NA, Duckett CP, McAninch JW. Indications for nonoperative management of renal stab wounds. J Urol 1999;161:768.
199. Chouhan JD, Winer AG, Johnson C, et al. Contemporary evaluation and management of renal trauma. Can J Urol 2016;23:8191.
200. Master VA, McAninch JW. Operative management of renal injuries: parenchymal and vascular. Urol Clin North Am 2006;33:21.
201. Brown MF, Graham JM, Mattox KL, et al. Renovascular trauma. Am J Surg 1980;140:802.
202. Carroll PR, McAninch JW, Klosterman P, et al. Renovascular trauma: risk assessment, surgical management, and outcome. J Trauma 1990;30:547.
203. Ivatury RR, Zubowski R, Stahl WM. Penetrating renovascular trauma. J Trauma 1989;29:1620.
204. Knudson MM, Harrison PB, Hoyt DB, et al. Outcome after major renovascular injuries: a Western Trauma Association multicenter report. J Trauma 2000;49:1116.
205. Heyns CF, Van Vollenhoven P. Selective surgical management of renal stab wounds. Br J Urol 1992;69:351.
206. Watts RA, Hoffbrand BI. Hypertension following renal trauma. J Hum Hypertens 1987;1:65.

Surgical Management of Abdominal Trauma
Hollow Viscus Injury

Jamie J. Coleman, MD[a], Ben L. Zarzaur, MD, MPH[b],*

KEYWORDS

- Blunt abdominal trauma • Penetrating abdominal trauma • Hollow viscus injury

KEY POINTS

- Hollow viscus injury due to blunt trauma is infrequent, yet difficult to diagnose.
- Computed tomography scans are a commonly used diagnostic tool in hemodynamically stable patients with blunt and penetrating trauma, but they do have limitations.
- Appropriate operative management of hollow viscus injury is imperative in improving patient outcomes and preventing complications, such as the development of enterocutaneous fistulae.

INTRODUCTION

Injuries to the stomach, duodenum, small intestine, and colon are common in penetrating trauma and relatively rare in blunt trauma. Violation of the peritoneum occurs in between 20% and 80% of patients with penetrating trauma, depending on the type of weapon used.[1,2] Conversely, hollow viscus injuries are found in approximately 1% or less of blunt trauma admissions.[3,4] The most common site of injury in both blunt and penetrating trauma is the small intestine.[3,5]

Although hollow viscus injuries do not often contribute to hemodynamic instability, they are associated with significant morbidity and mortality. Injuries to the colon, and subsequent contamination, have been cited as the most significant risk factor toward the development of a surgical site infection.[6,7] However, morbidity rates directly related to gastric and small bowel injuries are also high, and have been reported up to 27%.[8] Furthermore, the presence of multiple hollow viscus injuries and concomitant gastric and colon injuries, for example, has been shown to have a synergistic, additive effect on the rate of postoperative surgical site infections.[9]

The authors have no relevant disclosures.
[a] Department of Surgery, Indiana University School of Medicine, 1604 North Capitol Avenue, Office B242, Indianapolis, IN 46202, USA; [b] Department of Surgery, Indiana University School of Medicine, Indianapolis, IN, USA
* Corresponding author. 720 Eskenazi Avenue, H-2 Room 431, Indianapolis, IN 46202.
E-mail address: bzarzaur@iupui.edu

Surg Clin N Am 97 (2017) 1107–1117
http://dx.doi.org/10.1016/j.suc.2017.06.004
0039-6109/17/© 2017 Elsevier Inc. All rights reserved.

surgical.theclinics.com

The diagnosis of hollow viscus injuries, particularly in blunt trauma, can be difficult, and a delay in diagnosis can significantly increase the morbidity, mortality, and difficulty in management.[10,11] Operative management varies by the organ that is injured, as well as its severity. The American Association for the Surgery of Trauma (AAST) Organ Injury Scale is most commonly used to diagnose severity, and injuries are assigned a grade of I to V.[12]

DIAGNOSIS

As previously mentioned, the diagnosis of injury to the gastrointestinal tract can be difficult, particularly in blunt trauma. Symptoms vary depending on what organ was injured because a perforated stomach tends to produce significant signs of peritonitis, due to the low pH of its contents, in comparison with full-thickness injuries to the small bowel, which may take a longer time to produce significant signs and symptoms. The retroperitoneal position of portions of the colon can also hinder the development of classic peritonitis. To add to the difficulties, clinical examination of injured patients, many of whom have multisystem trauma, can be unreliable at best.

Historically, before the advent and widespread use of computed tomography (CT) scans in trauma patients, diagnostic peritoneal lavage (DPL) was a commonly used diagnostic tool in the evaluation of patients with both blunt and penetrating trauma. DPL is a very sensitive tool for possible intra-abdominal injury. Patients often underwent exploratory laparotomy for solid organ injury, even if they were hemodynamically stable. Due to the frequency of patients undergoing exploratory laparotomy during this time period, hollow viscus injuries were often diagnosed intraoperatively, and delays in the diagnosis of these injuries were uncommon.[13] As CT scans became the diagnostic imaging of choice, more and more patients began undergoing nonoperative management with periods of observation for solid organ injuries. Currently, studies have shown that more than two-thirds of patients with trauma to the spleen or liver are managed nonoperatively, including some patients with grades IV and V injuries.[13-17] This has led to a significantly larger proportion of patients who never undergo a laparotomy. Thus, the ability to diagnosis hollow viscus injury relies primarily on physical examination and CT scan findings.

The sensitivity and specificity of CT scan in the diagnosis of hollow viscus injury have varied widely in the literature, especially in determining which injuries require operative intervention. The sensitivity has been reported in ranges between 55% and 95%, with specificity between 48% and 92%.[5,18,19] In particular, false-negative rates in CT scans of patients with small bowel injury have been reported as high as 15%.[20] There are numerous pitfalls in the interpretation of CT scans for hollow viscus injury because there are numerous signs suggestive of but not specific to bowel injury. These signs include irregular contrast enhancement of the bowel, bowel wall thickening, mesenteric abnormality, and fluid inside the abdomen without an associated solid organ injury.[19,21]

The finding of free intraperitoneal fluid without findings of a solid organ injury remains a particular challenge to the surgeon. When a decision is made to operate on a patient solely for this radiographic finding, the rates of therapeutic laparotomy have varied widely, from 27% to 54%.[13,22,23] Due to this wide variation, few centers recommend immediate exploration for free intra-abdominal fluid without additional signs or symptoms of bowel perforation. Traditionally, the finding of pneumoperitoneum on CT scan has prompted immediate operative exploration. With the increasing sensitivity of CT scanners, an increased incidence of clinically insignificant pneumoperitoneum has been described in blunt trauma patients. In the series reported by

Marek and colleagues,[24] 78% of subjects with blunt abdominal trauma and pneumo-peritoneum detected by CT scan were without an identified gastrointestinal perfora-tion. In addition, no combination of radiologic findings has been shown to consistently predict bowel perforation.[25] These factors have combined to make bowel and mesenteric injuries the most commonly missed abdominal injury.[5] Some centers have advocated the use of repeat CT scans in the evaluation of patients for blunt bowel injury, particularly in patients with significant head trauma.[25]

Early reports of delays less than 12 to 24 hours in the diagnosis of small bowel in-juries showed limited, if any, increase in morbidity and mortality.[26–28] However, more recent literature has shown increased mortality directly related to a missed hol-low viscus injury in delays of less than 8 hours.[10,11] The morbidity of a negative lapa-rotomy, which has been reported between 8% and 40%, should be taken into account, and this information used in the counseling of patients in regard to operative intervention.[29–32]

CT also plays a role in the evaluation of patients with penetrating trauma to the torso who are hemodynamically stable. CT scans were originally found in the late 1980s to be highly sensitive and specific in patients with stab wounds to the back and flank, allowing for nonoperative management in most patients.[33,34] Since then, several in-vestigators have examined the use of triple contrast CT (oral, intravenous, and rectal contrast) in hemodynamically stable patients with both stab and gunshot wounds to the abdomen, back, and flank. Himmelman and colleagues[35] showed a 100% sensi-tivity of CT scans for retroperitoneal injury in subjects with penetrating trauma to the back and flank. In subjects with gunshot wounds to the abdomen, not just the back and flank, Munera and colleagues[36] found CT scans with triple contrast to be 96% ac-curate in detecting injury. Reflecting these findings, the latest practice management guideline from the Eastern Association for the Surgery of Trauma states "abdomino-pelvic CT should be strongly considered as a diagnostic tool" in hemodynamically sta-ble patients with penetrating abdominal trauma.[37]

Despite its limitations, CT remains the diagnostic method of choice for both blunt and penetrating mechanisms of injury; however, great care should be taken in the evaluation of patients with concern for hollow viscus injury. Oral and rectal contrasts have been shown to improve accuracy in hemodynamically stable patients with pene-trating trauma and can be used unless the administration of contrast would delay a diagnosis. Diligent physical examination, laboratory studies, and repeat imaging are all used as adjuncts in determining a patient's need for operation.

Stomach and Small Intestine

To fully evaluate a gastric injury, the stomach should be mobilized and the posterior wall inspected after opening the gastrocolic ligament in its avascular portion. The importance of full mobilization of the stomach cannot be overemphasized. The entire anterior wall of the stomach should be stretched so that there are no folds in the wall. One can accomplish this by grasping the nasogastric tube and pulling inferiorly on the stomach. Use of malleable or ribbon retractors can aid in visualization of the cardia and the gastroesophageal junction. Similar techniques can be used to visualize the posterior wall of the stomach. After entering the lesser sac, malleable or ribbon retrac-tors can be used in combination with traction on the stomach via the nasogastric tube to fully examine the posterior gastric wall. The other areas to examine closely for a missed injury are the greater and lesser curves. Full visualization of these areas may require dissection of the omentum from the wall greater curvature.

Repair of the injury depends on the severity. Grades I and II lacerations are repaired primarily, in 1 or 2 layers, after wound edges have been debrided back to healthy tissue, if needed. Grade III injuries, although larger, can be treated in the same manner, or closed with the use of a surgical stapler. Regardless of grade, care should be taken if the injury nears the pylorus so as not to occlude or narrow its lumen. If a wound involves or is directly adjacent to the pylorus, a pyloroplasty should be performed.[1] More extensive injuries with greater tissue loss or devascularization of the stomach, AAST grade IV, may require resection. Reconstruction may then be performed, depending on the amount of resection needed, with a Billroth I (antrectomy with gastroduodenostomy), Billroth II (antrectomy with gastrojejunostomy), or Roux-en-Y gastrojejunostomy or esophagojejunostomy. If a nonanatomic reconstruction is performed, vagotomy should accompany the resection to prevent the formation of a marginal ulcer.

The evaluation of the small bowel for injury should begin with evisceration of the small bowel. The ligament of Treitz is then identified and the small bowel inspected on both sides, in small segments, until its termination at the cecum. Care must be taken in order not to miss small perforations or lacerations. Mural and mesenteric hematomas should be noted and reassessed for expansion. Careful attention should be paid to the very proximal small bowel and the distal ileum because these are 2 locations where injuries can be missed due to the anatomy. To fully visualize the proximal small bowel at the ligament of Treitz, it is often necessary to combine a full Kocher maneuver with a Cattel maneuver. The Cattel maneuver involves mobilization of the avascular plane along the small bowel mesentery. Using these maneuvers, the surgeon can fully visualize the proximal jejunum at the ligament of Treitz. Further, these maneuvers can provide for tension-free repairs when the injury is close to the ligament of Treitz. Another area where injuries to the small bowel can be missed is along the mesenteric border. It is important to investigate all hematomas in the small bowel mesentery to be sure that there are no injuries on the mesenteric side.

Partial-thickness injuries should be closed with interrupted silk sutures in a seromuscular layer. Full-thickness small bowel injuries are treated similarly to the stomach in that grades I and II injuries should be repaired primarily after appropriate debridement, in 1 or 2 layers, running or interrupted. The repair should be performed in a tension-free manner and in a transverse fashion to prevent stenosis or narrowing of the small intestine. Multiple injuries are preferably repaired individually, unless the proximity does not allow for adequate closure. Options for multiple adjacent grades I or II injuries are to either combine them to allow for adequate repair or to treat them as higher grade injuries with resection. Grades III, IV, and V injuries are treated with resection of the injured and/or devascularized segments. Although there has been debate about the best method for performing an intestinal anastomosis, data have shown complication rates between stapled and hand sewn techniques to be similar in the setting of trauma.[1,38,39] Handsewn anastomoses can be performed in either 1 or 2 layers, in an interrupted or running fashion. Care should be taken to avoid the creation of a narrow or stenotic anastomosis. When a stapled anastomosis is performed, the surgeon should be knowledgeable about the stapler itself, which height of staples should be used, and what length of time the stapler should be applied before transection to allow for tissue edema to disperse. The resultant enterotomy after a stapled anastomosis is created can be closed either primarily with suture or a noncutting stapler. When either technique is used, adequate debridement of nonviable tissues must be performed before closure. In addition, attention must be paid to the creation of an anastomosis that is without tension. If the patient's hemodynamic or physiologic status requires damage control principles, then small bowel injuries should be quickly closed or resected to prevent ongoing contamination and anastomosis delayed. Reanastomosis should take place as soon as the patient becomes hemodynamically stable and physiologically optimized, preferably within 48 hours. Cothren and colleagues[40] have demonstrated a significant trend in the increased rate of leak with increasing fascial closure day. Other risk factors for the development of anastomotic leak and enterocutaneous fistula in the setting of abbreviated laparotomy include resuscitation volumes of more than 5 L within the first 48 hours of hospitalization and an increasing number of explorations.[41]

Duodenum

The duodenum is largely protected due to its primary location in the retroperitoneum and injuries are rare, accounting for less than 5% of all abdominal injuries.[42–44] In sharp contrast to its rarity, morbidity and mortality rates for injuries to the duodenum are high and range up to 65% and 47%, respectively.[45–48] These high rates are secondary to concomitant injuries, which are common due to the proximity of the duodenum with the pancreas and major vascular structures, and there is a higher incidence of leak in the duodenum compared with the remainder of the small intestine. Due to these factors, repair of duodenal injuries remains a considerable challenge to the surgeon.

Regardless of injury mechanism, surgical options in regard to the repair of duodenal injuries include primary repair, repair with intraluminal drain placement (triple tube therapy), pyloric exclusion, and Roux-en-Y duodenojejunostomy. Pancreaticoduodenectomy has also been used, but its use is typically limited to combined pancreatic and duodenal injuries with significant tissue loss. The choice of operative approach is determined by the stability of the patient and the severity of injury.

Grades I and II hematomas of the duodenum are more common in children but do occur in adults. These injuries are typically identified on CT scan, and typical symptoms include delayed gastric emptying or even gastric outlet obstruction. Treatment is usually nonoperative, with obstruction managed with gastric decompression and intravenous hydration. If, however, the hematoma is encountered at the time of laparotomy, most investigators recommend not opening the hematoma and treating the patient with gastric decompression and distal feeding access either through a nasojejunal tube or tube jejunostomy. Most patients with duodenal hematomas symptomatically resolve within 3 weeks. If a patient remains completely clinically obstructed after 10 to 14 days, re-evaluation should be performed either with CT scan or an upper gastrointestinal fluoroscopy. On re-evaluation, if the patient's hematoma has worsened or is showing no signs of improvement, operative intervention can be considered. Evacuation of the hematoma can be accomplished either with a laparoscopic or open approach after thorough mobilization of the duodenum, then simply closed in a transverse fashion after meticulous hemostasis.[44,49]

Grades I and II lacerations of the duodenum require exploratory laparotomy and should be managed with simple closure in a transverse fashion. The transverse closure is essential to prevent narrowing of the duodenal lumen. When performing a primary repair of the duodenum, necrotic and severely damaged edges should be debrided to ensure wound edges are clean. In addition, thorough mobilization of the duodenum needs to be performed to allow for adequate examination of the back wall and a tension-free repair. This technique is successful for up to 85% of duodenal injuries.[43,44,50] A diligent search for a wound on the pancreatic side of the duodenum should be carried out when there is a high suspicion of this type of injury. Wounds on the pancreatic side of the duodenum can be difficult to identify and repair. Occasionally, it is necessary to expand a laceration on the anterior or lateral border of the duodenum to fully visualize the injury on the medial duodenal border. Using this technique, it is possible to repair the medial wall of the duodenum from the inside.

Care should be taken, though, to identify the ampulla and to be sure it is not included in the repair. Extraluminal drains have been shown by some investigators to be associated with an increased risk of duodenal leak, and routine use is not recommended unless an associated pancreatic leak is suspected.[46,51]

Grade III injuries also should be evaluated for primary repair after mobilization and adequate debridement. If an end-to-end duodenoduodenostomy can be performed without undue tension, then this is a viable surgical option. Due to the duodenum's relatively short mesentery and attachments to the common bile duct and pancreas, this often is not possible. Other surgical repair options for this grade of injury include a Roux-en-Y duodenojejunostomy in which a limb of jejunum is anastomosed to the defect in the duodenum. If significant tissue loss necessitates resection of a portion of duodenum, the distal segment should be closed primarily and reconstruction performed to the proximal segment with an end-to-end Roux-en-Y duodenojejunostomy. Another operative approach if the injury is proximal to the ampulla, as outlined in the Western Trauma Association's algorithm for the management of duodenal injuries, is to perform a Billroth II (antrectomy and gastrojejunostomy).[44,49]

The most severe injuries, those that meet AAST criteria for grades IV or V, are typically combined pancreatic and duodenal injuries involving lacerations greater than 75% circumference, disruption of the ampulla or the distal common bile duct, and/or devascularization of the duodenum. Even in these severe injuries, emerging evidence has shown primary repair to be safe, with similar rates of sepsis and mortality as gastroenterostomy and pyloric exclusion but with a shorter hospital length of stay.[50-53] When primary repairs are tenuous or concern for dehiscence is high, adjuncts to primary repair include pyloric exclusion and triple-tube drainage. Pyloric exclusion was first described in 1977 by Vaughan and colleagues.[54] This operation entails closure of the pylorus, either by a noncutting stapler or suture, followed by a gastrojejunostomy. This is designed to protect a duodenal suture line or duodenostomy tube by diversion of gastric contents. The closure of the pylorus will spontaneously open over time, usually within 6 to 12 weeks.[49] However, the rate and time to spontaneous opening can vary widely and is largely unknown.[47,51,55] In 1979, Drs Stone and Fabian[55] described a different technique of suture line protection that is now commonly known as triple tube or triple ostomy. This technique involves repair of the duodenal injury in addition to placement of a nasogastric tube, feeding jejunostomy, and retrograde jejunostomy. Increased morbidity related to complications of the jejunostomies has been reported, yet advocates of this approach cite benefits to the diversion of bile and gastric and pancreatic secretions, and lowered intraluminal pressure.[46,48]

In duodenal injuries that are associated with disruptions of the pancreatic head and/or a nonintact ampulla, complex reconstructions are required. However, most of these patients have associated injuries and significant blood loss. Damage control principles should be applied, and the initial operation should focus solely on hemorrhage and contamination control. Reconstruction should occur when a patient is hemodynamically stable and physiologically improved. Options for reconstruction in this delayed setting include reimplantation of the common bile duct into a Roux-en-Y jejunal limb or a Whipple procedure (pancreaticoduodenectomy).[44,49]

Colon

In the first part of the twentieth century, injuries to the colon were often fatal. As surgical techniques improved and the development of antibiotics occurred, there was marked improvement in survival. One of the key principles of management of colon injuries was the creation of an ostomy instead of primarily repairing the injury.

Exteriorization of the injury via an ostomy was standard management until the early 1970s when several investigators reported their experience with primary repair of colon injuries. The controversy continued until 1979 when Drs Stone and Fabian[55] reported the results of their randomized trial of primary repair compared with colostomy for colon injuries. In this study, the investigators performed obligatory colostomy on subjects who were in shock at the time of arrival, who lost more than 1000 mL of blood, and who had more than 2 injured intra-abdominal organs, significant peritoneal soilage, delayed operation, destructive colon injury, or significant abdominal wall loss. There were 139 subjects who did not meet these criteria and who were randomized. The group randomized to primary closure had a lower rate of superficial and deep organ space infections. Morbidity was 10 times greater for the subjects randomized to colostomy compared with those who had a primary closure performed. After publication of this study, the pendulum swung in favor of primary repair. Multiple studies were conducted in the 1990s that supported the increasing use of primary repair with, at worst, equivalent morbidity rates and septic complications.[9,56–58] These findings led to the Eastern Association for the Surgery of Trauma to update their practice management guideline in 1998 to support primary repair for nondestructive colon wounds as standard of care in patients without peritonitis.[59] The practice guidelines further stated that the only patients who will benefit from diversion are those with destructive colon wounds and hemodynamic instability and/or significant comorbidities.[59]

Current management of colon injuries is primarily driven by whether or not the injury is deemed destructive at the time of laparotomy. The AAST injury grading scale for the colon can be used to help stratify management of these injuries. Grade I injuries are serosal injuries only. Grade II injuries are single-wall injuries. Grade III injuries involve less than 25% of the colon wall. Together, these make up nondestructive injuries. Most of these can be managed with primary repair. For serosal injuries, seromuscular interrupted suture should be used to close the defect in a transverse fashion. For grades II to III injuries, the edges should be debrided back to good tissue. Repair is usually accomplished in 2 layers if hand sewn. The surgeon can also use a noncutting stapler to close some injuries, but care should be taken not to narrow the lumen of the colon.

There is more controversy regarding the appropriate management of patients with destructive colon injuries. These include AAST grades IV and V injuries in which more than 25% of the colon wall is injured. Also, patients with blunt injury to the colon with more than 50% of the wall involved in a serosal tear or a large mesenteric defect are often included with those who have destructive injuries. For destructive injuries, resection and anastomosis, or resection and colostomy, are the most common management approaches. Some centers use physiologic criteria to stratify patients into those who are primarily anastomosed and those who are managed with a colostomy. The group from Memphis recently reported their experience using a defined management algorithm in patients with colon injuries from penetrating trauma.[60] In their defined algorithm, full-thickness injuries are classified as nondestructive or destructive. Nondestructive colon injuries undergo primary repair. In patients with destructive lesions, those with hemodynamic instability, comorbidities, or have received greater than 6 units of blood undergo diversion. Patients with destructive lesions without these features undergo resection and anastomosis. In their recent study, they compare the morbidity and mortality of patients using this algorithm to patients treated before the initiation of the algorithm. They found, despite an increased incidence of destructive colon injuries, that patients experienced a decreased rate of abscess formation and colon-related mortality.

Another criterion to consider is the location of the anastomosis. The splenic flexure is a known area of the colon that is particularly vulnerable to ischemia. In 2 autopsy studies, the ascending branch of the left colic and the left branch of the middle colic arteries were found to have either a tenuous or incomplete connection in approximately half of sujects.[61,62] Feliciano and colleagues[63] reported on their series of 217 subjects. They found 7 subjects who developed a suture line failure. All 7 had injuries in the watershed area of the colon: the splenic flexure and distal transverse colon. The investigators theorized that the more frequent breakdown of anastomoses on the left side occurred because several of these were in watershed areas of the colon. Based on this information, if the surgeon can perform an anatomic resection and anastomosis then this would be the preferred choice. If not, avoiding an anastomosis in the colon watershed areas is likely a prudent course of action.

With the advent of damage control or abbreviated laparotomy as standard of care in severely injured patients with hemodynamic and physiologic instability, more patients are now being left in intestinal discontinuity. Although small bowel anastomoses are necessary at the time of reoperation, controversy exists as to whether a patient with a colonic injury should undergo an anastomosis or diversion. In a multicenter trial, Tatebe and colleagues[64] hypothesized delayed colonic anastomoses after an abbreviated laparotomy were not associated with an increased rate of complications. Of the 267 subjects enrolled in the study, those who underwent an anastomosis after a damage control laparotomy did not have an increased rate of intra-abdominal abscess formation, surgical site infection, suture line failures, or enterocutaneous fistulae. Eighty percent of subjects with a colonic injury who underwent an abbreviated laparotomy were managed with the use of a stoma. In conclusion, delayed anastomosis of a colon injury is a viable option in most patients. However, clinical judgment should consider the patient's overall health before injury and physiologic status at the time of reoperation to aid in the determination of whether an ostomy remains the best course of action.

SUMMARY

Hollow viscus injuries present a unique challenge to surgeons. These injuries are associated with significant morbidity and mortality and can be difficult to diagnose due to additional injuries and the limitations of current imaging modalities. The operative repair of these injuries is affected by the patient's physiologic and hemodynamic status, and can be technically difficult due to anatomic location. Overall, clinical suspicion should remain high in both hemodynamically unstable and stable patients, and great consideration given to timing and technique of operative repair.

REFERENCES

1. Diebel LN. Stomach and small intestine. In: Mattox KL, Moore EE, Feliciano DV, editors. Trauma. 7th edition. New York: McGraw Hill; 2013. p. 581–602.
2. Edelman DA, White MT, Tyburski JG, et al. Factors affecting prognosis in patients with gastric trauma. Am Surg 2007;73(1):48–53.
3. Watts DD, Fakhry SM, EAST Multi-Institutional Hollow Viscus Injury Research Group. Incidence of hollow viscus injury in blunt trauma: an analysis from 275,557 trauma admissions from the East multi-institutional trial. J Trauma 2003;54(2):289–94.
4. Coimbra R, Pinto MC, Aguiar JR, et al. Factors related to the occurrence of postoperative complications following penetrating gastric injuries. Injury 1995;26(7): 463–6.

5. Khan I, Bew D, Elias DA, et al. Mechanisms of injury and CT findings in bowel and mesenteric trauma. Clin Radiol 2014;69(6):639–47.

6. Causey MW, Rivadeneira DE, Steele SR. Historical and current trends in colon trauma. Clin Colon Rectal Surg 2012;25(4):189–99.

7. O'Neill PA, Kirton OC, Dresner LS, et al. Analysis of 162 colon injuries in patients with penetrating abdominal trauma: concomitant stomach injury results in a higher rate of infection. J Trauma 2004;56(2):304–12 [discussion: 12–3].

8. Salim A, Teixeira PG, Inaba K, et al. Analysis of 178 penetrating stomach and small bowel injuries. World J Surg 2008;32(3):471–5.

9. Jacobson LE, Gomez GA, Broadie TA. Primary repair of 58 consecutive penetrating injuries of the colon: should colostomy be abandoned? Am Surg 1997; 63(2):170–7.

10. Fakhry SM, Brownstein M, Watts DD, et al. Relatively short diagnostic delays (<8 hours) produce morbidity and mortality in blunt small bowel injury: an analysis of time to operative intervention in 198 patients from a multicenter experience. J Trauma 2000;48(3):408–14 [discussion: 14–5].

11. Malinoski DJ, Patel MS, Yakar DO, et al. A diagnostic delay of 5 hours increases the risk of death after blunt hollow viscus injury. J Trauma 2010;69(1):84–7.

12. Moore EE, Cogbill TH, Malangoni MA, et al. Organ injury scaling, II: pancreas, duodenum, small bowel, colon, and rectum. J Trauma 1990;30(11):1427–9.

13. Fakhry SM, Watts DD, Luchette FA, et al. Current diagnostic approaches lack sensitivity in the diagnosis of perforated blunt small bowel injury: analysis from 275,557 trauma admissions from the EAST multi-institutional HVI trial. J Trauma 2003;54(2):295–306.

14. Stassen NA, Bhullar I, Cheng JD, et al. Nonoperative management of blunt hepatic injury: an Eastern Association for the Surgery of Trauma practice management guideline. J Trauma Acute Care Surg 2012;73(5 Suppl 4):S288–93.

15. Stassen NA, Bhullar I, Cheng JD, et al. Selective nonoperative management of blunt splenic injury: an Eastern Association for the Surgery of Trauma practice management guideline. J Trauma Acute Care Surg 2012;73(5 Suppl 4): S294–300.

16. Scarborough JE, Ingraham AM, Liepert AE, et al. Nonoperative management is as effective as immediate splenectomy for adult patients with high-grade blunt splenic injury. J Am Coll Surg 2016;223(2):249–58.

17. van der Wilden GM, Velmahos GC, Emhoff T, et al. Successful nonoperative management of the most severe blunt liver injuries: a multicenter study of the research consortium of new England centers for trauma. Arch Surg 2012;147(5):423–8.

18. Atri M, Hanson JM, Grinblat L, et al. Surgically important bowel and/or mesenteric injury in blunt trauma: accuracy of multidetector CT for evaluation. Radiology 2008;249(2):524–33.

19. Bhagvan S, Turai M, Holden A, et al. Predicting hollow viscus injury in blunt abdominal trauma with computed tomography. World J Surg 2013;37(1):123–6.

20. Malhotra AK, Fabian TC, Katsis SB, et al. Blunt bowel and mesenteric injuries: the role of screening computed tomography. J Trauma 2000;48(6):991–8 [discussion: 998–1000].

21. Tan KK, Liu JZ, Go TS, et al. Computed tomography has an important role in hollow viscus and mesenteric injuries after blunt abdominal trauma. Injury 2010; 41(5):475–8.

22. Brasel KJ, Olson CJ, Stafford RE, et al. Incidence and significance of free fluid on abdominal computed tomographic scan in blunt trauma. J Trauma 1998;44(5): 889–92.

23. Rodriguez C, Barone JE, Wilbanks TO, et al. Isolated free fluid on computed tomographic scan in blunt abdominal trauma: a systematic review of incidence and management. J Trauma 2002;53(1):79–85.

24. Marek AP, Deisler RF, Sutherland JB, et al. CT scan-detected pneumoperitoneum: an unreliable predictor of intra-abdominal injury in blunt trauma. Injury 2014; 45(1):116–21.

25. Walker ML, Akpele I, Spence SD, et al. The role of repeat computed tomography scan in the evaluation of blunt bowel injury. Am Surg 2012;78(9):979–85.

26. Kafie F, Tominaga GT, Yoong B, et al. Factors related to outcome in blunt intestinal injuries requiring operation. Am Surg 1997;63(10):889–92.

27. Allen GS, Moore FA, Cox CS Jr, et al. Hollow visceral injury and blunt trauma. J Trauma 1998;45(1):69–75 [discussion: 75–8].

28. Sherck JP, Oakes DD. Intestinal injuries missed by computed tomography. J Trauma 1990;30(1):1–5 [discussion: 5–7].

29. McNutt MK, Chinapuvvula NR, Beckmann NM, et al. Early surgical intervention for blunt bowel injury: the bowel injury prediction score (BIPS). J Trauma Acute Care Surg 2015;78(1):105–11.

30. Renz BM, Feliciano DV. Unnecessary laparotomies for trauma: a prospective study of morbidity. J Trauma 1995;38(3):350–6.

31. Hasaniya N, Demetriades D, Stephens A, et al. Early morbidity and mortality of non-therapeutic operations for penetrating trauma. Am Surg 1994;60(10):744–7.

32. Lowe RJ, Boyd DR, Folk FA, et al. The negative laparotomy for abdominal trauma. J Trauma 1972;12(10):853–61.

33. Fletcher TB, Setiawan H, Harrell RS, et al. Posterior abdominal stab wounds: role of CT evaluation. Radiology 1989;173(3):621–5.

34. Meyer DM, Thal ER, Weigelt JA, et al. The role of abdominal CT in the evaluation of stab wounds to the back. J Trauma 1989;29(9):1226–8 [discussion: 1228–30].

35. Himmelman RG, Martin M, Gilkey S, et al. Triple-contrast CT scans in penetrating back and flank trauma. J Trauma 1991;31(6):852–5.

36. Munera F, Morales C, Soto JA, et al. Gunshot wounds of abdomen: evaluation of stable patients with triple-contrast helical CT. Radiology 2004;231(2):399–405.

37. Como JJ, Bokhari F, Chiu WC, et al. Practice management guidelines for selective nonoperative management of penetrating abdominal trauma. J Trauma 2010; 68(3):721–33.

38. Witzke JD, Kraatz JJ, Morken JM, et al. Stapled versus hand sewn anastomoses in patients with small bowel injury: a changing perspective. J Trauma 2000;49(4): 660–5 [discussion: 665–6].

39. Kirkpatrick AW, Baxter KA, Simons RK, et al. Intra-abdominal complications after surgical repair of small bowel injuries: an international review. J Trauma 2003; 55(3):399–406.

40. Burlew CC, Moore EE, Cuschieri J, et al. Sew it up! A Western Trauma Association multi-institutional study of enteric injury management in the postinjury open abdomen. J Trauma 2011;70(2):273–7.

41. Bradley MJ, Dubose JJ, Scalea TM, et al. Independent predictors of enteric fistula and abdominal sepsis after damage control laparotomy: results from the prospective AAST open abdomen registry. JAMA Surg 2013;148(10):947–54.

42. Kelly G, Norton L, Moore G, et al. The continuing challenge of duodenal injuries. J Trauma 1978;18(3):160–5.

43. Asensio JA, Feliciano DV, Britt LD, et al. Management of duodenal injuries. Curr Probl Surg 1993;30(11):1023–93.

44. Malhotra A, Biffl WL, Moore EE, et al. Western Trauma Association critical decisions in trauma: diagnosis and management of duodenal injuries. J Trauma Acute Care Surg 2015;79(6):1096–101.
45. Ordonez C, Garcia A, Parra MW, et al. Complex penetrating duodenal injuries: less is better. J Trauma Acute Care Surg 2014;76(5):1177–83.
46. Schroeppel TJ, Saleem K, Sharpe JP, et al. Penetrating duodenal trauma: a 19-year experience. J Trauma Acute Care Surg 2016;80(3):461–5.
47. Martin TD, Feliciano DV, Mattox KL, et al. Severe duodenal injuries. Treatment with pyloric exclusion and gastrojejunostomy. Arch Surg 1983;118(5):631–5.
48. Ivatury RR, Nallathambi M, Gaudino J, et al. Penetrating duodenal injuries. Analysis of 100 consecutive cases. Ann Surg 1985;202(2):153–8.
49. Biffl WL. Duodenum and pancreas. In: Mattox KL, Moore EE, Feliciano DV, editors. Trauma. 7th edition. New York: McGraw-Hill; 2013. p. 603–19.
50. Siboni S, Benjamin E, Haltmeier T, et al. Isolated blunt duodenal trauma: simple repair, low mortality. Am Surg 2015;81(10):961–4.
51. Velmahos GC, Constantinou C, Kasotakis G. Safety of repair for severe duodenal injuries. World J Surg 2008;32(1):7–12.
52. DuBose JJ, Inaba K, Teixeira PG, et al. Pyloric exclusion in the treatment of severe duodenal injuries: results from the National Trauma Data Bank. Am Surg 2008; 74(10):925–9.
53. Seamon MJ, Pieri PG, Fisher CA, et al. A ten-year retrospective review: does pyloric exclusion improve clinical outcome after penetrating duodenal and combined pancreaticoduodenal injuries? J Trauma 2007;62(4):829–33.
54. Vaughan GD 3rd, Frazier OH, Graham DY, et al. The use of pyloric exclusion in the management of severe duodenal injuries. Am J Surg 1977;134(6):785–90.
55. Stone HH, Fabian TC. Management of duodenal wounds. J Trauma 1979;19(5): 334–9.
56. Chappuis CW, Frey DJ, Dietzen CD, et al. Management of penetrating colon injuries. A prospective randomized trial. Ann Surg 1991;213(5):492–7 [discussion: 497–8].
57. Sasaki LS, Allaben RD, Golwala R, et al. Primary repair of colon injuries: a prospective randomized study. J Trauma 1995;39(5):895–901.
58. Berne JD, Velmahos GC, Chan LS, et al. The high morbidity of colostomy closure after trauma: further support for the primary repair of colon injuries. Surgery 1998; 123(2):157–64.
59. Pasquale M, Fabian TC. Practice management guidelines for trauma from the Eastern Association for the surgery of trauma. J Trauma 1998;44(6):941–56 [discussion: 956–7].
60. Sharpe JP, Magnotti LJ, Weinberg JA, et al. Adherence to a simplified management algorithm reduces morbidity and mortality after penetrating colon injuries: a 15-year experience. J Am Coll Surg 2012;214(4):591–7 [discussion: 597–8].
61. Griffiths JD. Surgical anatomy of the blood supply of the distal colon. Ann R Coll Surg Engl 1956;19(4):241–56.
62. Meyers MA. Griffiths' point: critical anastomosis at the splenic flexure. Significance in ischemia of the colon. AJR Am J Roentgenol 1976;126(1):77–94.
63. Dente CJ, Patel A, Feliciano DV, et al. Suture line failure in intra-abdominal colonic trauma: is there an effect of segmental variations in blood supply on outcome? J Trauma 2005;59(2):359–66 [discussion: 366–8].
64. Tatebe L, Jennings A, Tatebe K, et al. Traumatic colon injury in damage control laparotomy - a multicenter trial: is it safe to do a delayed anastomosis? J Trauma Acute Care Surg 2017;82(4):742–9.

Surgical Management of Musculoskeletal Trauma

Daniel J. Stinner, MD[a,b,*], Dafydd Edwards, FRCS (Tr&Orth)[a,c]

KEYWORDS

- Extremity trauma • Limb salvage • Limb reconstruction
- Damage control orthopedics • Early total care • Early appropriate care

KEY POINTS

- Extremity injuries account for more than 50% of the total costs to society for nonfatal injuries.
- Communication between the orthopedic surgeon, trauma team leader, and other surgical services is paramount to optimize outcomes.
- Damage control orthopedics (DCO) is reserved for the physiologically unstable or borderline patient.
- Early total care (ETC) is often ideal for the management of stable trauma patients with isolated extremity injuries.
- Early appropriate care refers to the decision to apply either DCO or ETC depending on the patient's physiologic status and response to resuscitation.

SOCIETAL BURDEN OF EXTREMITY TRAUMA

Injuries remain a leading cause of death in people younger the age of 65 years. When considering years of potential life lost, it ranks higher than malignant neoplasms, heart disease, and cerebrovascular disease. However, deaths are truly just the tip of the iceberg. For every trauma-related death there are 13 hospital discharges and 140 emergency department visits related to injury or trauma.[1] With advances in automobile safety and improvements in acute resuscitation strategies, lives are being saved, but that comes at a cost for both the patient and society. When evaluating societal costs due to injury, 20% can be attributed to medical and related costs, another 35% are due to productivity losses due to death, and 45% are due to productivity losses

Disclosure: The opinions or assertions contained herein are the private views of the authors and are not to be construed as official or as reflecting the views of the Department of the Army, the Department of Defense, or the UK Ministry of Defense.
^a Royal School of Mines, Centre for Blast Injury Studies, Imperial College London, Prince Consort Road, Kensington, London SW7 2BP, UK; ^b US Army Institute of Surgical Research, San Antonio, TX, USA; ^c Royal Centre for Defence Medicine, Birmingham, UK
* Corresponding author. Royal School of Mines, Centre for Blast Injury Studies, Imperial College London, Prince Consort Road, Kensington, London SW7 2BP, UK.
E-mail address: Daniel.stinner@gmail.com

Surg Clin N Am 97 (2017) 1119–1131
http://dx.doi.org/10.1016/j.suc.2017.06.005
surgical.theclinics.com

due to disability. When looking specifically at the comprehensive costs on society of nonfatal injuries, upper limb injuries account for 16% and lower limb injuries account for 38%, attributing well more than 50% of the total costs on society for nonfatal injuries to the extremities.[2] Furthermore, of those working before an injury from a moderate to high-energy force with an orthopedic injury with an Abbreviated Injury Scale (AIS) of 3 or more, only 58% have returned to work at 1 year.[3] This gives orthopedic surgeons the opportunity to have a significant impact on minimizing this burden by doing their part to optimize outcomes of those with extremity injuries.

NEED FOR A COORDINATED NATIONAL TRAUMA SYSTEM TO OPTIMIZE OUTCOMES

Having an established and optimized trauma system is essential to improve the outcomes of those who sustain high-energy extremity trauma. Research clearly demonstrates that those sustaining severe lower-limb injuries benefit from treatment at a trauma center.[4,5] Interestingly enough, although the total number of trauma centers is increasing throughout the United States, the number of severe orthopedic injuries seen at these centers seems to be decreasing, which ultimately results in less trauma volume per orthopedic surgeon.[6] The American College of Surgeons Committee on Trauma has recognized this dilemma and has published a position statement outlining several guidelines for the optimization of a regional trauma system, which seeks to best serve the needs of the injured patient.[7] In addition, through the establishment of a coordinated National Trauma System, which may be on the horizon in the United States, outcomes of extremity trauma patients are likely to improve.[8]

TRAUMA-RELATED MORTALITY

In the developed world, trauma is the most common cause of death in those younger than the age of 44 years and is most commonly due to road traffic accidents. Donald Trunkey[9] described a predictable trimodal distribution of death in 1983.

Acute or Primary Mortality

The casualties that belong in this group are ones that have sustained injuries that are incompatible with life. Typical injuries include severe head injuries, major hemorrhage, high cervical vertebra (C3 and above) and spinal cord injuries, airway obstruction, or mediastinal and cardiac disruption. Casualties often succumb to these injuries within seconds because they are not amenable to medical intervention regardless of the timeline.

Secondary Mortality

Death in the second peak usually occurs within minutes to hours and is potentially preventable by early and appropriate medical intervention. Examples of early or acute injuries in this group are intracranial hemorrhage, pneumothorax, cardiac tamponade, hemothorax, intra-abdominal hemorrhage, pelvic fracture, or long bone fracture, in particular femoral fractures. All of these are characterized by the need for early invasive medical intervention to stabilize the casualty before physiologic disruption and organ failure occurs. For the orthopedic surgeon, interventions include pelvis and long bone stabilization; however, it is important for them to be aware that patients with these injuries often require significant resuscitation.

Tertiary Mortality

Thirty percent of all trauma-related deaths occur within days or weeks following the injury.[10] The triggering of multiorgan failure and subsequent death is usually on a continuum and starts with potentially reversible physiologic dysfunction usually caused by sepsis or cardiorespiratory failure. This concept of multiple, progressive or sequential systems failure was first described in 1975 by Baue.[10] The term multiorgan dysfunction syndrome has been adopted to describe this condition and is characterized by the failure of at least 2 organs.

The goal of the orthopedic surgeon is to attempt to prevent secondary or tertiary deaths and subsequently minimize morbidity related to musculoskeletal injury. Typically, mortality in the secondary peak can be minimized by stabilization of fractures to the pelvis and long bones. Stabilization of such injuries not only helps with the reduction of blood loss but also deceases the pain stimuli, reducing the analgesia and anesthetic requirement, which can help with the regulation and normalization of physiology. Furthermore, stabilization of the long bones can also minimize the risk of pulmonary complications due to fat emboli and inability to mobilize.

ADVANCED TRAUMA LIFE SUPPORT

During the primary survey, the orthopedic surgeon can assist in the management of musculoskeletal injuries that have a direct impact on the primary survey or injuries that are diagnosed during primary investigations. Overtly fractured limbs impeding assessment, the fractured pelvis with hemodynamic instability, and open long bone fractures with ongoing hemorrhage are all indications for the early intervention by the orthopedic surgeon. As the orthopedic surgeon identifies these injuries, they must stay in continual communication with the trauma team leader because they may affect resuscitation strategies.

Restoring gross length and alignment of fractures and stabilizing long bone and/or pelvic ring fractures with splints and/or a pelvic binder can minimize further blood loss, bone and soft tissue trauma, and reduce patient pain and analgesia requirement. However, it should be noted that resuscitation and the primary survey always take precedence over splinting of extremity fractures.

Of note, missed extremity injuries, especially in the hand and foot, can occur in more than 8% of trauma patients, which emphasizes the importance of repeat assessment.[11] A low threshold for a high index of suspicion of spinal injuries should also be considered in an unconscious patient and triple immobilization should be maintained until formal clinical evaluation is possible. If this is not possible due to a persistent unconscious or anesthetized patient, spine-specific imaging, computed tomography (CT), and MRI should be performed before removal of the immobilization. Adjuncts to the secondary survey include further radiographic imaging. It is now commonplace to perform a trauma protocol CT scan that may replace the need for other radiographs.[12]

ORTHOPEDICS IN THE EMERGENCY DEPARTMENT: EARLY INTERVENTIONS CAN IMPROVE OUTCOMES

Although the orthopedic surgeon may not be directly involved in the primary survey of the severely injured patient, their acute management of several conditions can have a dramatic effect on the patient's overall outcome.

Major Hemorrhage

The patient who presents in major hemorrhage is often in extremis. In the setting of major hemorrhage from an extremity injury, the main goal for the orthopedic surgeon is to assist in the so-called Stop the Bleed. This is initially managed by direct pressure, whether manual or via a pressure bandage. Failure to control hemorrhage through direct pressure should result in tourniquet application.[13,14] Because tourniquet use is more common prehospital, a patient may arrive with a tourniquet in place. Caution should always be taken when removing a tourniquet and it is advisable to have another ready to use proximally on removal or ensure it is removed in a controlled environment to ensure more harm is not inflicted. In the setting of a traumatic amputation, a tourniquet should be applied if hemorrhage control is needed and then it can be reassessed in the operating room.

Open Fractures

Open fractures involve a direct communication of the injured bone with the environment and are often the reflection of a high-energy injury. Not only does the potential for contamination worsen the injury burden but the high energy indicates severe damage to the local soft tissues, both leading to wound complications and an increased potential for infection. Open fractures are commonly classified by 2 different systems. The more commonly used Gustilo-Anderson Classification and the newer Orthopaedic Trauma Association's Open Fracture Classification (**Boxes 1** and **2**).[15,16] The most important predictor of infection following open fracture seems to be timeliness of antibiotic administration, with antibiotics given more than 60 minutes after injury being an independent risk factor for infection.[17] Typically, a first-generation cephalosporin is recommended with additional broader coverage only in certain scenarios.[18] Surgical debridement and irrigation should be performed within 24 hours, and ideally sooner depending on the level of contamination. The type of fixation, which can be either temporary or definitive, depends of the level of soft tissue injury and contamination. When required, wound coverage should be performed within 5 to 7 days.[17,19]

Femur Fractures

In the presence of hemodynamic instability and physiologic parameters that indicate hypovolemic shock, the assessment of circulation and hemorrhage involves the examination of the lower extremity for swelling. Even in the context of a closed femoral fracture, blood loss can be as much as 2.2 L.[20,21] Furthermore, 40% of isolated femoral fractures require blood transfusion.[22] In such situations it is advocated that skeletal immobilization of long bone fractures be performed during the primary survey.

Box 1
Gustilo-Anderson open fracture classification

Type 1

Wound is ≤1 cm with minimal soft tissue injury

Type 2

Wound is greater than 1 cm in length, moderate soft tissue injury

Type 3

- Extensive soft tissue injury, degloving, or periosteal stripping, but soft tissue closure is possible
- Extensive soft tissue injury with periosteal stripping, requires flap coverage
- Associated with an arterial injury requiring repair

From Gustilo RB, Mendoza RM, Williams DN. Problems in the management of type III (severe) open fractures: a new classification of type III open fractures. J Trauma 1984;24(8):743.

Box 2
Orthopaedic Trauma Association open fracture classification

Skin
1. Can be approximated
2. Cannot be approximated
3. Extensive degloving

Muscle
1. No muscle in area, no appreciable muscle necrosis, some muscle injury with intact muscle function
2. Loss of muscle but the muscle remains functional, some localized necrosis in the zone of injury that requires excision, intact muscle-tendon unit
3. Dead muscle, loss of muscle function, partial or complete compartment excision, complete disruption of a muscle-tendon unit, muscle defect does not approximate

Arterial
1. No injury
2. Artery injury without ischemia
3. Artery injury with distal ischemia

Contamination
1. None or minimal contamination
2. Surface contamination (easily removed; not embedded in bone or deep soft tissues)
3a. Imbedded in bone or deep soft tissues
3b. High-risk environmental conditions (eg, barnyard, fecal, dirty water)

Bone loss
1. None
2. Bone missing or devascularized but still some contact between proximal and distal fragments
3. Segmental bone loss

From Agel J, Evans AR, Marsh JL, et al. The OTA open fracture classification. J Orthop Trauma 2013;27(7):379–84; with permission.

The femur can be immobilized with in-line traction bucks or skeletal traction until early operative skeletal stabilization is performed.[23]

Pelvic Ring Injuries

Because of the energy needed to create a pelvic ring injury, they are often associated with hemodynamic instability, head injuries, thoracoabdominal injuries, and long bone fractures. In fact, pelvic fractures resulting in blood loss and hypovolemia have a mortality rate between 3% and 20%.[24] With increasing fracture severity, that is, more posterior pelvic disruption, the pelvic venous plexus, and internal iliac vessels are at an increased risk of injury and subsequent uncontrolled hemorrhage. Fluid resuscitation and hemorrhage control are vital. Many trauma centers have an algorithm based on the facility's capabilities to direct management, which involves stabilization of the pelvic ring injury at a minimum, for example, pelvic binder initially followed by external fixation.

Compartment Syndrome

Acute compartment syndrome (ACS) occurs when there is progressive myoneural ischemia due to the accumulation of fluid within a confined myofascial space or prolonged elevated pressure due to an external source such as a crush injury. ACS is considered a surgical emergency because irreversible muscle necrosis can begin within 6 hours of injury. Clinical examination findings of ACS consist of the 5 Ps:

pain out of proportion, pallor, paresthesia, pulselessness, and paralysis in the setting of a swollen extremity. The extremity often feels tight and the soft tissues are less compressible than the contralateral limb. ACS remains a clinical diagnosis; however, tools to measure intramuscular pressure and tissue oxygenation can be used to confirm the clinical diagnosis, which can be extremely useful in making the diagnosis in the obtunded patient. When obtaining intramuscular pressure measurements, a difference of less than 30 mm Hg from the diastolic blood pressure is concerning for ACS. Once ACS is diagnosed, emergent fasciotomies are performed to relieve the pressure and prevent further myoneural ischemia.

Vascular Injury

A vascular injury should be suspected if the injured extremity shows signs of pallor, reduced temperature, prolonged capillary refill, and reduced pulses. Before further examination, gross limb length and alignment should be obtained and the limb re-examined. The ankle-brachial index should be obtained if a vascular injury is suspected with a value of 0.90 or lower having a high positive predictive value for an associated vascular injury.[25] Re-establishment of the blood supply to the limb is an emergency because muscle necrosis begins to occur within 6 hours of injury. Close coordination with the vascular surgeon is vital because each surgical plan depends on the other. The sequence of the surgical procedure must be discussed to maximize care and minimize the ischemia time and risk of further injury to the patient and vascular repair if skeletal stabilization is done after the vascular repair.

Major Joint Dislocations

The close proximity and tethering of neurovascular structures to joints places them at significant risk of injury in joint dislocation. Localized soft-tissue swelling, distal extremity edema, abnormal neurology or the signs of vascular compromise are all markers for a high index of suspicion of a major joint dislocation. Expedient joint relocation and stabilization in a splint or traction may be necessary. Unlike most dislocations, a hip dislocation is considered an orthopedic emergency and should be reduced immediately on recognition because an increased time to reduction is associated with subsequent development of avascular necrosis.[26]

SCORING SYSTEMS: ARE THEY RELIABLE?

The decision to perform limb salvage or an amputation remains difficult. Scoring systems, such as the Mangled Extremity Severity Score (MESS)[27] and Limb Salvage Index (LSI),[28] have been developed to help guide surgeons in their decision-making process. However, the decision to salvage or amputate a limb often requires more factors to be considered than those commonly used in the scoring systems. As a result, their utility came into question and, in 2001, Bosse and colleagues[29] found that, out of all scoring systems evaluated, the MESS; the LSI; the Predictive Salvage Index; the Nerve Injury, Ischemia, Soft-Tissue Injury, Skeletal Injury, Shock, and Age of Patient Score; and the Hannover Fracture scale-98, none were able to predict the need for amputation in a large, multicenter prospective observational study. In 2008, Ly and colleagues[30] followed the same set of patients and found that the same scoring systems also lacked the ability to predict outcome and patient recovery following high-energy lower extremity trauma. Scoring systems also do not seem to have utility when treating severe combat injuries, as demonstrated by Sheean and colleagues.[31]

Other clinical examination findings have been considered in the decision-making process, such as the presence of plantar sensation on presentation. In fact, the absence of plantar sensation has historically been a primary reason for orthopedic and general surgeons to consider acute amputation.[32] However, an analysis performed by Bosse and colleagues[33] of subjects presenting without plantar sensation compared with matched controls following high-energy trauma demonstrated no difference in outcomes between groups at 2 years. Therefore, the treating surgeon should use all factors that are available in helping to make the decision and not hang their hat on 1 scoring system or 1 primary clinical examination finding. In addition, when time permits, that is, the patient is not in extremis, it is always helpful to confer with colleagues, other members of the trauma team, and, when able, the patient before the decision is made to amputate or salvage a severely injured extremity because there may be other factors to consider.

WHEN SHOULD IT BE FIXED?

One of the frequent discussions among orthopedic and general surgeons revolves around the appropriate timing to stabilize fractures. Although the discussion is often short and indications for urgent operative stabilization in those with isolated extremities is rather clear, the discussion can be longer and may involve multiple services in the polytrauma patient because more factors must be considered to ensure that the surgical intervention does not increase patient morbidity. Ideally, the right surgery is performed for each patient, personally tailored to their physiologic status. The term used to describe this is the application of early appropriate care (EAC). However, to apply EAC, what constitutes appropriate care must be understood. To do so, it is helpful to understand both sides of the historical argument between early total care (ETC) and damage control orthopedics (DCO), which can be used to selectively provide appropriate care, depending on the patient's clinical status and response to resuscitation. Although most research evaluating optimal timing of fracture fixation is centered on the femur, the principles can be applied to fractures of other long bones and the pelvic ring.

Early Total Care

Patients with unstable fractures of the femur, pelvis, acetabulum, and spine are often forced into a recumbent position, which predisposes them to pulmonary complications and prolonged systemic inflammation. Early stabilization of these injuries can lead to improved pain relief and mobility. Several studies have clearly demonstrated the benefits of ETC. Harvin and colleagues[34] published their decade of experience comparing femur fractures definitively stabilized with intramedullary nails before and after 24 hours. After adjusting for anatomic (Injury Severity Score [ISS]) and physiologic (Revised Trauma Score) indices, early fracture fixation was independently associated with a reduction in pulmonary complications by nearly 60%. It was also associated with a reduction in ventilator days, hospital length of stay, and overall hospital charges. These results are similar to those demonstrated by Vallier and colleagues,[35] who compared definitive fixation of unstable femur, acetabulum, pelvis, and thoracolumbar fractures performed before and after 24 hours. After adjusting for age and ISS, days in the intensive care unit and total hospital stay were lower with early fixation. In addition, there were greater than 10% fewer overall complications (24% vs 35.8%), and lower rates of acute respiratory distress syndrome (ARDS), pneumonia, and sepsis in those undergoing early versus delayed fixation.

As this evidence suggests, early definitive treatment may be safely used for patients with multiple injuries. However, ETC is not ideal for all patients because there is a clear subset of patients who benefit from DCO.

Damage Control Orthopedics

As the pendulum swung toward ETC, it was realized that not all patients did well having their fractures undergo definitive stabilization early. In fact, some types of patients seemed to do quite poorly with ETC. It became apparent that in certain patients, particularly those with pulmonary or head injuries, a less aggressive approach to fracture fixation might be needed. Trauma causes a sustained response of the immune system and the early hyperinflammatory response is often followed by a hypoinflammatory stage. In the polytrauma patient, extended surgery, which can lead to increased blood loss, hypothermia, and surgical trauma, can result in an excessive inflammatory reaction, which has been termed the second hit. In these patients, extensive surgical procedures can overwhelm the immune system, which can trigger a pulmonary complication, such as ARDS, or multiple organ failure.[36]

One alternative is delayed fracture care, that is, splinting or traction, of unstable fractures and performing surgical skeletal stabilization days to weeks later. Before the advent of modern surgical skeletal stabilization techniques, this was the norm. There are, however, significant disadvantages to delayed fracture care. In patients without adequate stabilization, in the case of the femur this would usually involve some form of skeletal traction, patients cannot be mobilized. As a result, they are at an increased risk for pulmonary complications and pressure ulcers. With the advancement in surgical skeletal stabilization techniques, there was a shift toward aggressive early stabilization of extremity fractures but, as alluded to earlier, ETC is not appropriate for everyone. Thus, the emergence of DCO.

DCO involves doing the necessary surgical interventions to stabilize the fracture to minimize excessive blood loss, improve pain, and promote mobilization. This usually involves procedures such as external fixation of long bone fractures or unstable pelvic ring injuries. Through the placement of external fixation in the acute period, that is, avoiding open and often lengthy and/or bloody surgical procedures, the second hit is theoretically avoided and definitive reconstruction can occur at a later point after the patient's physiologic parameters have improved. The benefits of this strategy on the immune system have been demonstrated by Pape and colleagues.[37] In a prospective, randomized, multicenter study, 35 polytrauma subjects (ISS >16) with a diaphyseal femur fracture were randomized to either ETC or DCO, and serum inflammatory markers were trended over time. In those with ETC (intramedullary nail), there was a sustained increase in serum inflammatory markers, which was not seen in the DCO group following both the initial external fixation and subsequent conversion to definitive fixation with an intramedullary nail.

In a retrospective study, Harwood and colleagues[38] compared the Systemic Inflammatory Response Syndrome (SIRS) Score and Marshall multiorgan dysfunction score of subjects with femur fractures treated with either ETC or DCO. It was not surprising that the DCO group had more severe injuries based on the new ISS, and more head and thoracic injuries. Despite this, they had a smaller, shorter postoperative SIRS and did not suffer significantly more pronounced organ failure than the ETC group. Interestingly, those in the DCO group who underwent conversion to an intramedullary nail when their SIRS score was raised suffered the most pronounced subsequent inflammatory response and organ failure, which emphasizes the impact that the second hit can have and the importance of planning the definitive fixation based on physiologic improvement.

Early Appropriate Care: When to Choose Early Total Care Versus Damage Control Orthopedics

What is very clear is that stable patients should be treated with ETC, whereas unstable patients should undergo DCO. The challenge has been defining the appropriate clinical indications to perform DCO or ETC in the borderline patient. Various definitions of the borderline patient have been made to include that by Pape and colleagues,[37] who define it by the following: ISS greater than 40, multiple injuries (ISS >20) in combination with thorax trauma, multiple injuries in combination with severe abdominal or pelvic injury, hemorrhagic shock at the moment of administration, moderate or severe head trauma, radiographic evidence of pulmonary contusion, bilateral femur fractures, or a body temperature below 35°C.[36] D'Alleyrand and O'Toole[39] have proposed 3 common indicators for DCO of borderline patients that they use at the R. Adams Cowley Shock Trauma Center in Baltimore, MD: (1) closed head injury, (2) poor response to resuscitation in the first 12 hours, and (3) poor respiratory status at the time of fracture treatment.

It is helpful to know where these indications have come from and what defines an appropriate response to resuscitation to safely apply them. One increasingly used method of assessing response to resuscitation is trending lactate levels. In patients undergoing definitive fixation of a femur fracture with an intramedullary nail within 24 hours of injury, admission lactate is significantly associated with pulmonary complications when other factors such as age, Glasgow Coma Scale, and AIS were controlled. However, preoperative lactate was not found to be a risk factor.[40] A median preoperative lactate of 2.8 mmol/L was not associated with increased pulmonary complications, as opposed to previous publications.[41] These results are similar to those seen by Vallier and colleagues[35,42] in which admission lactate, in addition to the severity of the abdominal and thoracic injuries, contribute most to the development of pulmonary morbidity. It is likely that the trend in lactate, that is, a lactate level improving and approaching 2.5 mmol/L, demonstrates an adequate response to resuscitation and, therefore, can lead to safe application of ETC. On the contrary, in those with closed head injuries, severe abdominal, or severe thoracic injuries, DCO should be considered.

This was also demonstrated in a review by Vallier and colleagues[42] of subjects with pelvis, acetabulum, spine, and/or proximal or diaphyseal femur fractures treated surgically. Pulmonary complications occurred in 12% of subjects with 8.2% developing pneumonia. Lactate levels were greater with pulmonary complications and were the single most specific predictor of complications. An uncomplicated course was associated with absence of a chest injury and definitive fixation within 24 or 48 hours. The investigators concluded that complications can be minimized when isolated fractures are treated on early and, when patients have injuries to other body systems and/or severe hemorrhage, DCO may be advisable to optimize outcomes.

In summary, if the patient demonstrates any physiologic signs of end-organ hypoperfusion, DCO should be pursued. It is also important for the orthopedic surgeon to communicate with both the general surgeon and the anesthetist so that care is optimized. This allows the treatment plan to be altered in an effort to optimize the patient's outcomes if the patient's physiologic parameters change throughout the resuscitation process or surgical procedure.

SUMMARY

Severe extremity injuries are not only a challenge to treat but doing so results in high resource utilization and often high levels of levels of disability.[3,43] The decision to pursue DCO versus ETC may lead to a shorter hospital stay and fewer complications, but there is likely more that surgeons can do optimize patient outcomes throughout the entire care continuum beyond the decisions made or actions taken within the first few hours following injury. The best available data comparing outcomes of limb salvage and amputees from the Lower Extremity Assessment Project (LEAP) Study Group found no difference in outcomes between groups at both 2 and 7 years. They did, however, identify several predictors of poor outcome, regardless of group, to include a poor social support network and low self-efficacy.[3,44] This concept of self-efficacy and social support network is something that many orthopedic surgeons have not paid much attention to in the past. Multiple studies have highlighted the importance of various factors in a patient's overall recovery process, such as access to vocational and mental health support.[45] In addition, certain psychological factors play a significant role in predicting pain following trauma.[46,47] It is important that orthopedic surgeons and members of the trauma team take their level of care a step further beyond saving life and limb, and take these factors into consideration when attempting to optimize patient outcomes.

REFERENCES

1. WISQARS (Web-based Injury Statistics Query and Reporting System), Injury Center, CDC. Available at: https://www.cdc.gov/injury/wisqars/index.html. Accessed March 2, 2017.
2. Miller TR, Pindus NM, Douglass JB, et al. Databook on nonfatal injury: incidence, costs, and consequences. Washington, DC: Urban Institute Press; 1995.
3. MacKenzie EJ, Bosse MJ, Pollak AN, et al. Long-term persistence of disability following severe lower-limb trauma. Results of a seven-year follow-up. J Bone Joint Surg Am 2005;87(8):1801–9.
4. Mackenzie EJ, Rivara FP, Jurkovich GJ, et al. The impact of trauma-center care on functional outcomes following major lower-limb trauma. J Bone Joint Surg Am 2008;90(1):101–9.
5. Morshed S, Knops S, Jurkovich GJ, et al. The impact of trauma-center care on mortality and function following pelvic ring and acetabular injuries. J Bone Joint Surg Am 2015;97(4):265–72.
6. Sielatycki JA, Sawyer JR, Mir HR. Supply and demand analysis of the orthopaedic trauma surgeon workforce in the United States. J Orthop Trauma 2016;30(5): 278–83.
7. American College of Surgeons Committee on Trauma. Statement on trauma center designation based upon system need. Bull Am Coll Surg 2015;100(1):51–2. Available at: http://www.ncbi.nlm.nih.gov/pubmed/25626271. Accessed March 2, 2017.
8. Stinner DJ, Johnson AE, Pollak A, et al. "Zero preventable deaths and minimizing disability" – the challenge set forth by the national academies of sciences, engineering, and medicine. J Orthop Trauma 2017. http://dx.doi.org/10.1097/BOT. 0000000000000806.
9. Trunkey DD. Trauma. Accidental and intentional injuries account for more years of life lost in the U.S. than cancer and heart disease. Among the prescribed remedies are improved preventive efforts, speedier surgery and further research. Sci Am 1983;249(2):28–35. Available at: http://www.ncbi.nlm.nih.gov/pubmed/6623052. Accessed March 2, 2017.
10. Baue AE. Multiple, progressive, or sequential systems failure. A syndrome of the 1970s. Arch Surg 1975;110(7):779–81. Available at: http://www.ncbi.nlm.nih.gov/pubmed/1079720. Accessed March 2, 2017.
11. Giannakopoulos GF, Saltzherr TP, Beenen LFM, et al. Missed injuries during the initial assessment in a cohort of 1124 level-1 trauma patients. Injury 2012;43(9): 1517–21.

12. Huber-Wagner S, Lefering R, Qvick L-M, et al. Effect of whole-body CT during trauma resuscitation on survival: a retrospective, multicentre study. Lancet 2009;373(9673):1455–61.

13. Brodie S, Hodgetts TJ, Ollerton J, et al. Tourniquet use in combat trauma: UK military experience. J R Army Med Corps 2007;153(4):310–3. Available at: http://www.ncbi.nlm.nih.gov/pubmed/18619170. Accessed March 2, 2017.

14. Kragh JF, Walters TJ, Baer DG, et al. Survival with emergency tourniquet use to stop bleeding in major limb trauma. Ann Surg 2009;249(1):1–7.

15. Gustilo RB, Anderson JT. Prevention of infection in the treatment of one thousand and twenty-five open fractures of long bones: retrospective and prospective analyses. J Bone Joint Surg Am 1976;58(4):453–8. Available at: http://www.ncbi.nlm.nih.gov/pubmed/773941. Accessed March 2, 2017.

16. Agel J, Evans AR, Marsh JL, et al. The OTA open fracture classification. J Orthop Trauma 2013;27(7):379–84.

17. Lack WD, Karunakar MA, Angerame MR, et al. Type III open tibia fractures. J Orthop Trauma 2014;29(1):1.

18. Murray CK, Obremskey WT, Hsu JR, et al. Prevention of infections associated with combat-related extremity injuries. J Trauma 2011;71(2 Suppl 2):S235–57.

19. D'Alleyrand J-CG, Manson TT, Dancy L, et al. Is time to flap coverage of open tibial fractures an independent predictor of flap-related complications? J Orthop Trauma 2014;28(5):288–93.

20. Powers WF, Hensley CD. Circulating blood volume changes incident to major orthopedic surgery. J Am Med Assoc 1959;169(6):545–7. Available at: http://www.ncbi.nlm.nih.gov/pubmed/13620501. Accessed March 2, 2017.

21. Clarke R, Topley E, Flear CT. Assessment of blood-loss in civilian trauma. Lancet 1955;268(6865):629–38. Available at: http://www.ncbi.nlm.nih.gov/pubmed/14354953. Accessed March 2, 2017.

22. Lieurance R, Benjamin JB, Rappaport WD. Blood loss and transfusion in patients with isolated femur fractures. J Orthop Trauma 1992;6(2):175–9. Available at: http://www.ncbi.nlm.nih.gov/pubmed/1602337. Accessed March 2, 2017.

23. Even JL, Richards JE, Crosby CG, et al. Preoperative skeletal versus cutaneous traction for femoral shaft fractures treated within 24 hours. J Orthop Trauma 2012;26(10):e177–82.

24. Giannoudis PV, Grotz MRW, Tzioupis C, et al. Prevalence of pelvic fractures, associated injuries, and mortality: the United Kingdom perspective. J Trauma 2007;63(4):875–83.

25. Mills WJ, Barei DP, McNair P. The value of the ankle-brachial index for diagnosing arterial injury after knee dislocation: a prospective study. J Trauma 2004;56(6):1261–5. Available at: http://www.ncbi.nlm.nih.gov/pubmed/15211135. Accessed March 2, 2017.

26. Sahin V, Karakas E, Aksu S, et al. Traumatic dislocation and fracture-dislocation of the hip: a long-term follow-up study. J Trauma 2003;54(3):520–9.

27. Johansen K, Daines M, Howey T, et al. Objective criteria accurately predict amputation following lower extremity trauma. J Trauma 1990;30(5):568–72 [discussion: 572–3]. Available at: http://www.ncbi.nlm.nih.gov/pubmed/2342140. Accessed March 2, 2017.

28. Russell WL, Sailors DM, Whittle TB, et al. Limb salvage versus traumatic amputation. A decision based on a seven-part predictive index. Ann Surg 1991;213(5):473–80 [discussion: 480–1]. Available at: http://www.ncbi.nlm.nih.gov/pubmed/2025068. Accessed March 2, 2017.

29. Bosse MJ, MacKenzie EJ, Kellam JF, et al. A prospective evaluation of the clinical utility of the lower-extremity injury-severity scores. J Bone Joint Surg Am 2001; 83-A(1):3–14. Available at: http://www.ncbi.nlm.nih.gov/pubmed/11205855.

30. Ly TV, Travison TG, Castillo RC, et al. Ability of lower-extremity injury severity scores to predict functional outcome after limb salvage. J Bone Joint Surg Am 2008;90(8):1738–43.

31. Sheean AJ, Krueger CA, Napierala MA, et al, Skeletal Trauma and Research Consortium (STReC). Evaluation of the mangled extremity severity score in combat-related type III open tibia fracture. J Orthop Trauma 2014;28(9):523–6.

32. MacKenzie EJ, Bosse MJ, Kellam JF, et al. Factors influencing the decision to amputate or reconstruct after high-energy lower extremity trauma. J Trauma 2002;52(4):641–9. Available at: http://www.ncbi.nlm.nih.gov/pubmed/11956376. Accessed March 2, 2017.

33. Bosse MJ, McCarthy ML, Jones AL, et al. The insensate foot following severe lower extremity trauma: an indication for amputation? J Bone Joint Surg Am 2005;87(12):2601–8.

34. Harvin JA, Harvin WH, Camp E, et al. Early femur fracture fixation is associated with a reduction in pulmonary complications and hospital charges: a decade of experience with 1,376 diaphyseal femur fractures. J Trauma Acute Care Surg 2012;73(6):1442–8.

35. Vallier HA, Super DM, Moore TA, et al. Do patients with multiple system injury benefit from early fixation of unstable axial fractures? The effects of timing of surgery on initial hospital course. J Orthop Trauma 2013;27(7):405–12.

36. Lichte P, Kobbe P, Dombroski D, et al. Damage control orthopedics: current evidence. Curr Opin Crit Care 2012;18(6):647–50.

37. Pape HC, Grimme K, van Griensven M, et al, EPOFF Study Group. Impact of intramedullary instrumentation versus damage control for femoral fractures on immunoinflammatory parameters: prospective randomized analysis by the EPOFF Study Group. J Trauma 2003;55(1):7–13.

38. Harwood PJ, Giannoudis PV, van Griensven M, et al. Alterations in the systemic inflammatory response after early total care and damage control procedures for femoral shaft fracture in severely injured patients. J Trauma 2005;58(3): 446–52.

39. D'Alleyrand JCG, O'Toole RV. The evolution of damage control orthopedics. Current evidence and practical applications of early appropriate care. Orthop Clin North Am 2013;44(4):499–507.

40. Richards JE, Matuszewski PE, Griffin SM, et al. The role of elevated lactate as a risk factor for pulmonary morbidity after early fixation of femoral shaft fractures. J Orthop Trauma 2016;30(6):312–8.

41. Crowl AC, Young JS, Kahler DM, et al. Occult hypoperfusion is associated with increased morbidity in patients undergoing early femur fracture fixation. J Trauma 2000;48(2):260–7. Available at: http://www.ncbi.nlm.nih.gov/pubmed/10697084. Accessed March 2, 2017.

42. Vallier HA, Wang X, Moore TA, et al. Timing of orthopaedic surgery in multiple trauma patients: development of a protocol for early appropriate care. J Orthop Trauma 2013;27(10):543–51.

43. Masini BD, Waterman SM, Wenke JC, et al. Resource utilization and disability outcome assessment of combat casualties from operation Iraqi freedom and operation enduring freedom. J Orthop Trauma 2009;23(4):261–6.

44. Bosse MJ, MacKenzie EJ, Kellam JF, et al. An analysis of outcomes of reconstruction or amputation after leg-threatening injuries. N Engl J Med 2002;347(24): 1924–31.
45. Archer KR, Castillo RC, MacKenzie EJ, et al, LEAP Study Group. Perceived need and unmet need for vocational, mental health, and other support services after severe lower-extremity trauma. Arch Phys Med Rehabil 2010;91(5):774–80.
46. Vranceanu A-M, Bachoura A, Weening A, et al. Psychological factors predict disability and pain intensity after skeletal trauma. J Bone Joint Surg Am 2014; 96(3):e20.
47. Castillo RC, Wegener ST, Heins SE, et al. Longitudinal relationships between anxiety, depression, and pain: results from a two-year cohort study of lower extremity trauma patients. Pain 2013;154(12):2860–6.

Surgical Management of Vascular Trauma

Pedro G.R. Teixeira, MD[a], Joe DuBose, MD[b,c,d,e],*

KEYWORDS

- Vascular trauma • Trauma care • Hemorrhage

KEY POINTS

- Vascular injuries remain among the most challenging entities encountered in the setting of trauma care.
- Improvements in diagnostic capabilities, resuscitation approaches, vascular techniques, and prosthetic device options have afforded considerable advancement in the care of these patients.
- This evolution in care capabilities continues — most recently in the form of endovascular treatment modalities.
- Despite advances, however, uncontrolled hemorrhage due to major vascular injury remains one of the most common causes of death after trauma.
- Successful management of vascular injury requires the timely diagnosis and control of bleeding sources; to facilitate this task, trauma providers must appreciate the capabilities and limitations of diagnostic imaging modalities.
- Above all else, trauma providers must understand when and how to most effectively apply these strategies.

INTRODUCTION AND GENERAL CONSIDERATIONS

Vascular injuries remain among the most challenging entities encountered in the setting of trauma care. Although described since the earliest eras of surgical history, it has only been in the latter half of the twentieth century that significant progress has been made in the management of these injuries. Improvements in diagnostic capabilities, resuscitation approaches, vascular techniques, and prosthetic device options

[a] Department of Surgery and Perioperative Care, University Medical Center Brackenridge, Dell Medical School, University of Texas at Austin, 1501 Red River Street, Austin, TX 78712, USA; [b] Uniformed Services University of the Health Sciences, 4301 Jones Bridge Road, Bethesda, MD 20814, USA; [c] David Grant Medical Center, 101 Bodin Cir, Travis Air Force Base, Fairfield, CA 94535, USA; [d] Division of Vascular Surgery, University of California, Davis, 2315 Stockton Blvd, Davis, CA 95817, USA; [e] Division of Trauma, Acute Care Surgery and Surgical Critical Care, University of California, Davis, 2315 Stockton Blvd, Davis, CA 95817, USA
* Corresponding author. Division of Trauma, Acute Care Surgery, University of California, 2315 Stockton Blvd, Davis, CA 95817, USA
E-mail address: jjd3c@yahoo.com

Surg Clin N Am 97 (2017) 1133–1155
http://dx.doi.org/10.1016/j.suc.2017.05.001
0039-6109/17/Published by Elsevier Inc.
surgical.theclinics.com

have afforded considerable advancement in the care of these patients. This evolution in care capabilities continues — most recently in the form of endovascular treatment modalities. Despite these advances, however, uncontrolled hemorrhage due to major vascular injury remains one of the most common causes of death after trauma.

Successful management of vascular injury requires the timely diagnosis and control of bleeding sources. To facilitate this task, trauma providers must appreciate the capabilities and limitations of diagnostic imaging modalities. They must also prove facile in the effective emergent control of these injuries and understand the appropriate role of both initial and definitive management strategies. Above all else, they must understand when and how to most effectively apply these strategies.

Entire textbooks have been dedicated to the topic of vascular trauma. The limited context of this article strives to emphasize key topics pertinent to the contemporary care of vascular injuries. Key principles are reviewed, with additional comment on injuries at specific locations and injury in unique populations.

INITIAL EVALUATION

Patient presentation is an important consideration in the choice of diagnostic strategies that might be used in the evaluation of suspected vascular injuries. For patients presenting with active hemorrhage, the diagnosis is straightforward and no additional evaluation is required. As a general principle, the presence of a hard sign of vascular injury (**Table 1**) warrants immediate operation for exploration and earliest possible control of vascular hemorrhage. Patients who present with soft signs (see **Table 1**) suggestive of occult vascular injury, however, benefit from additional diagnostic imaging. A variety of imaging options are available, each with important capabilities and limitations to consider.

Duplex Ultrasonography

Duplex ultrasonography can be performed at the bedside. This imaging modality does, however, require effective training for utilization and likely has limited applicability in most acute trauma settings. Images may be obscured by the presence of associated hematoma, soft tissue injury, and bony injuries. When adequate images are attainable, however, color flow duplex and spectral waveform analysis combine to provide invaluable information (**Fig. 1**). This tool is also useful for follow-up of injuries treated nonoperatively and for postoperative evaluation of vascular injury repairs.

Computed Tomographic Angiography

Modern Computed Tomographic angiography (CTA) has emerged as the modality of choice for the diagnosis of vascular injury for the majority of stable trauma patients with vascular injuries — even at peripheral arterial injury locations.[1-3] This modality

Table 1	
Signs of vascular injury	
Hard Signs	**Soft Signs**
Active pulsatile bleeding	Diminished pulses distal to the injury site
Absent pulses distal to the injury site	Stable, small hematoma
Expanding or pulsatile hematoma	Proximity to major vessels
Bruit or thrill at the injury site	Peripheral nerve deficit
Unexplained shock	History of hemorrhage at scene
	Suspicious pattern of fracture or dislocation

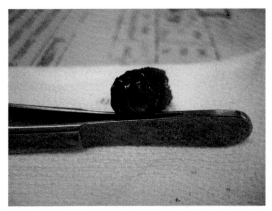

Fig. 1. Gross back-table photo of a dissection of the superficial femoral artery detected by duplex ultrasound evaluation.

is generally more rapid than traditional angiography to obtain at most centers, is widely available, and yields high-resolution imaging that can be used for management planning. It is important to consider, however, that optimal imaging requires a contrast load — which may be detrimental to patients with impaired renal function at presentation. Additionally, although rapidly obtained, CTA images require time to obtain that may not be afforded in patient who has aggressive hemorrhage and instability. Despite these concerns, CTA has emerged as the modality of choice for vascular imaging after trauma at most centers.

Traditional Angiography

Once the mainstay of vascular imaging, traditional digital subtraction angiography has now largely been replaced by CTA. In specific instances, however, this modality remains an integral tool of evaluation — particularly when foreign metal objects in proximity to vascular structures result in scatter artifacts that obscure CTA images. One classic scenario where this may occur is that of a shotgun blast injury at relatively close range — resulting in focused metallic burden that defies optimal CTA imaging of nearby vascular structures. In addition, the resources and expertise that must be mustered for optimal employment of traditional angiography may take considerably more time than modern CT-based imaging.

Intravascular Ultrasound

Although not used aggressively in a majority of centers, intravascular ultrasound (IVUS) bears mention as an emerging technology for the imaging of large vessel injuries.[4] This technology has already demonstrated potential in the effective characterization of blunt thoracic aortic injuries and can serve to provide key information regarding optimal sizing of endovascular covered stent grafts for these injuries. Although additional study is required, IVUS demonstrates some promise in select applications of this kind after vascular injuries.

EMERGENT MANAGEMENT — DAMAGE CONTROL SURGERY

Although definitive surgical treatment of vascular trauma remains the ultimate objective of care for patients requiring surgery, there are important caveats to consider. Vascular repairs can prove technically demanding and time-consuming affairs. Patients with physiologic depletion due to hemorrhage may require the employment of abbreviated damage control approaches that permit stabilization of the patient. In this fashion, a second intervention can be undertaken in a more controlled setting and under circumstances that permit an optimal definitive repair. Similarly, damage control approaches may be optimal in situations that demand expedient conduct of more critical procedures. For example, a shunt can be used to restore temporary perfusion to a distal limb so that a craniectomy can be conducted to prevent herniation in the setting of severe traumatic brain injury.

A variety of vascular damage control adjuncts have been described. Each has utility in specific situations but also potential pitfalls. An exhaustive discussion of the application of these adjuncts is not permissible here, but each warrant mention as a potential tool of emergent vascular trauma care.

Ligation

As a general rule, all major named arteries should be repaired or reconstructed if at all possible. In the setting of damage control, however, ligation may be considered for specific vessels if the conduct of repair will compromise the ability of the patient to survive operation. It must be recognized, for example, that the principle of "life over limb" applies in specific settings. Specific anatomic redundancies of the vascular system and collateral pathways for distal perfusion may also afford ligation as a simple answer for the patient in extremis. Applicable situations of this type include ligation of the radial artery in an upper extremity that has dominant ulnar perfusion to the palmar arch or ligation of the peroneal artery in the setting of an intact tibial artery outflow to the plantar arch.

In more drastic situations, ligation of the carotid artery has been described without residual ischemic sequela — provided the patient has an intact circle of Willis. Ligation of the subclavian artery has also been described, with preservation of upper extremity perfusion. Although ligation in these more extreme situations has been espoused an effective means of salvaging life, modern experience has suggested that the liberal use of temporary arterial vascular shunts may prove a more appropriate damage control intervention for injuries to these vessels.

A majority of venous injuries should be ligated in the setting of damage control, whereas in stable patients formal repair of simple injuries is advisable. The decision to repair venous injuries that require an interposition graft should be made on a case-by-case basis and should be considered advisable in larger venous structures. As with arterial injury, temporary vascular shunts can be used for larger venous injuries as a temporizing measure.

Temporary Vascular Shunts

Endoluminal temporary shunts should be used in damage control situations that involve injuries to moderate-sized arteries (ie, popliteal and visceral) but can be effectively used in a variety of venous and arterial vessels of varying sizes.[5] Commercially available shunts used in elective vascular surgery are ideally suited for this purpose. Careful insertion of the shunt is required to prevent additional vessel trauma and distal dissection. Prior to insertion, the injured vessel should be débrided and all thrombus removed both proximally and distally. A Rummel tourniquet using either umbilical tapes or silastic vessel loops can be used to secure the shunts and prevent dislodgment during patient movement (**Fig. 2**).

Temporary Balloon Occlusion

Growing experience with the utilization of endovascular technologies in the trauma setting has demonstrated that balloon occlusion for proximal vascular control can

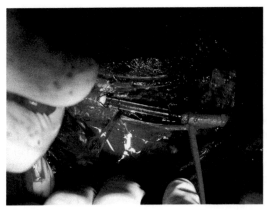

Fig. 2. Vascular shunt of the superficial femoral artery used in damage control setting.

prove useful in a variety of settings. Endovascular balloon positioning and inflation can be used either as a bridge to definitive endovascular repair of traumatic injuries or in a hybrid approach to facilitate open exposure and surgical repair. The use of endovascular balloon occlusion in a hybrid fashion may prove particularly useful when vascular injuries occur at anatomic sites that represent challenging surgical exposures, including axillosubclavian and iliac artery injuries occurring in the junctional region between the torso and the extremities.

Recent evidence also suggest that there may be a role for early Resuscitative Endovascular Balloon Occlusion of the Aorta (REBOA) for patients who present to the trauma center with significant hemorrhage at noncompressible sites.[6] Although additional study is required on the topic, early evidence suggests that REBOA is a feasible alternative to traditional aortic occlusion via resuscitative thoracotomy for patients in extremis due to bleeding from these sources.[7]

DEFINITIVE REPAIR

Definitive vascular repair may take place after stabilization of a patient after damage control utilization or as initial treatment in patients who are stable enough to tolerate the time required for repair at the first operation. The modern era of care affords a variety of potential definitive solutions to most vascular injury problems. The choice of repair must be made with careful consideration of the potential role of each approach.

Primary Repair

Primary repair of both venous and arterial injuries can be considered for clean lacerations of vessels. It may also be entertained when, after appropriate débridement, the gap between the proximal and distal ends of the vessel can be mobilized to come together in a tension-free fashion. Traditional dogma has often espoused 2 cm as the maximal gap that can be bridged to achieve this goal. In practice, however, even a smaller gap between anastomotic ends can prove problematic at select anatomic locations. A safe principle for utilization is to strongly consider an interposition graft when any tension is anticipated with attempted primary repair.

Specific suture size and repair technique are dictated by vessel size and location. Repair with interrupted suture may prove the least likely to result in an anastomotic stricture when addressing smaller arteries. The adjunctive utilization of vascular pledgets may prove useful in specific large vessel repairs, particularly when conducting tenuous repairs of large, thin-walled venous structures.

Autogenous versus Prosthetic Conduit

Interposition repair using autogenous reversed saphenous vein grafts remains a standard of vascular injury repair for appropriately sized vessels (**Fig. 3**). These native vessels are considered a lower risk for potential infection and are familiar to the majority of trauma and vascular surgeons. Size mismatch, however, frequently makes this option an impossibility in the trauma setting. In addition, adequate vein may not be available for a variety of reasons, and there is a concern of possible delayed aneurysmal conversion of these grafts. Finally, saphenous vein harvest can take additional time to perform.

Prosthetic Conduits

Prosthetic grafts are an effective and durable alternative when used in surgical fields that are not compromised by gross contamination. For vessels greater than 4 mm to 6 mm in diameter, a prosthetic graft is also an advisable solution to avoid the size mismatch that can be problematic with saphenous vein utilization. Prosthetic utilization also obviates time that is required for vein harvest. When prosthetic is selected as the interposition conduit after vascular injury, expanded polytetrafluoroethylene (ePTFE) is preferred due to its higher resistance to infection.[8]

Endovascular Stent Grafts

For stable patients, emerging endovascular capabilities have demonstrated considerable promise a specific anatomic locations of vascular injury. The treatment of blunt thoracic vascular injury with thoracic endovascular aortic repair (TEVAR) has, for example, proved superior to traditional open repair techniques.[9,10] The potential of endovascular repair at other anatomically challenging locations, such as the axillosubclavian region, has also been recently demonstrated.[11,12] Although additional study is required to determine the optimal role of endovascular stent grafts in the treatment of vascular injuries at other locations, early incorporation of providers with endovascular skillsets may prove useful in determining the repair options for these injuries.

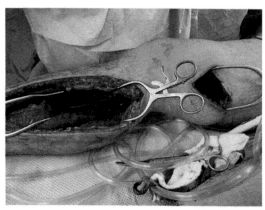

Fig. 3. Saphenous vein interposition graft repair of a popliteal artery injury.

Intraoperative Anticoagulation

The use of systemic heparinization is ubiquitous to elective vascular surgery and may be beneficial for the operative management of vascular injuries after vascular control and during reconstruction. The use of this adjunct has been shown to improve outcomes in select vascular injuries, including carotid and popliteal artery injuries.[12,13] The decision to use systemic heparinization does, however, require careful consideration and multidisciplinary discussion with the trauma team. Appropriate use requires patient stability, the absence of traumatic brain injury, or neurologic deficit and minimal associated blood loss from concomitant solid organ and musculoskeletal injuries. When heparin is contraindicated, the authors recommend liberal instillation of heparinized saline into the proximal and distal segments of the injured vessel at regular intervals during repair.

Postoperative Evaluation

After any vascular intervention or repair, restoration of perfusion should be confirmed appropriately. For patients with return of bounding distal pulses, physical examination may suffice. A multiphasic hand-held Doppler signal is a reassuring finding that should be sought when palpable pulses are not clearly appreciated or there is a discrepancy between sides for repairs of extremity vessels. Any discrepancy should likely be investigated with an intraoperative formal duplex examination or angiogram to confirm patency of repair and the absence of a missed additional injury. Even among patients who have clear demonstration of patency at the time of initial operation, significant vigilance must be maintained with serial examinations/Doppler utilization in a monitored setting postoperatively to guard against early loss of patency.

An additional question postoperatively remains the optimal role of postintervention anticoagulation or antiplatelet therapy. Although data to definitively guide management are currently lacking, the routine use of aspirin for most repairs should be considered long term, particularly in the setting of stent utilization or synthetic conduit repairs. More advanced antiplatelet medications should also be considered strongly in these 2 settings. The role of heparin, direct-thrombin inhibitors, or other agents has not been defined — but may be of use for repairs/interventions considered at high risk for thrombosis. In every instance the risk of antiplatelet or anticoagulation induced bleeding must be carefully weighed against the benefit of use — which requires careful consideration of individual risk for each patient. It is the authors' hope that additional data will accumulate in coming years to better guide these choices.

SPECIFIC INJURIES
Head and Neck/Cerebrovascular Injuries

The neck is classically divided into 3 distinct anatomic: zone I extends from the clavicles to the cricoid cartilage, zone II from the cricoid cartilage to the angle of the mandible, and zone III from the angle of the mandible to the base of the skull. Injuries in zone II are the most accessible for direct surgical exposure, which is performed through an anterolateral cervical exploration. Exposure of injuries in zone I usually requires median sternotomy for proximal control. Surgical exposure of injuries in zone III is challenging, which makes these lesions best treated with an endovascular approach.

Carotid arteries

Differently from blunt cerebrovascular injuries, which are in general treated with anticoagulation or antiplatelet therapy (**Fig. 4**), penetrating cerebrovascular injuries

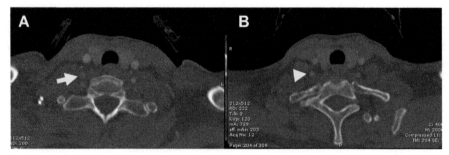

Fig. 4. CT scan demonstrating blunt injury of the right vertebral artery (*A*) Injury denoted by arrow, with complete resolution after 6 weeks on antiplatelet therapy. (*B*) Former location of injury indicated by arrowhead.

generally require surgical intervention. Unless hard signs of cerebrovascular injury are present, mandating surgical exploration, CT angiogram is imaging modality of choice for diagnosis.

Injuries to the external carotid artery with active bleeding are, in general, best managed by ligation or embolization (**Fig. 5**). Penetrating injuries to the internal and common carotid arteries are best managed by direct repair or reconstruction.[13,14] For those cases in which the tissue destruction is minimal, usually resulting from a stab wound, direct repair or patch may be applicable. In most instances, however, particularly with firearm injuries, arterial reconstruction is necessary.

The carotid sheath is exposed through an anterolateral neck incision. There is usually a significant hematoma that distorts the anatomy and may increase the risk of cranial nerve damage. After the carotid is exposed, proximal and distal control is obtained and the injury is carefully evaluated. All nonviable tissue should be débrided and a decision is made regarding the need to use an interposition graft. A reverse greater

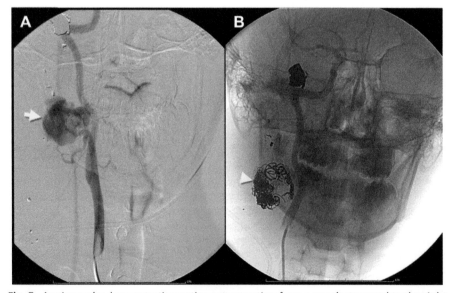

Fig. 5. Angiography demonstrating active extravasation from a gunshot wound to the right external carotid artery (*A*) indicated by arrow and after successful coil embolization (*B*) indicated by arrow head.

saphenous vein graft is the preferred conduit for carotid reconstruction **Fig. 6**; however, the repair can be done with ePTFE if time is of the essence or if no suitable autogenous conduit is available.

Perioperative shunting is usually not necessary for injuries of the common carotid artery particularly if there is adequate back bleeding from the distal stump.

For internal carotid injuries, the use of a temporary shunt, although not definitively supported by data, may have a role not only in decreasing the risk of cerebral ischemia during the reconstruction but also in maintaining cerebral perfusion while an autogenous conduit is harvested or while other associated life-threatening injuries are addressed.

Vertebral artery

Because of its trajectory through the vertebral foramen from the sixth to the first cervical vertebrae, exposure to the vertebral artery is exceedingly challenging and repair is not feasible in most situations. If exposure of the vertebral artery, however, becomes necessary to control active bleeding, it can be achieved by unroofing the vertebral transverse process foramen using a rongeur or pituitary forceps. Ligation of the proximal segment, before the artery becomes surrounded by the bony structures, can be performed and it is an acceptable approach. Angioembolization techniques are also attractive therapeutic modalities for injuries of the vertebral artery.

Internal jugular vein

Isolated penetrating injuries of the jugular vein can be safely managed nonoperatively[15]; however, neck exploration is usually necessary to address associated injuries. Unilateral internal jugular injuries are best managed with ligation if significant stenosis of the vein would result from an attempt to repair. In the rare occasion of bilateral internal jugular vein injuries, at least one of the veins must be repaired because bilateral ligation invariably results in cerebral venous congestion with high mortality, this being the only indication for extensive internal jugular vein reconstruction with patch or interposition graft.

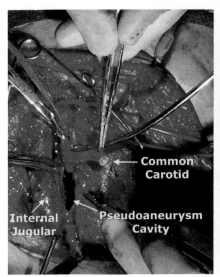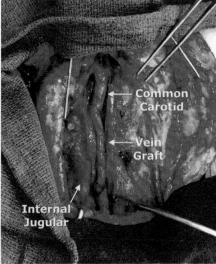

Fig. 6. Pseudoaneurysm of the right common carotid artery before and after repair with interposition graft using reverse greater saphenous vein.

Thoracic

Penetrating thoracic injuries

Penetrating thoracic vascular injuries are highly lethal and often present with exsanguination resulting in hemodynamic instability requiring immediate surgical exploration for resuscitation and hemostasis. Patients with thoracic penetrating wounds are managed according to the Advanced Trauma Life Support guidelines, usually involving a chest tube placement early during the primary survey and resuscitation phase. Hemodynamic instability and high-volume output from the chest tube are both indicators for thoracotomy. The decision regarding what incision to perform depends on the estimated injury trajectory and suspected vascular injury, side of high chest tube output, and need for open cardiac massage. It is also important to consider that not uncommonly more than one cavity may need to be explored, particularly if a transmediastinal or thoracoabdominal injury trajectory is suspected.

Injuries to the aortic arch branches are usually approached through a median sternotomy. This incision can also be extended through an anterolateral neck incision when additional exposure to the thoracic outlet is necessary (**Fig. 7**). Proximal left subclavian injuries may be challenging to control through a median sternotomy due to a more posterior location of this vessel. A left high thoracotomy through the second or third intercostal space provides optimal access and allows control of the proximal left subclavian artery. After proximal and distal control of the aortic arch, branch is obtained and hemostasis achieved, the next decision is how to best repair the vascular injury. Options include primary repair, patch, or reconstruction with an interposition graft. For the aortic arch branches, reconstruction with prosthetic grafts

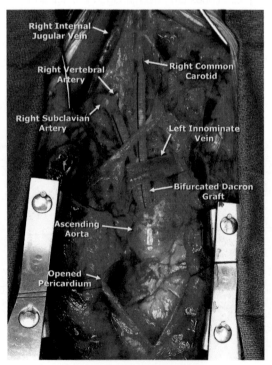

Fig. 7. Innominate artery injury repaired with an ascending aortic to right subclavian artery and right common carotid artery bypass using bifurcated Dacron graft.

(8–10 mm ePTFE or Dacron) is usually adequate due to the high patency rates of prosthetic grafts in these high-flow arterial beds.

All superior vena cava injuries should be repaired either primarily or using a venous or prosthetic patch. In those instances of destructive injuries to the superior vena cava requiring reconstruction with an interposition graft, large diameter (18–20 mm) ringed ePTFE grafts are the alternative of choice. These injuries, however, carry an exceedingly high mortality.

Penetrating injuries to the aortic arch are rarely survivable injuries. For those patients in whom repair is attempted, femoral cannulation and cardiopulmonary bypass may be necessary.

Blunt descending thoracic aortic injury

Thoracic aortic injury remains a major cause of mortality for victims of blunt trauma, with a majority of deaths occurring at the scene of the accident. For the select group of patients in whom exsanguination does not happen at the scene, significant changes have occurred in the way this injury is diagnosed and managed. CT scan has become the diagnostic imaging modality of choice and strict blood pressure control has significantly reduced the risk of rupture. This injury can, therefore, be addressed in a delayed fashion, after abnormal physiology is corrected and other immediately life-threatening injuries are treated. Ongoing progress in endovascular techniques have resulted in significant survival improvement and aortic stenting has now replaced open surgery as the preferred treatment modality.[16]

Currently, all patients with a diagnosis of blunt thoracic aortic injury should be considered candidates for endovascular repair. After strict blood pressure control is instituted in the ICU and associated life-threatening associated injuries are treated, endovascular aortic repair is performed using an endograft selected based on the initial chest CT scan (**Fig. 8**). IVUS can be used to confirm the location of the pseudoaneurysm and its distance from the aortic arch branches and to determine aortic diameters (**Fig. 9**). After deployment of the thoracic aortic endograft, completion angiogram is obtained to confirm complete exclusion of the pseudoaneurysm (**Fig. 10**). Coverage of the left subclavian artery by the endostent may be necessary to obtain adequate proximal seal (**Fig. 11**), which is usually well tolerated in trauma patients.[10,17,18] Stroke and spinal ischemia are the most important potential acute complications of left subclavian artery coverage. Myocardial infarction can also occur in patients with a history of left internal mammary coronary bypass. Subclavian steal syndrome and left arm claudication are both possible long-term sequelae of left subclavian artery ostial

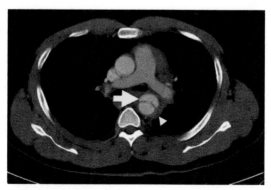

Fig. 8. Chest CT scan demonstrating descending thoracic aortic pseudoaneurysm (*arrow*) and mediastinal hematoma (*arrowhead*).

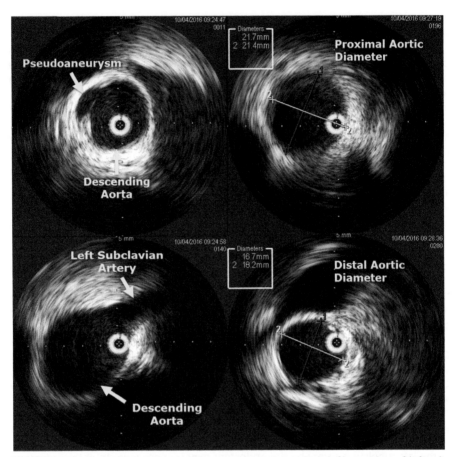

Fig. 9. IVUS during TEVAR, demonstrating pseudoaneurysm (*top left*), position of left subclavian artery (*bottom left*), and measurement of aortic diameters (*right top and right bottom*).

occlusion by the stent graft. If subclavian revascularization is needed, both carotid-subclavian bypass (**Fig. 12**) and subclavian-carotid transposition (**Fig. 13**) are acceptable surgical options.

A more expanded understanding of the natural history of blunt thoracic aortic injuries is evolving. Several groups have demonstrated that most Society for Vascular Surgery grade I and 2 injuries can likely be managed without repair and will not progress to aneurysm or rupture. Anticoagulation or antiplatelet use in these settings is under investigation, with the routine use of long-term aspirin used preferentially in some centers. When nonoperative management is selected, it is advisable that these injuries be referred after discharge to a vascular surgeon for long-term follow-up.

Lumbar drain is not used routinely but should be promptly placed in patients who develop symptoms of spinal ischemia, which is unusual in this setting.

Abdominal

Patients with penetrating abdominal vascular injuries are generally hemodynamic unstable on presentation and require immediate surgical exploration for hemostasis. Bleeding from retroperitoneal vascular injuries may remain contained and high level

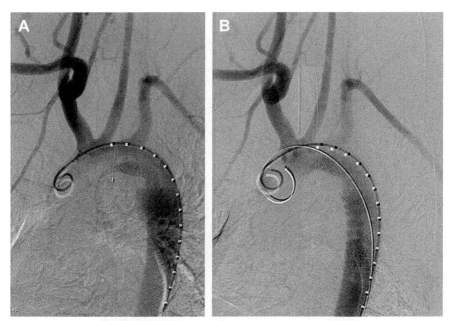

Fig. 10. Blunt descending thoracic aortic injury (*A*) before and (*B*) after endovascular repair.

of suspicion is necessary to identify those injuries in patients who arrive hemodynamically stable or who respond to initial volume resuscitation. The presence of peritonitis not only points to the presence of associated hollow viscus injury but also suggests the possibility of intra-abdominal vascular injury.[19]

Surgical exposure of the abdominal aorta and its visceral branches is challenging and major blood loss usually happens before hemostasis is achieved. The presence

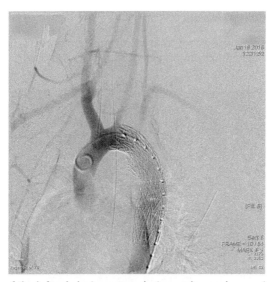

Fig. 11. Coverage of the left subclavian artery during endovascular repair of blunt descending thoracic aortic injury.

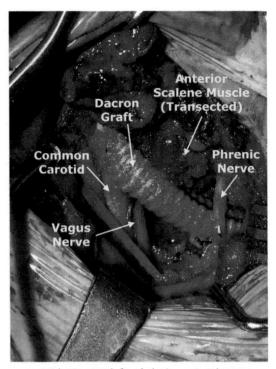

Fig. 12. Left common carotid artery to left subclavian artery bypass.

of associated intra-abdominal injuries aggravates this complex scenario. Successful treatment of patients with abdominal vascular injuries is not possible without strict adherence to damage control principles and keen knowledge of surgical anatomy. Early blood product resuscitation with balanced ratios and protocolized massive transfusion strategies are also important contributors to improve the outcomes for this patient population. In contrast to peripheral vascular injuries, abdominal vascular injuries cannot be temporarily controlled by external pressure. Immediate abdominal exploration with expedited assessment of the injury burden is paramount. This

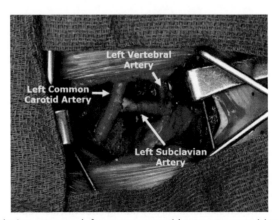

Fig. 13. Left subclavian artery to left common carotid artery transposition.

information should be promptly used in conjunction with the patient's hemodynamic and physiologic condition to decide if damage control operation should be performed. This decision must be made as early as possible. Abdominal vascular injuries are usually associated with additional intra-abdominal injuries. Associated injuries not only increase the complexity of the procedure but may also result in enteric contamination of the vascular repairs. Autologous conduits are preferable for intra-abdominal vascular reconstructions, notably in the presence of enteric contamination. Adherence to the basic principles of nonviable tissue débridement and gentle balloon catheter thromboembolectomy of both inflow and outflow prior to vascular repair is important.

The retroperitoneum is systematically compartmentalized into 4 anatomic zones (a single zone 1, paired lateral zone 2s, and a distal zone 3), with implications for the surgical approach to abdominal vascular injuries:

- Zone I: central area of the retroperitoneum, from the aortic hiatus to the sacral promontory. The aorta with its major branches (celiac artery, superior mesenteric artery [SMA], renal arteries, and inferior mesenteric artery), the inferior vena cava (IVC), and the superior mesenteric vein (SMV).
- Zone II: located laterally, it includes the kidneys and hilar renal vessels.
- Zone III: located in the space of the pelvic retroperitoneum and contains the iliac arteries and veins.

Zone I

Exploration is indicated for all hematomas encountered in zone I to rule out the possibility of major vascular injuries, regardless of the injury mechanism. Prior to entering the hematoma, proximal aortic control is essential. This can be accomplished through 1 of 3 maneuvers:

1. Left anterolateral thoracotomy and control of distal thoracic aorta in the chest (thoracic aorta cross-clamp). This maneuver is appropriate for patients who progress to cardiac arrest prior to laparotomy. In this situation the left anterolateral thoracotomy is used both for resuscitative purposes as well as for placement of an aortic cross-clamp. The left thoracotomy may also be necessary when a massive zone I hematoma extends proximally into the aortic hiatus. If an aortic injury is suspected at the level of the aortic hiatus, a thoracophrenolaparotomy can be quickly performed by extending the laparotomy into a low left thoracotomy at the level of the eighth or ninth intercostal space and dividing the diaphragm toward the hiatus. This maneuver is rarely performed in the trauma setting but provides adequate exposure for proximal control and definitive repair of an aortic injury at the thoracoabdominal transition.
2. Control the distal thoracic aorta through the esophageal hiatus (supraceliac aortic control). Placement of a vascular clamp across the supraceliac aorta may be challenging due to the dense connective and neurovascular tissue surrounding the aorta at this level. Direct compression of the proximal abdominal aorta against the spine at the level of the hiatus using an aortic compression device is a better alternative if an additional surgical assistant is available to hold pressure until definitive hemostasis is obtained. Another alternative is to cross-clamp the distal thoracic aorta, which is accessible through the esophageal hiatus, a location where the artery is relatively free from the aforementioned dense periaortic tissue, facilitating the exposure and placement of a vascular clamp. The gastrohepatic ligament is divided and the hepatic left lateral segment is mobilized to the patient's right. The esophagus is circumferentially mobilized and retracted to the left with a Penrose drain. The right diaphragmatic crus is divided at the 2-o'clock position

and the aorta is bluntly dissected on each side, allowing placement of a DeBakey or Cooley aortic aneurysm clamp.

3. Left medial visceral rotation. This maneuver allows exposure of the proximal abdominal aorta and visceral branches. First, the white line of Toldt on the left is divided and the left colon is mobilized away from the lateral abdominal wall. The dissection plane at the retroperitoneum is carried out anteriorly to the Gerota fascia leaving the left kidney in place. The dissection is extended in a cephalad direction. The splenophrenic ligament is divided and an en bloc medial rotation of the spleen, pancreas, colon, and small bowel is performed. This exposes the proximal abdominal aorta as it travels across the aortic hiatus. Exposure of the celiac axis, SMA, and left renal artery is achieved. If an injury to the posterior aspect of the aorta is suspected, the same maneuver (described previously) is performed, but instead of staying anterior to the left kidney, the plane of dissection extends posterior to the left kidney, which is included in the en bloc medial visceral rotation.

Visceral branches

Celiac Artery The celiac artery emerges anteriorly from the aorta and trifurcates into left gastric, common hepatic, and splenic arteries. In addition to the medial visceral rotation, described previously, the celiac trunk and its branches can also be approached through the lesser sac. This exposure, however, requires division of the median arcuate ligament and the celiac ganglion, which may not be straightforward in the trauma setting. If properly performed however, excellent exposure of the supraceliac aorta and celiac trunk is accomplished.

A rich network of collaterals makes ligation of the celiac trunk the treatment of choice when an injury is encountered in this location. Ligation of the celiac branches, including the common hepatic artery, can also be performed with negligible risk of visceral ischemia. Injuries to the proper hepatic artery that is distal to the gastroduodenal artery should be repaired.

Superior Mesenteric Artery, Superior Mesenteric Vein, and Portal Vein Surgical approach to the SMA is determined by the segment of the artery requiring exposure. As described previously, a left visceral rotation maneuver provides adequate exposure to the retropancreatic SMA segment. The SMA segment caudal to the inferior pancreatic border is best exposed through the root of the mesentery by retracting the transverse colon cephalad, dividing the ligament of Treitz and mobilizing the duodenum to the right. Transection of the pancreas is a well described maneuver to obtain expedited exposure to the retropancreatic segment of the mesenteric vessels. This maneuver, however, must be used very parsimoniously because the possibility of a pancreatic leak at the area of vascular reconstruction has significant morbidity implications.

Unless irreversible bowel necrosis has already occurred, injuries to the SMA generally require repair or reconstruction. Ligation of this artery invariably results in bowel ischemia, more significant if the ligation is performed proximal to the middle colic artery, which usually results in extensive ischemia to the entire small bowel and right colon. Autogenous conduits are preferable for SMA reconstructions, but prosthetic grafts can be used if enteric contamination is not present. Most cases of SMA reconstruction in should be managed with a temporary abdominal closure and planned second look to confirm graft patency and bowel viability.

For unstable patients, the use of a damage control temporary SMA shunt should be considered because complex prolonged reconstructions may result in further deterioration of the patient physiologic condition.

Injuries to the SMA and portal vein are highly lethal. Although ligation is a viable strategy, mortality associated with this maneuver is exceedingly high[20] and, unless the hemodynamic condition of the patient is prohibitive, these injuries should be repaired. If primary repair is expected to result in significant stenosis, the vein should be reconstructed either with a venous patch or an interposition graft. The internal jugular vein remains the best conduit for an interposition graft at the SMV/portal vein location.

Inferior Vena Cava Injuries to the IVC are usually associated with significant blood loss and are highly lethal. Quick exposure to the IVC is achieved with a Cattell-Braasch maneuver extended with kocherization of the duodenum and full mobilization of the duodenopancreatic complex. This exposes the entire extent of the IVC from the common iliac veins confluence to where the cava becomes retrohepatic. Direct sponge-stick compression above and below the IVC injury is effective for temporary bleeding control, which allows assessment of the extension of the injury and definitive repair. Immediate control is also important to avoid air embolism. Primary repair without significant stenosis can be accomplished in a majority of cases. If greater than 50% stenosis is expected with primary repair, ligation should be performed and is generally well tolerated in the infrarenal segment. Complex infrarenal IVC reconstructions have limited indication, only for patients with isolated IVC injury and normal hemodynamic condition. Repair of juxtarenal IVC injuries can be facilitated by division of the left renal vein adjacent to the IVC, which is safe because the venous outflow from the left kidney is maintained through the left renal vein tributaries (lumbar, gonadal, and adrenal veins). Ligation of the right renal vein results in hemorrhagic infarct of the right kidney.

Ligation of the suprarenal IVC is associated with high risk of renal failure. IVC injuries at this level should be repaired primarily or using a patch. If reconstruction is necessary, a large diameter (18–20 mm) externally supported polytetrafluoroethylene graft is the graft with best patency rates.[21,22]

Zones I and II

Proximal renal artery exposure is achieved by division of the ligament of Treitz and mobilization of the duodenum to the right. The left renal vein is identified and usually needs to be mobilized to allow exposure of the aortic segment where the renal arteries originate.

The management of renovascular injuries is determined by the duration of warm ischemia, hemodynamic status of the patient, and condition of the contralateral kidney. Active bleeding from a renal hilum is best managed by nephrectomy in a hemodynamically unstable patient, but renovascular reconstruction should be considered for a hemodynamically stable patient with less than 6 hours of warm renal ischemia.

Zone III

Hematomas from penetrating trauma in zone III should be explored to rule out injuries to the iliac vessels. Proximal control prior to hematoma exploration is obtained at the distal aorta level or at the common iliac level in cases of smaller unilateral hematomas. For injuries at the level of the external iliac arteries, distal control may need to be performed at the thigh and division of the inguinal ligament may be necessary. Iliac arterial reconstruction is routinely performed with prosthetic grafts. If a patient's hemodynamic condition allows, an endovascular repair with covered stent can be attempted in those institutions equipped with a hybrid operating room. If enteric contamination is present, the cavity should be extensively irrigated and an omental flap should be used to cover the area of arterial reconstruction.

Injuries to the iliac veins are managed with ligation if simple primary repair without stenosis is not possible.

Zone III hematomas secondary to blunt trauma are not explored unless they are expanding in the operating room. Angioembolization is the modality of choice for management of ongoing pelvic bleeding from blunt trauma. For those patients, however, who require exploration of a pelvic hematoma to control massive hemorrhage, the utility of internal iliac artery ligation and pelvic packing has been described.[23]

Peripheral Vascular Injuries

Peripheral vascular injuries occur due to blunt and penetrating mechanisms at equal frequencies, although the mortality rate associated with blunt injury is typically higher and mortality is increased with more proximal injuries.[24,25] In the upper extremity, the forearm vessels are the most commonly injured. In the lower extremity, the popliteal artery is the most commonly injured after blunt mechanisms, whereas the superficial femoral is the most common penetrating location of vascular injury. Amputation rates after vascular injury tend to be higher after blunt trauma and are more common at the level of the forearm for the upper extremity and the popliteal level for lower extremity.[25]

Although patients with hard signs require immediate surgical intervention, patients with soft signs concerning for vascular trauma should undergo a wrist to ankle brachial index of the injured extremity. An index of less than 0.9 is suggestive of a vascular injury and warrants additional investigation.[26] CTA has emerged as the preferred imaging modality in most trauma centers. Patients with documented arterial injuries consisting of small intimal tears, downstream intimal flaps, pseudoaneurysm (<5 mm), and small arteriovenous fistulas can be safely observed.[27] Formal angiography may prove useful as an adjunct of intervention in the operating room — as such, patients with vascular injury should be placed on an operative table capable of accommodating fluoroscopic imaging intraoperatively.

There are several general rules that should be applied to the operative treatment of all peripheral vascular injuries. Preparation of the effected extremity should be circumferential, with consideration of preparing for potential saphenous vein harvest from the contralateral extremity. The applicability of tourniquets, temporary balloon occlusion, and rapid proximal open exposure and vessel control should be considered early.

Once vascular control has been obtained, the decision to use damage control principles, as discussed previously, should be evaluated. Liberal utilization of temporary vascular shunts, in particular, is invaluable for the purpose in extremity vascular injury. For definitive repair, the saphenous vein is generally the conduit of choice for interposition repairs in extremity vascular trauma. If this choice is not available, ePTFE is preferred although there is a greater risk for infection. Wide débridement of wound contamination and nonviable tissue should be undertaken, with special attention paid to the coverage of a vascular repair with viable soft tissue.

For stable patients with few associated injuries, the decision to repair major venous injuries is predicated on the extent of injury. Primary or patch repair should be performed ideally. If a more complex venous repair at this location is required, ligation is likely indicated. A majority of venous ligations are well tolerated in the extremities with postoperative elevation and cautious compression.

A low threshold should exist for performance of prophylactic fasciotomies — particularly in the lower extremities and with prolonged ischemia, significant resuscitation needs, or associated musculoskeletal injury. In every instance, all 4 compartments of the lower extremity should be liberally decompressed.

Specific Peripheral Vascular Injuries

Subclavian/axillary

Among the most challenging of peripheral exposures, it is useful to appreciate the routes to proximal control of subclavian and axillary injuries. Proximal control of subclavian injuries medial to the anterior scalene may require a high anterior thoracotomy. Proximal control of axillary arteries medial to the pectoralis minor muscle may require supraclavicular exposure and control of the subclavian artery.

Selected subclavian/axillary injuries can be managed by endovascular covered stents in stable patients (**Fig. 14**). When an open interposition repair is required, an 8-mm ePTFE graft is a useful conduit in most patients. Brachial plexus injuries are not uncommon with injuries at these locations.

Brachial artery

During exposure of the brachial artery, care must be taken to avoid injury to the median nerve as it runs medial in the brachial sheath. If distal exposure of the brachial artery distal to the flexure of the elbow is required, an S-shaped incision can be carried across the antecubital fossa and onto the forearm. The brachial artery lends itself to mobilization with dissection and exposure, facilitating an end-to-end anastomosis in a majority of instances. For the remainder, autogenous vein interposition is recommended.

Ulnar/radial arteries

In the setting of an isolated occlusive vessel injury to either the ulnar or radial arteries, assessment for a patent palmar arch by an Allen test should be performed. If the palmar arch is patent, surgical repair is not necessary. Isolated arteriovenous fistula and pseudoaneurysms can be treated by endovascular embolization or ligation, provided palmar arch patency is preserved. Injuries to both vessels require repair of the ulnar artery at a minimum, because it is most commonly the dominant source of palmar arch arterial supply. Selected patients may require radial repair as well — all predicated on palmar arch anatomy.

Femoral arteries

Exposure of the femoral arteries is obtained through a slightly oblique incision extended longitudinally. The inguinal ligament can be divided if additional proximal exposure is required. The common femoral artery is commonly repaired with a short segment interposition of ePTFE graft or via vein patch. All profunda femoris artery

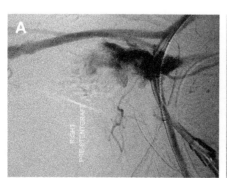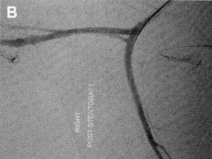

Fig. 14. (A) Before and (B) after arteriogram images of a penetrating injury to the left subclavian artery repaired with an endovascular stent graft.

injuries should be optimally repaired. Ligation of this vessel is only acceptable in the extremes of damage control for unstable patients with multiple injuries. The superficial femoral artery is best repaired with interposition saphenous vein graft (**Fig. 15**). These injuries are rarely amenable to end-to-end or patch repair.

Popliteal artery

Blunt popliteal arteries are commonly associated with tibial plateau fractures and posterior knee dislocations (**Fig. 16**). Missed injuries and injuries not promptly repaired have high rates of amputation. Medial exposure of the retrogeniculate popliteal is accomplished with separate incisions above and below the knee, preserving the musculotendinous attachments of the semimembranosis and semitendinosis tendons whenever possible. Select short segment popliteal injuries in the retrogeniculate location may be repaired through a posterior approach.

A majority of popliteal artery injuries can be repaired with either an end-to-end repair or a saphenous vein interposition. Associated venous injuries should be performed if primary or patch repair is possible. Prophylactic, 4-compartment lower extremity fasciotomy should be strongly considered for occlusive popliteal injuries with prolonged warm ischemic time (4–6 hours).

Tibial/peroneal

Surgical repair of an isolated single-vessel tibial artery injury is not indicated. For patients with multiple injuries, at least one tibial (anterior or posterior) should be repaired. Interposition or bypass repairs using saphenous vein are usually required.

Special Population — Pediatric Patients

In young children, supracondylar humerus fractures are associated with high risk for brachial artery injury. If a radial pulse or strong Doppler signal is not restored after reduction of these fractures, brachial artery exploration should be performed.

The vessels of young children are small and prone to vasospasm during the manipulation required for repair. Topical or intra-arterial nitroglycerine or papaverine may prove helpful for treatment of this arterial vasospasm.

For extremity arterial injuries, a limb with normal neurologic function and distal arterial Doppler signals can be managed nonoperatively. Long-term follow-up is required,

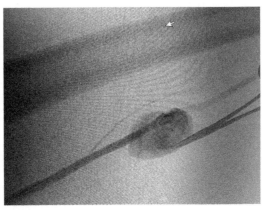

Fig. 15. Pseudoaneurysm of the superficial femoral artery after a stab wound. This injury was repaired with a reversed saphenous vein interposition graft.

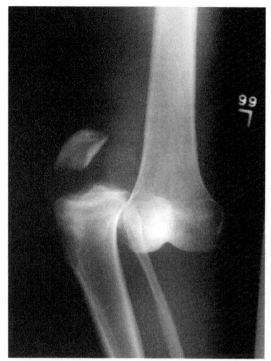

Fig. 16. Plain radiograph of a posterior knee dislocation.

however, due to the risk of stunted limb growth with age. When required, pediatric arterial repairs should be performed with interrupted anastomotic sutures.

REFERENCES

1. Branco BC, Linnebur M, Boutrous ML, et al. The predictive value of multidetector CTA on outcomes in patients with below-the-knee vascular injury. Injury 2015; 46(8):1520–6.

2. Inaba K, Branco BC, Menaker J, et al. Evaluation of multidetector computed to-mography for penetrating neck injury: a prospective multicenter study. J Trauma Acute Care Surg 2012;72(3):576–83 [discussion: 583–4].

3. Inaba K, Branco BC, Reddy S, et al. Prospective evaluation of mutlidetector computed tomography for extremity vascular trauma. J Trauma 2011;70(4): 808–15.

4. Azizzadeh A, Valdes J, Miller CC 3rd, et al. The utility of intravascular ultrasound compared to angiography in the diagnosis of blunt traumatic aortic injury. J Vasc Surg 2011;53(3):608–14.

5. Rasmussen TE, Clouse WD, Jenkins DH, et al. The use of temporary vascular shunts as a damage control adjunct in the management of wartime vascular injury. J Trauma 2006;61(1):8–12 [discussion: 12–5].

6. DuBose JJ, Scalea TM, Brenner M, et al, AAST AORTA Study Group. The AAST prospective Aortic Occlusion for Resuscitation in Trauma and Acute Care Surgery (AORTA) registry: Data on contemporary utilization and outcomes of aortic

occlusion and resuscitative balloon occlusion of the aorta (REBOA). J Trauma Acute Care Surg 2016;81(3):409–19.

7. Biffle WL, Fox CJ, Moore EE. The role of REBOA in the control of exsanguinating torso hemorrhage. J Trauma Acute Care Surg 2015;78(5):1054–8.

8. Back MR. Local complications: graft infections. In: Cronenwett J, Johnston KW, editors. Rutherford's vascular surgery. 8th edition. Atlanta (GA): Elsevier Press; 2014. p. 654–72.

9. Demetriades D, Velmahos GC, Scalea TM, et al. Diagnosis and treatment of blunt thoracic aortic injuries: changing perspectives. J Trauma 2008;64(6):1415–8 [discussion: 1418–9].

10. DuBose JJ, Leake SS, Brenner M, et al, Aortic Trauma Foundation. Contemporary management of outcomes of blunt thoracic aortic injury: a multicenter retrospective study. J Trauma Acute Care Surg 2015;78(2):360–9.

11. Branco BC, DuBose JJ. Endovascular solutions for the management of penetrating trauma: an update on REBOA and axillo-subclavian injuries. Eur J Trauma Emerg Surg 2016;42(6):687–94.

12. Branco BC, Bourtrous ML, DuBose JJ, et al. Outcome comparison between open and endovascular management of axillosubclavian arterial injuries. J Vasc Surg 2016;63(3):702–9.

13. Kuehne JP, Weaver FA, Papanicolaou G, et al. Penetrating trauma of the internal carotid artery. Arch Surg 1996;131:942–8.

14. Weaver FA, Yellin AE, Wagner WH, et al. The role of arterial reconstruction in penetrating carotid injuries. Arch Surg 1988;123:1106–11.

15. Inaba K, Munera F, McKenney MG, et al. The nonoperative management of penetrating internal jugular vein injury. J Vasc Surg 2006;43(1):77–80.

16. Demetriades D, Velmahos GC, Scalea TM, et al. Operative repair or endovascular stent graft in blunt traumatic thoracic aortic injuries: results of an American Association for the Surgery of Trauma Multicenter study. J Trauma Acute Care Surg 2008;64(3):561–70 [discussion: 570–1].

17. Azizzadeh A, Ray HM, Dubose JJ, et al. Outcomes of endovascular repair for patients with blunt traumatic aortic injury. J Trauma Acute Care Surg 2014;76(2): 510–6.

18. McBride CL, Dubose JJ, Miller CC, et al. Intentional left subclavian artery coverage during thoracic endovascular aortic repair for traumatic aortic injury. J Vasc Surg 2015;61(1):73–9.

19. Brown CV, Velmahos GC, Neville AL, et al. Hemodynamically "stable" patients with peritonitis after penetrating abdominal trauma: identifying those who are bleeding. Arch Surg 2005;140(8):767–72.

20. Asensio JA, Petrone P, Garcia-Nuñez L, et al. Superior mesenteric venous injuries: to ligate or to repair remains the question. J Trauma 2007;62:668–75.

21. Quinones-Baldrich W, Alktaifi A, Eilber F, et al. Inferior vena cava resection and reconstruction for retroperitoneal tumor excision. J Vasc Surg 2012;55:1386–93.

22. Bower TC, Nagorney DM, Cherry KJ Jr, et al. Replacement of the inferior vena cava for malignancy: an update. J Vasc Surg 2000;31:270–81.

23. DuBose J, Inaba K, Barmparas G, et al. Bilateral internal iliac artery ligation as a damage control approach in massive retroperitoneal bleeding after pelvic fracture. J Trauma 2010;69:1507–14.

24. Wagner WH, Caulkins E, Weaver FA, et al. Blunt popliteal artery trauma: 100 consecutive cases. J Vasc Surg 1988;7:736–43.

25. Weaver FA, Yellin AE, Bauer M, et al. Is arterial proximity a valid indication for arteriography in penetrating extremity trauma? A prospective analysis. Arch Surg 1990;125:1256–60.
26. Schwartz MR, Weaver FA, Bauer M, et al. Refining the indications for arteriography in penetrating extremity trauma: a prospective analysis. J Vasc Surg 1993;17:116–22.
27. Johansen KM, Lynch K, Paun M, et al. Non-invasive vascular tests reliably exclude occult arterial trauma. J Trauma 1991;31:515–22.

Evidence-Based Care of Geriatric Trauma Patients

Steven E. Brooks, MD[a,b,*], Allan B. Peetz, MD[c]

KEYWORDS

- Geriatric trauma • Geriatric • Frailty • Acute care surgery • Surgical critical care

KEY POINTS

- The doubling of the geriatric population over the next 20 years will challenge the existing health care system.
- Care of geriatric trauma patients will be of paramount importance to the health care discussion in America.
- Geriatric trauma patients warrant special consideration because of altered physiology and decreased ability to tolerate the stresses imposed by trauma.
- In spite of increased risk for worsened outcomes, geriatric trauma patients are less likely to be triaged to a designated trauma center.
- There must be, with either patients or surrogate decision makers, an exploration regarding patient goals of care and a discussion about what patients would consider meaningful outcomes.

INTRODUCTION: WHY *GERIATRIC* TRAUMA?

The United States is experiencing an exponential increase in its older adults unlike any that has ever occurred. With the aging of the baby boomer generation, the geriatric, commonly defined as those aged 65 and older, are the most rapidly growing segment of the US population.[1] According to the Census Bureau this age group will nearly double in 2 decades, from 39.6 million in 2009 to 72.1 million in the year 2030.[2,3] Although trauma is the number one cause of death in those aged 44 years and younger, it is also

The authors have no commercial relationships or financial interests to disclose.
[a] Geriatric Trauma Unit, Division of Trauma, Surgical Critical Care, Acute Care Surgery, Department of Surgery, John A. Griswold Trauma Center, Texas Tech University Health Sciences Center, 3601 4th Street MS 8312, Lubbock, TX 79430, USA; [b] Pediatric Intensive Care Unit, Division of Trauma, Surgical Critical Care, Acute Care Surgery, Department of Surgery, John A. Griswold Trauma Center, Texas Tech University Health Sciences Center, 3601 4th Street MS 8312, Lubbock, TX 79430, USA; [c] Emergency General Surgery, Division of Trauma, Surgical Critical Care, Vanderbilt University Medical Center, Medical Arts Building Suite 404, 1211 21st Avenue South, Nashville, TN 37212, USA
* Corresponding author. Department of Surgery, Texas Tech University Health Science Center, 3601 4th Street MS 8312, Lubbock, TX 79430.
E-mail address: Steven.Brooks@ttuhsc.edu

the fifth leading cause of death when all age groups are considered.[4] The doubling of the geriatric population will challenge the existing health care system, both numerically and monetarily.

Why do we assign the term *geriatric* to trauma patients aged 65 years and older? *Geriatric trauma* patients have significantly higher mortality and poorer functional outcomes after major injury.[3,5–7] Although they are injured less frequently than their younger counterparts, trauma is the fourth leading cause of death in those aged 55 to 64 years.[4] Trauma is still the ninth leading cause of mortality in patients aged 65 years and older.[4] Rather than having a derogatory connotation, the term *geriatric* represents the statistically significant inflection point in patients' morbidity and mortality for a given injury compared with a younger patient.

Thirty-day mortality, a traditional outcome measure, is a poor metric in geriatric populations. Quality care may be associated with survival to discharge, but in the older population there exists high mortality within 2 months of discharge in geriatric trauma survivors.[8–10] Those who do survive are often debilitated and institutionalized, an outcome that many would deem unsuccessful or even unacceptable.

In the year 2000, the number of persons aged 65 years and older represented just more than 12% of the US population. By the year 2050, this group will increase to more than 20%.[11] In addition to growing numerically, these older patients are living longer and more active lives. Those aged 80 years and older, the *oldest old* category, will increase to nearly 20 million persons by the year 2030.[4] The changing composition of trauma patients reflects this growth. In a 2008 study, geriatric trauma patients accounted for 14% of all trauma-related emergency department (ED) visits. These data are consistent with both published and unpublished data at level 1 university trauma centers, such as Vanderbilt University (Nashville, Tennessee) and Texas Tech University (Lubbock, Texas), which showed an increasing percentage of geriatric trauma patients from 10% to 20% over a 10-year period.[3]

The fiscal impact of geriatric trauma care is undeniable and significant. The present political climate has ushered in an era of unprecedented attention to the economics of health care. Geriatric trauma accounts for 33% of all trauma health care expenditures in the United States, or $9 billion per year.[12] The future cost of geriatric trauma will be integral to the health care discussion in America. The increasing number of geriatric and *oldest old* geriatric trauma patients will have serious financial implications for not only future trauma care but also for the entire US health care system.

PHYSIOLOGY IN GERIATRIC TRAUMA PATIENTS

The evolution of clinical care in geriatric trauma originated with a dramatic shift in thought process about the physiology of the geriatric. In 1984 Harborview Medical Center published a review of 100 trauma patients older than 70 years that reported an 85% survival rate but noted that 88% did not return to their previous level of independence. The article stated that, "...what impact preexisting disease has on survival following injury has not been adequately studied."[13] In a 1986 study, Horst described 39 consecutive trauma patients more than 70 years of age and concluded, "[Mortality in the geriatric patient] should not differ substantially from other age groups."[14] These studies, in addition to others published in the 1980s, failed to detect outcome differences between geriatric trauma patients and younger cohorts. The paradigm shift in recognizing these differences would not occur until the end of that decade.

In 1990, Scalea and colleagues[15] published an article that stated, "To our knowledge, no one has described managing geriatric trauma patients any differently than younger patients...diffuse blunt trauma is a very different disease process in the geriatric trauma patient. Older patients sustaining this type of injury are at considerably higher risk than younger patients."[15] The first step toward improving geriatric trauma care was acknowledging the outcome differences in geriatric injured patients and connecting those outcomes to differences to physiology.

PREEXISTING CONDITIONS: COMORBIDITIES AND CHRONIC ILLNESS

Geriatric trauma patients may have many or all of the comorbidities that portend poorer outcomes in trauma:

- Decreased vision and hearing
- Slower reflexes
- Poorer balance
- Impaired motor and/or cognitive function
- Decreased muscle mass and/or strength
- Decreased bone density
- Decreased joint flexibility

Additionally, 80% of geriatric trauma patients have at least 1 or more chronic diseases, such as hypertension, arthritis, heart disease, pulmonary disease, cancer, diabetes, or history of stroke.[4] These preexisting illnesses, when combined with the altered physiology of increased age described later, make geriatric trauma patients less able to tolerate the stress of trauma.

CENTRAL NERVOUS SYSTEM CHANGES IN THE GERIATRIC

The central nervous system in geriatric patients may be impaired because of cortical atrophy and plaque buildup in the cerebrovascular vessels. Clinical implications include decrements in all 5 sensations in addition to cognitive decline. Decreased cerebellar function and associated worsening of balance add to risk of falls.[4] The combination of polypharmacy and acute injury may exacerbate agitation and delirium in geriatric trauma patients.[16]

CARDIOVASCULAR CHANGES WITH AGING

Geriatric patients have altered cardiovascular physiology, with cardiac function declining by 50% between 20 and 80 years of age.[17] Patients in this age group will experience 30% of all myocardial infarctions and 60% of all associated deaths.[18] The cardiac muscle and conductive pathways are replaced with fat and fibrous tissue, predisposing the heart to arrhythmias. This stiffer heart is also more likely to have diastolic dysfunction, or inadequate ability to relax, decreasing its effectiveness as a pump. The heart's first compensatory behavior for improving cardiac output in class II hemorrhagic shock, tachycardia, might be stultified by beta-blocker medications.[19] The stiffer, fibrous heart limits increasing cardiac output via stroke volume. With the two mechanisms for improving cardiac output diminished, geriatric patients compensate by increasing systemic vascular resistance, resulting in a deceptively acceptable blood pressure.

Understanding the cardiac changes and resultant difference in compensation promotes better pattern recognition for patients in danger with respect to vital signs. A 2010 review of more than 4000 trauma patients found a significant mortality increase in geriatric patients whose heart rates were greater than 90 beats per minute, an association not seen until a heart rate of 130 in younger patients.[20] They also found that mortality markedly increased with a systolic blood pressure less than 110 in geriatric patients but not until a systolic blood pressure of less than 95 in young patients.

Importantly, vital signs are less predictive of mortality in geriatric trauma patients.[21] Additionally, the cardiovascular physiology and vital signs concerning in the younger population are not the same as those in geriatric trauma patients. Heart rate greater than 90 beats per minute or blood pressure less than 110 mm Hg should promote concern in the trauma surgeon.

PULMONARY AND THORACIC CHANGES WITH AGING

Geriatric patients are particularly vulnerable to pulmonary disease. Lower respiratory tract pathology is the third leading cause of death and significant disability in persons aged 65 and older.[22] Anatomic changes of the geriatric include kyphosis, or narrowing of the intervertebral disc spaces, leading to narrowing of the intercostal spaces and altering the angle and insertion of intercostal muscles.[23] Decreasing skeletal muscle mass and strength, loss of type II fast twitch muscle fibers, weaker diaphragmatic inspiratory effort, gradual reduction in lung elastic recoil, reduction in alveolar surface area, decreased ATP reserve, and reduced response to hypoxia and hypercapnia contribute to an increasingly ineffective pulmonary system in the geriatric.[22]

Physiologic considerations include the decreasing minimal alveolar concentration of inhalational agents by 6% per decade after 40 years of age.[22] Neuromuscular blocking agents may have an increased duration of action due to preexisting hepatic or renal disease. These patients have a more rigid chest wall, more compliant lungs that generate less elastic recoil, and parenchymal changes that lead to air trapping and hyperinflation. These physiologic differences lead to increased residual volume by 5% to 10% per decade and decline of both forced expiratory volume in the first second of expiration and forced vital capacity by up to 30 mL per year.[24]

Geriatric patients are at increased risk for postoperative pulmonary complications, including aspiration, pneumonia, atelectasis, bronchospasm, pleural effusion, and pulmonary embolism.[22] These risks are related to age-acquired decrease in cough reflex, decreased mucociliary epithelium function, decreased response to foreign antigen, and increased oropharyngeal colonization with microorganisms.[25] The anatomic and physiologic changes of age all contribute to a pulmonary system that is less able to tolerate acute traumatic injury.

RENAL CHANGES IN THE GERIATRIC

Anatomic changes of the renal parenchyma include glomerulosclerosis, a gradual replacement of glomerular tissue with fibrous tissue, causing a loss of 30% to 50% of cortical glomeruli by 70 years of age.[26] Additionally, intimal thickening of both the afferent and efferent renal arterioles occurs secondary to atherosclerosis and atrophy of smooth muscle media.[27] Perhaps the most profound renal anatomic change with aging is the decreased ability to preserve the renovascular reflex, termed *renovascular dysautonomy*.[28] This diminished ability to maintain hemostasis lessens the renal capacity for preserving its own function in both hypotensive and hypertensive states. The sum of these anatomic and physiologic alterations in geriatric renal function results in higher risk or acute kidney injury (AKI) and also failure to recover function after AKI.[29]

GASTROINTESTINAL SYSTEM IN THE GERIATRIC

Nutritional status of geriatric trauma patients is integral in predicting surgical risk. Malnutrition has been associated with increased postoperative morbidity, perioperative mortality, hospital length of stay (LOS), and decreased quality of life.[30–32] Unfortunately, malnutrition is reportedly as high as 40% to 50% in hospital and nursing home settings.[33] Fortunately, these are modifiable risk factors when nutritional interventions are applied smartly. Recommended interventions include a brief nutritional assessment on admission using one of several available screening tools, ensuring that the prescribed diet is actually the one delivered to patients, and regular reassessment in the hospital for nutritional intolerance (nausea, emesis, pain, difficulty chewing or swallowing, or impaired bowel function).[34]

MECHANISMS OF INJURY IN THE GERIATRIC

Ground-level falls (GLFs), accounted for 2.1 million ED visits among those aged 65 years and older in 2008.[11] This staggering figure is almost 10 times more common than motor vehicle crashes, the second leading cause of trauma in older adults.[35] Nearly 1 in 3 geriatric persons will have a GLF each year, and emergency medical services will respond to between 5 and 10 times more calls than for motor vehicle crashes.[36] Six percent of GLF patients will sustain a fracture, and 10% to 30% of these patients will have polytrauma.[36] Most importantly, mortality in GLF patients is reported as high as 7%, underscoring that GLFs are not benign.[36]

Although the third most common mechanism is (geriatric) pedestrian versus auto, geriatric patients are especially vulnerable to violent assault (the fourth most common mechanism), resulting in 10% of geriatric trauma admissions. Significantly, these geriatric victims of violence are 5 times more likely to die as a result of their attack when compared with younger victims.[37]

TREATMENT OF SPECIFIC INJURIES
Traumatic Brain Injury

Traumatic brain injury (TBI) is an epidemic problem in the geriatric trauma population, prompting more than 80,000 ED visits each year.[17,38] Geriatric TBI patients have greater morbidity and mortality compared with younger TBI patients.[39] The aging baby boomer generation has increased the prevalence of atrial fibrillation and other conditions requiring anticoagulation. In 2004, there were 31 million outpatient prescriptions for warfarin in the United States, a 45% increase from the prior 6 years.[40] Use of this therapy increases the risk of intracerebral hemorrhage (ICH) 7- to 10-fold.[41] The past decade has also given rise to irreversible anticoagulants, adding an additional degree of difficulty to the management of anticoagulation-associated ICH. Unfortunately, 1-month mortality following ICH approaches 40%, and only 12% to 39% of patients after an ICH regain independent function, underscoring the need for additional improvement in geriatric TBI treatment.[42]

The initial key to improved care in geriatric TBI is a high index of suspicion for injury and a low threshold for performing a computerized tomography (CT) scan to confirm the diagnosis. One study of geriatric, mild TBI patients reported a 14.3% incidence of acute pathologic changes on CT.[17] There were no reliable clinical predictors of pathology identified; therefore, liberal use of head CT was recommended. Inability to rapidly diagnose ICH results in profound increases in morbidity and mortality, as coagulopathy reversal and neurosurgical interventions are delayed.[43]

Patients on anticoagulation (AC) or antiplatelet (AP) therapy have presented with delayed ICH, thereby prompting some trauma services to perform repeat CT scans after an initial negative scan. Docimo and colleagues[44] attempted to answer the question of whether head trauma patients on AC or AP, who presented with an initial CT negative for ICH, needed a second scan for delayed ICH. In this retrospective study, 2 of 168 patients (1.9%) presented with delayed hemorrhage, and both were on warfarin and had an international normalized ratio (INR) greater than 2.[44] Based on review of prior literature and the conclusions of their study, the investigators noted the risk of delayed ICH was associated with the use of warfarin and, therefore, recommended the following[44]:

1. Patients on warfarin or warfarin/aspirin combo receive repeat head CT.
2. Patients on preinjury aspirin or clopidogrel should have a period of observation and clinical evaluation, followed by repeat head CT only for neurologic changes.

Ivascu and colleagues[43,45,46] published results of an aggressive protocol for TBI patients on AC, describing one of the most significant mortality improvements in the trauma literature. The protocol, which ensured rapid CT of the head, initiation of INR correction for patients with coagulopathy on warfarin (Coumadin) within 2 hours, and correction of INR to less than 1.6 within 4 hours of admission, resulted in a 75% decrease in mortality for posttraumatic intracranial hemorrhage in geriatric patients.

Blunt Thoracic Injury and Rib Fractures

Acute chest trauma, cardiopulmonary injury or thoracic skeletal insult, accounts for 25% of blunt trauma mortality.[47] Pulmonary contusions are the most common blunt thoracic trauma injury and may occur in up to 75% of patients.[47] Contusions may be an isolated injury, but trauma patients with severe thoracic skeletal trauma (such as flail chest) nearly always have concomitant pulmonary contusions.[47] This information prompts the trauma surgeon to consider the combination of rib fractures and pulmonary contusions as an injury constellation with inseparable pathophysiology, a thought process that has implications for optimal treatment.

Bulger and colleagues[48] published a seminal article describing geriatric trauma patients as having twice the mortality and thoracic morbidity of younger patients with a similar injury. The study described 3 to 4 rib fractures as the break point for pneumonia when compared with younger trauma patients, conferring a 31% risk of pneumonia in geriatric patients compared with 17% in younger patients.[48] When geriatric trauma patients sustain 6 rib fractures, risk of pneumonia skyrockets to worse than 50%. Mortality was also significantly worse at 3 rib fractures; nearly 1 in 5 geriatric patients died, with mortality increasing in geriatric trauma patients to 33%.[48]

In addition to the correlation between rib fractures and pneumonia/mortality, there is also a correlation between rib fractures and solid organ injury. Splenic injury is increased 1.7 times and liver injury 1.4 times, and 50% of patients with blunt cardiac injury have rib fractures.[48] The key is recognition that rib fractures in the geriatric are a marker for increased mortality, morbidity, and concomitant polytraumatic injury.

Rib fracture morbidity is predominantly explained by chest wall pain that limits pulmonary function. Pain first leads to chest wall splinting, decreased recruitment of alveoli, and development of atelectasis. This series of events, coupled with inadequate cough for clearing of secretions, increases the risk of pulmonary infection. The objective measures of a forceful cough and the ability to inhale 15 mL/kg with incentive spirometry are useful in denoting adequate pain control in these patients.[49]

Bulger and colleagues[48,50] demonstrated a significant drop in overall mortality across all age groups when patients received an epidural catheter for analgesia. These conclusions were supported by a National Trauma Data Bank study of nearly 65,000 rib fracture patients.[51]

Evidence-based guidelines for minimizing thoracic morbidity and mortality in geriatric trauma patients with rib fractures include

1. Use of an optimal, multimodal analgesia regimen and aggressive chest physiotherapy should be applied to minimize the likelihood of respiratory failure and ensuing ventilator support.[47]

2. Consider epidural analgesia as a key part of that multimodal analgesia regimen.[51]
3. There should be early consideration of open reduction and internal fixation of rib fractures in selected patients.[52–60] Evidence-based indications for surgical stabilization of rib fractures have been recently summarized in the literature.[60–64]

ORTHOPEDIC INJURIES

Orthopedic fractures confer significant risk to the geriatric population. In a 2015 study of more than 25,000 US geriatric trauma patients in 127 hospitals, Maxwell and colleagues[65] found that 56% had a major operative procedure. Thirty-six percent of patients had femoral neck fractures, the most common injury. Eighteen percent of the patients fractured either the neck or trunk. Twenty-one percent had either lower extremity fractures or upper extremity fractures. Fractures of the hip, spine, proximal humerus, and wrist are disproportionally represented in geriatric trauma patients.[66] Considerations for optimal care include preoperative risk evaluation, acute operative management, timing of operation, and functional outcomes.

Fractures from low-energy mechanisms (ie, GLFs) are termed *fragility fractures*.[66] Patients with such fractures should be evaluated for osteopenia, the treatment for which has been shown to lower secondary fracture risk.[66] In higher-energy fractures, the skin, muscle, and tendon integrity alterations with age predispose soft tissue damage. Surrounding blood supply to the healing bone may be compromised. Importantly, only one long bone fracture places geriatric trauma patients in the high-risk category, implicating fractures as a significant cardiovascular stressor and underscoring the need for potential preoperative risk modification whenever possible.

Aggressive effort at early definitive repair has been shown in numerous studies to decrease risk of major medical complications.[67–69] Early operative intervention has also been proven to reduce mortality. Earlier mobility after repair also lowers risk of pneumonia, bed sores, and pressure ulcers.[67–69] One study of geriatric trauma hip fracture patients showed that those who received definitive repair after 48 hours had more than double the risk of death in the ensuing year.[70] The principal tenants for fracture management are restoration of patients' expected function expeditiously, preventing progressive decline, and avoiding decreased quality of life.

ABDOMINAL INJURIES

Although blunt trauma management has become increasingly nonoperative in hemodynamically stable patients, geriatric trauma patients warrant careful consideration. For example, in case of a splenic injury, older patients are more likely to fail nonoperative management.[71] Additionally, geriatric trauma patients compensate differently during acute hemorrhage (see physiology section earlier). University of Southern California studied penetrating trauma in the geriatric trauma population and found that 50% of the geriatric patients who died had normal vital signs.[72] Those vital signs that would alarm the trauma surgeon in younger patients do not apply to geriatric trauma patients.[20] The decision for nonoperative management weighs heavily on the trauma surgeon, as mortality increases when this management fails, more so than in younger patients.[17]

CRITICAL CARE TRIAGE AND INTENSIVE CARE UNIT DELIRIUM MANAGEMENT

Because preventable complications in the geriatric dramatically worsen outcomes, improving triage by placing appropriate geriatric patients in the intensive care unit (ICU) may be the first step in morbidity and mortality improvement. A study of more than 22,500 trauma patients (including more than 7100 geriatric trauma patients) revealed that geriatric patients had significantly lower ICU admission rates compared with younger patients with similar injury severity.[73] Studies at both Baltimore Shock Trauma in Maryland and the University of Southern California at Los Angeles have shown improved outcomes with earlier trauma team activation and intensive monitoring in the geriatric.[15,74] Nathens and colleagues[75] demonstrated an improved mortality after trauma, which was most pronounced in geriatric trauma patients, in critical care units led by surgeon intensivists. Although comprehensive critical care of geriatric trauma patients is outside the scope of this article, tremendous advances in ICU delirium management have been described in the recent literature.[16,76]

Delirium is an acute brain dysfunction leading to prolonged cognitive dysfunction after critical illness.[77] The cardinal features of delirium are inattention and confusion that represent the brain temporarily failing.[78] The association between delirium duration and adverse outcomes, such as prolonged mechanical ventilation, prolonged hospitalization, persistent cognitive impairment, and increased 1 year post–critical illness mortality, has been well documented.[79] Delirium is not only a significant risk factor for morbidity and mortality in the ICU but its management also affects the trajectory of trauma patients' recovery as far out as 1 year after hospital discharge.[79] Only one episode of delirium puts ICU patiens at 3 times the risk for death in the ensuing 6 months.[80]

Unfortunately, up to 80% of ICU patients will be diagnosed with delirium; in 2 out of 3 of these patients, the diagnosis will go unrecognized.[77–80] Additionally, increased delirium duration is independently associated with greater disability in activities of daily living (ADLs) and worsening motor-sensory function at 1 year after ICU discharge.[79] One year after critical illness, 25% of patients will have cognitive dysfunction similar in severity to that seen in mild Alzheimer disease and 33% will have impairment commensurate with moderate TBI.[77] One in 3 patients will also have physical disabilities in ADLs a year after critical illness.[79] Delirium increases hospital costs by $2500 per patient leading to $6.9 billion of Medicare expenditures annually.[81] The full extent of clinical and financial consequences has only been recognized in the past decade.

A road map for integrated, evidence-based, patient-centered protocols for preventing and treating pain, agitation, and delirium in critically ill patients exists in the 2013 clinical practice guidelines published in *Critical Care Medicine*.[16] These guidelines detail evidence-based recommendations for assessment and treatment of pain, depth of sedation, monitoring of sedation and brain function, detecting and monitoring delirium, risk factors for delirium, and delirium prevention and treatment.

CREATION OF A DEDICATED GERIATRIC TRAUMA UNIT

Mangram and colleagues[82,83] published 1 year of data following creation of a geriatric trauma unit for patients aged 60 years and older. The G-60 unit, as it was named, showed improvement in multiple morbidities, such as pneumonia, respiratory failure, and urinary tract infection. The G-60 also demonstrated mortality improvement.[82,83] Decreases were seen in ED LOS, average ED to operative management time, surgical critical care unit LOS, and average hospital LOS.[82,83] In spite of dramatic improvements in morbidity, mortality, and time-based secondary outcomes, hospitals throughout the country have not readily created similar specialized units to care for geriatric trauma patients.

Dr Mangram previously hypothesized that such a unit might promote significant cost savings. Texas Tech University, a level 1 regional trauma and burn center in West Texas that admits more than 850 geriatric trauma patients annually, created a similar Geriatric Trauma Unit (GTU) and has affirmed this financial benefit (largely due to decreased ICU admissions and shorter hospital LOS).[84] Suggested goals for a geriatric trauma service include

1. Patients should be seen by the surgical service in less than 2 hours.
2. Patients should be admitted to the GTU in less than 4 hours.
3. Definitive surgical repairs occur within 48 hours.
4. Consultation of primary care physician or geriatrician should occur within 24 hours of admission for multidisciplinary management.
5. There should be evidence-based practice and optimal care for all traumatically injured patients (eg, prompt correction of coagulopathy TBI patients with therapeutic anticoagulation).
6. Discharge within 5 days with safe disposition planning.

OTHER CONSIDERATIONS IN GERIATRIC TRAUMA
Triage

Although geriatric trauma patients are at greater risk for adverse outcomes when compared with younger counterparts, they are actually less likely to receive care at trauma centers.[75,85,86] A retrospective 10-year study in Maryland of more than 26,000 patients showed that undertriage was significantly more likely in patients older than 65 years.[37] This finding is in spite of evidence that when surgical intensivists lead critical care in trauma centers, in-hospital mortality is greatly reduced.[75] The mortality reduction is most pronounced in geriatric patients with comorbidities and decreased physiologic reserve.[75] Geriatric patients in designated trauma centers are also less likely to experience preventable adverse events.[85] Yet nearly half of injured older adults, especially those in older age groups and also female sex, are admitted to non-designated trauma centers.[65] Literature supports a lower threshold for trauma activation for injured patients aged 65 years and older; geriatric patients with at least one Abbreviated Injury Scale score of 3 or greater or those with a base deficit of −6 or less should be treated at trauma centers staffed by surgical intensivists.[1]

Frailty

Physical frailty is a syndrome describing diminished strength and endurance and decreased physiologic function and is a marker for physiologic age versus chronologic age.[87] Physical frailty prevalence among geriatric trauma patients ranges from 44% to 78%.[5,88] Rogers noted that undertriaged geriatric GLF patients had higher mortality than higher acuity patients who were evaluated as activated traumas.[89] Studies such as these emphasize the need for assessment tools that identify physical frailty.

More than 30 instruments have been created to assess for frailty. Maxwell assessed 188 patients using the Vulnerable Elders Survey, Barthel Index, and the Life Space Assessment and concluded that screening injured older adults for frailty is both feasible and desirable for providing efficient and effective care interventions.[88]

ETHICAL DECISIONS IN GERIATRIC TRAUMA

Complex ethical dilemmas are often the rule rather than the exception in caring for geriatric trauma patients. Futility provides some of these dilemmas, such as in the case of an 89-year-old, frail woman after a GLF, devastating subdural hematoma, and 72-hour history of GCS less than 8 whose family members want everything done. Other dilemmas are created when treatments for acute trauma exacerbate preexisting conditions and create myriad of unwanted side effects, such as in the case of a 72-year-old gentleman with a history of advanced chronic obstructive pulmonary disease, who after sustaining multiple rib fractures in a motor vehicle crash, requires pain medications that exacerbate his underlying dementia and lung disease.

Unfortunately, such patients and their ethical dilemmas are commonplace in the American trauma system. Geriatric patients account for at least 15% of our trauma patients and a disproportionate number of our trauma-related deaths.[90] Traumatically injured geriatric patients, even when highly functional and independent before trauma, are less likely to discharge home when compared with a younger patient with the same injuries.[91]

The ethical problems of geriatric trauma patients center around 4 main principles: autonomy, beneficence, nonmaleficence, and justice.[8] Debating these principles may promote insight into the philosophic underpinnings of humanity, but it rarely produces solutions for patient care in the acute setting. Asking yourself whether you are respecting a patient's autonomy is about as impractical a question as it is stilted language.

Trauma surgeons are often less interested in theoretic principle as they are with deciding the right thing to do for the patient immediately under their care. Ideally, they treat patients in accordance with best practice, evidence-based care. Although the evolution and advancement of this evidence-based care may result in keeping more patients alive, this lower mortality does not necessarily lead to restoring quality of life. Prolonged hospital LOS, protracted post–acute care recovery, and significant permanent disability in these geriatric patients suggest that geriatric trauma management has tremendous room for improvement. Although the disparate outcomes seen in geriatric trauma patients are not the result of an inattention to ethical standards, proper application of these standards may go a long way toward improving care for geriatric traumatically injured patients.

The first step in navigating the moral dilemmas posed in geriatric trauma care is through improved communication when interacting with geriatric patients and their surrogates.[92–96]

Communication that determines patients' goals of care and clarifies their definition of quality of life is a key ingredient for treatment and care. If communication is poor and these definitions are poorly defined, physicians may presume inaccurately and direct care toward an outcome that patients and/or family members deem unwanted or unacceptable.

THE 4 MAIN PRINCIPLES OF MEDICAL ETHICS
Autonomy

Autonomy is the ability of a person to make a decision freely. Accomplishing this requires informing, rather than coercing, patients. Patients must have the capacity to reasonably comprehend their options and also rationally use the information. Such capacity may be compromised in the geriatric population.

Dementia is the most common cognitive disorder of the geriatric and can affect patients' ability to make autonomous decisions. Evaluating capacity is not always straightforward. Determining capacity must include an understanding of patients' deficits and ability to comprehend the consequences of the decision being made. Mildly demented patients may have capacity to consent to an arterial line placement but may not have the capacity to determine code status. The assessment of capacity is a crucial component of any trauma surgeon's duty when treating geriatric patients. Although detailing an examination of capacity is outside the scope of this article, the trauma surgeon should identify a surrogate decision maker when capacity is diminished.

Surrogates are individuals who speak for patients. Strictly speaking, surrogates are individuals who perform the duties of substituted judgment. Surrogates provide substituted judgment through consistently communicating patients' values. In doing so, surrogates effectively restore the patients' voice.

The trauma surgeon should facilitate, whenever possible, the surrogates' ability to communicate patient values. This facilitation is often difficult in the trauma milieu as patients' devastating injury or in extremis condition may necessitate communication under temporal duress. Although the ability to do this might be included in what some refer to as *the art of medicine*, there are guidelines to effectively improve communication of patients' values.

Beneficence

The principle of beneficence describes the duty of a trauma surgeon to make decisions that improve patients' well-being. This responsibility is particularly difficult in the geriatric population, whereby survival can be subordinate to quality of life after discharge.[8–10,90,97,98] That which is beneficent toward geriatric trauma patients depends on patients' value system and what patients would consider a meaningful outcome. The beneficent trauma surgeon understands the importance of this as the foundation for goals of care, enabling the surgeon to determine the intended benefit of potential treatment options.

Goals of Care

Defining patients' or surrogates' goals of care may promote understanding and agreement between patient (or surrogate) and physician regarding the plan of care. Schwarze and colleagues[96] assert that a question posed to surrogates regarding what patients would *want* is flawed in that it emphasizes treatments (life support or comfort care) rather than promoting a discussion of the value of different outcomes.[96]

Instead, Schwarze and colleagues promote the use of words, such as *say* or *think*, to prompt families to deliberate, weigh options, and evaluate trade-offs from the patients' perspective.[96] For example, asking a family member to tell you what his or her mother would say about living with a TBI and multiple broken bones in her pelvis and legs causes the family member to consider a loved one's values, what the patient has said in the past, and the kinds of experiences the patient has previously enjoyed.[96] The physician poses these questions with an equipoise and empathy, thereby enabling rational medical decision-making and prompting morally relevant and clinically useful answers.[96,99] The defined goals of care may be used as a foundation for subsequent decision-making regarding appropriate interventions and treatment of geriatric trauma patients.

Nonmaleficence

The most famous directive, *first, do no harm*, from *The History of Epidemics* in the *Hippocratic corpus*, is often easier said than done. This principle is especially difficult for surgeons whose care often involves the administration of a planned and deliberate trauma inherent in surgery. For injured geriatric patients, nonmaleficence describes a mindful and realistic approach to proposed treatments. Geriatric patients die more frequently after trauma.[90] Geriatric trauma patients also have permanent, life-changing deficits more often than younger patients.[90] One may assert that harm has been done when a treatment results in survival but leaves patients in an unacceptably debilitated state. Realistic expectations of that which might be achieved from various treatment options enable an informed decision-making process for patients or surrogates.

Justice

Justice, the principle that defines the distribution of resources, addresses how the medical needs of the many in society must be balanced against the needs of the few or the individual. In an excellent review of ethical issues in geriatric trauma care, Cocanour[8] simplifies the idea of justice for the trauma surgeon by highlighting what the health care team should consider when evaluating its clinical application: "The healthcare team must consider four main areas when evaluating justice: fair distribution of scarce resources, competing needs for those resources, rights and obligations, and potential conflicts with established legislation."[8] Consideration of resources and balancing the needs of the many with those of the few or the individual serves to protect vulnerable populations, such as geriatric trauma patients.

COMMUNICATION WHEN CARING FOR GERIATRIC TRAUMA PATIENTS

Communication is paramount in uncovering patients' definition of a meaningful outcome. Communication inadequacies in health care commonly generate ethical consults in clinical care.[100] Surgeons are susceptible to having inadequate or poor end-of-life conversations because of time constraints, inadequate communication training, the complexity of clinical prognostication, and a tendency to overestimate prognosis.[92] Cooper defines 9 elements for structured communication with patients in an emergency setting in order to maximize best possible outcomes and minimize harms:

1. Formulating prognosis
2. Creating a personal connection
3. Disclosing information regarding the acute problem in the context of the underlying illness
4. Establishing a shared understanding of patients' condition
5. Allowing silence and dealing with emotion
6. Describing surgical and palliative treatment options
7. Eliciting patients' goals and priorities
8. Making a treatment recommendation
9. Affirming ongoing support for patients and families

Overall, effective communication is predicated on the clinician's ability to effectively and sincerely affirm a commitment to patients' well-being.

MULTIDISCIPLINARY APPROACHES TO GERIATRIC TRAUMA: GERIATRICS CONSULTATION, SUPPORTIVE (PALLIATIVE) CARE, AND ETHICS CONSULT SERVICES

Geriatrics Service Consultation

Geriatric consultation services provide a specialized approach to care of geriatric patients. The consultants may help navigate the unique problems posed to geriatric patients and provide a more complete approach to their care. The addition of a geriatric consult service may lead to more effective in-hospital care and better outcomes.[91,97]

Lenartowicz and colleagues[91] studied a compulsory geriatric consult service for trauma patients older than 60 years and found that, consistent with prior literature, the trauma team followed most of the recommendations from the geriatric consultants. These recommendations resulted in treatment changes and improved outcomes, including decreased incidence of delirium and discharge to long-term care facilities for patients admitted from home.[91]

Palliative/Supportive Care Consultation

Similar to those for geriatricians, consulting a palliative care or supportive care service may also benefit geriatric trauma patients. These experts not only mange pain and symptoms but are also trained to communicate proficiently regarding goals of care and end-of-life concerns. Use of this specialized training profoundly effects delivery and type of care, especially when communication is poor or confrontational between surgeon and surrogate or when goals of care are unclear.

Ethics Consultation

Ethics consultation services (ECS) are nearly ubiquitous in hospitals across the United States.[100] Nearly 55% of US physicians order an ethical consultation, and up to 95% agree that the presence of this service is both useful and important.[100] A consulting ethicist with specialized training evaluates ethical aspects of patient care and provides practical guidance regarding that care and are supported by a hospital ethics committee that oversees the recommendations of the service. Ethics consults are most helpful after a specific question is defined. Examples of questions for which an ethics consult service might be helpful include

- Questions regarding who should serve as a health care proxy agent when the situation (or the law) is unclear
- Questions regarding who makes decisions in unbefriended, obtunded patients
- Questions regarding code status disagreements between patients/surrogates and the care team
- Questions regarding futility of care
- Questions regarding withdrawal or continuation of life-sustaining treatment.
- Questions regarding shared decision-making

Ethics consultations may be called when a surgeon ascertains that there is some ethical conflict or ambiguity. ECS may also assist in cases when hospital policies are unclear. The ethics consult service may be requested by patients, families, nurses, physicians, or anyone participating in patients' care. This accessibility enables the identifier of an ethical issue to ask the expertise of the ethics consult service without fear of reprisal or retribution.

REFERENCES

1. Calland JF, Ingraham AM, Martin N, et al. Evaluation and management of geriatric trauma: an Eastern Association for the Surgery of Trauma practice management guideline. J Trauma Acute Care Surg 2012;73(5 Suppl 4):S345–50.

2. Kerem Y, Watts H, Kulstad E. Evaluation of the revised trauma and injury severity scores in elderly trauma patients. J Emerg Trauma Shock 2012;5(2):131.

3. Brooks SE, Mukherjee K, Gunter OL, et al. Do models incorporating comorbidities outperform those incorporating vital signs and injury pattern for predicting mortality in geriatric trauma? J Am Coll Surg 2014;219(5):1020–7.

4. Grabo DJ, Braslow BM, Schwab CW. Current therapy of trauma and surgical critical care. In: Asensio JA, Trunkey D, editors. 2nd edition. Elsevier; 2016.

5. Joseph B, Pandit V, Zangbar B, et al. Superiority of frailty over age in predicting outcomes among geriatric trauma patients: a prospective analysis. JAMA Surg 2014;149(8):766–72.

6. Hashmi A, Ibrahim-Zada I, Rhee P, et al. Predictors of mortality in geriatric trauma patients. J Trauma Acute Care Surg 2014;76(3):894–901.

7. Pandit V, Rhee P, Hashmi A, et al. Shock index predicts mortality in geriatric trauma patients. J Trauma Acute Care Surg 2014;76(4):1111–5.

8. Cocanour CS. Ethics and the emergency care of the seriously ill and injured elderly patient. Curr Geri Rep 2016;5(1):55–61.

9. Bouras T, Stranjalis G, Korfias S, et al. Head injury mortality in a geriatric population: differentiating an "edge" age group with better potential for benefit than older poor-prognosis patients. J Neurotrauma 2007;24(8):1355–61.

10. Søreide K, Desserud KF. Emergency surgery in the elderly: the balance between function, frailty, fatality and futility. Scand J Trauma Resusc Emerg Med 2015;23(1):10.

11. Halaweish I, Alam HB. Changing demographics of the American population. Surg Clin North Am 2015;95(1):1–10.

12. Weir S, Salkever DS, Rivara FP, et al. One-year treatment costs of trauma care in the USA. Expert Rev Pharmacoecon Outcomes Res 2010;10(2):187–97.

13. Oreskovich MR, Howard JD, Copass MK, et al. Geriatric trauma: injury patterns and outcome. J Trauma 1984;24(7):565–72.

14. Horst HM, Obeid FN, Sorensen VJ, et al. Factors influencing survival of elderly trauma patients. Crit Care Med 1986;14(8):681–4.

15. Scalea TM, Simon HM, Duncan AO, et al. Geriatric blunt multiple trauma: improved survival with early invasive monitoring. J Trauma 1990;30(2):129–34 [discussion: 134–6].

16. Barr J, Fraser GL, Puntillo K, et al. Clinical practice guidelines for the management of pain, agitation, and delirium in adult patients in the intensive care unit. Crit Care Med 2013;41(1):263–306.

17. Mattox KL, Moore EE, Feliciano DV. Trauma. In: Mattox KL, Moore EE, Feliciano DV, editors. 7th edition. McGraw Hill; 2013.

18. Martin RS, Farrah JP, Chang MC. Effect of aging on cardiac function plus monitoring and support. Surg Clin North Am 2015;95(1):23–35.

19. Neideen T, Lam M, Brasel KJ. Preinjury beta blockers are associated with increased mortality in geriatric trauma patients. J Trauma 2008;65(5):1016–20.

20. Heffernan DS, Thakkar RK, Monaghan SF, et al. Normal presenting vital signs are unreliable in geriatric blunt trauma victims. J Trauma 2010;69(4):813–20.

21. Martin JT, Alkhoury F, O'Connor JA, et al. "Normal" vital signs belie occult hypoperfusion in geriatric trauma patients. Am Surg 2010;76(1):65–9.

22. Ramly E, Kaafarani HMA, Velmahos GC. The effect of aging on pulmonary function: implications for monitoring and support of the surgical and trauma patient. Surg Clin North Am 2015;95(1):53–69.

23. Culham EG, Jimenez HA, King CE. Thoracic kyphosis, rib mobility, and lung volumes in normal women and women with osteoporosis. Spine 1994;19(11):1250–5.

24. Knudson RJ, Slatin RC, Lebowitz MD, et al. The maximal expiratory flow-volume curve. Normal standards, variability, and effects of age. Am Rev Respir Dis 1976;113(5):587–600.

25. Janssens JP. Aging of the respiratory system: impact on pulmonary function tests and adaptation to exertion. Clin Chest Med 2005;26(3):469–84, vi–vii.

26. Abdel-Kader K, Palevsky PM. Acute kidney injury in the elderly. Clin Geriatr Med 2009;25(3):331–58.

27. Musso CG, Oreopoulos DG. Aging and physiological changes of the kidneys including changes in glomerular filtration rate. Nephron Physiol 2011; 119(Suppl 1):p1–5.

28. Baldea AJ. Effect of aging on renal function plus monitoring and support. Surg Clin North Am 2015;95(1):71–83.

29. Schmitt R, Coca S, Kanbay M, et al. Recovery of kidney function after acute kidney injury in the elderly: a systematic review and meta-analysis. Am J Kidney Dis 2008;52(2):262–71.

30. Kwag S-J, Kim J-G, Kang W-K, et al. The nutritional risk is a independent factor for postoperative morbidity in surgery for colorectal cancer. Ann Surg Treat Res 2014;86(4):206–11.

31. White JV, Guenter P, Jensen G, et al. Consensus statement of the Academy of Nutrition and Dietetics/American Society for Parenteral and Enteral Nutrition: characteristics recommended for the identification and documentation of adult malnutrition (undernutrition). J Acad Nutr Diet 2012;112:730–8.

32. Almeida AI, Correia M, Camilo M, et al. Nutritional risk screening in surgery: valid, feasible, easy! Clin Nutr 2012;31(2):206–11.

33. Vischer UM, Frangos E, Graf C, et al. The prognostic significance of malnutrition as assessed by the Mini Nutritional Assessment (MNA) in older hospitalized patients with a heavy disease burden. Clin Nutr 2012;31(1):113–7.

34. Nohra E, Bochicchio GV. Management of the gastrointestinal tract and nutrition in the geriatric surgical patient. Surg Clin North Am 2015;95(1):85–101.

35. Labib N, Nouh T, Winocour S, et al. Severely injured geriatric population: morbidity, mortality, and risk factors. J Trauma 2011;71(6):1908–14.

36. Spaniolas K, Cheng JD, Gestring ML, et al. Ground level falls are associated with significant mortality in elderly patients. J Trauma 2010;69(4):821–5.

37. Chang DC, Bass RR, Cornwell EE, et al. Undertriage of elderly trauma patients to state-designated trauma centers. Arch Surg 2008;143(8):776–81.

38. Thompson HJ, McCormick WC, Kagan SH. Traumatic brain injury in older adults: epidemiology, outcomes, and future implications. J Am Geriatr Soc 2006;54(10):1590–5.

39. Victorino GP, Chong TJ, Pal JD. Trauma in the elderly patient. Arch Surg 2003; 138(10):1093.

40. Le Roux P, Pollack CV, Milan M, et al. Race against the clock: overcoming challenges in the management of anticoagulant-associated intracerebral hemorrhage. J Neurosurg 2014;121(Suppl):1–20.

41. Bechtel BF, Nunez TC, Lyon JA, et al. Treatments for reversing warfarin anticoagulation in patients with acute intracranial hemorrhage: a structured literature review. Int J Emerg Med 2011;4(1):40.

42. van Asch CJ, Luitse MJ, Rinkel GJ, et al. Incidence, case fatality, and functional outcome of intracerebral haemorrhage over time, according to age, sex, and ethnic origin: a systematic review and meta-analysis. Lancet Neurol 2010;9(2): 167–76.

43. Ivascu FA, Janczyk RJ, Junn FS, et al. Treatment of trauma patients with intracranial hemorrhage on preinjury warfarin. J Trauma 2006;61(2):318–21.

44. Docimo S, Demin A, Vinces F. Patients with blunt head trauma on anticoagulation and antiplatelet medications: can they be safely discharged after a normal initial cranial computed tomography scan? Am Surg 2014;80(6):610–3.

45. Ivascu FA, Howells GA, Junn FS, et al. Rapid warfarin reversal in anticoagulated patients with traumatic intracranial hemorrhage reduces hemorrhage progression and mortality. J Trauma 2005;59(5):1131–7 [discussion: 1137–9].

46. Barbosa RR, Jawa R, Watters JM, et al. Evaluation and management of mild traumatic brain injury. J Trauma Acute Care Surg 2012;73:S307–14.

47. Simon B, Ebert J, Bokhari F, et al. Management of pulmonary contusion and flail chest: an Eastern Association for the Surgery of Trauma practice management guideline. J Trauma Acute Care Surg 2012;73(5 Suppl 4):S351–61.

48. Bulger EM, Arneson MA, Mock CN, et al. Rib fractures in the elderly. J Trauma 2000;48(6):1040–6 [discussion: 1046–7].

49. Todd SR, McNally MM, Holcomb JB, et al. A multidisciplinary clinical pathway decreases rib fracture–associated infectious morbidity and mortality in high-risk trauma patients. Am J Surg 2006;192(6):806–11.

50. Bulger EM, Edwards T, Klotz P, et al. Epidural analgesia improves outcome after multiple rib fractures. Surgery 2004;136(2):426–30.

51. Flagel BT, Luchette FA, Reed RL, et al. Half-a-dozen ribs: the breakpoint for mortality. Surgery 2005;138(4):717–25.

52. Nirula R, Allen B, Layman R, et al. Rib fracture stabilization in patients sustaining blunt chest injury. Am Surg 2006;72(4):307–9.

53. Fitzpatrick DC, Denard PJ, Phelan D, et al. Operative stabilization of flail chest injuries: review of literature and fixation options. Eur J Trauma Emerg Surg 2010; 36(5):427–33.

54. Khandelwal G, Mathur RK, Shukla S, et al. A prospective single center study to assess the impact of surgical stabilization in patients with rib fracture. Int J Surg 2011;9(6):478–81.

55. Girsowicz E, Falcoz P-E, Santelmo N, et al. Does surgical stabilization improve outcomes in patients with isolated multiple distracted and painful non-flail rib fractures? Interact Cardiovasc Thorac Surg 2012;14(3):312–5.

56. Bhatnagar A, Mayberry J, Nirula R. Rib fracture fixation for flail chest: what is the benefit? J Am Coll Surg 2012;215(2):201–5.

57. Slobogean GP, MacPherson CA, Sun T, et al. Surgical fixation vs nonoperative management of flail chest: a meta-analysis. J Am Coll Surg 2013;216(2): 302–11.e1.

58. Marasco SF, Davies AR, Cooper J, et al. Prospective randomized controlled trial of operative rib fixation in traumatic flail chest. J Am Coll Surg 2013;216(5): 924–32.

59. Doben AR, Eriksson EA, Denlinger CE, et al. Surgical rib fixation for flail chest deformity improves liberation from mechanical ventilation. J Crit Care 2014; 29(1):139–43.

60. Pieracci FM, Rodil M, Stovall RT, et al. Surgical stabilization of severe rib fractures. J Trauma Acute Care Surg 2015;78(4):883–7.

61. Majercik S, Vijayakumar S, Olsen G, et al. Surgical stabilization of severe rib fractures decreases incidence of retained hemothorax and empyema. Am J Surg 2015;210(6):1112–6.

62. Caragounis E-C, Olsén MF, Pazooki D, et al. Surgical treatment of multiple rib fractures and flail chest in trauma: a one-year follow-up study. World J Emerg Surg 2016;11:27.

63. Pieracci FM, Lin Y, Rodil M, et al. A prospective, controlled clinical evaluation of surgical stabilization of severe rib fractures. J Trauma Acute Care Surg 2016; 80(2):187–94.

64. Pieracci FM, Majercik S, Ali-Osman F, et al. Consensus statement: surgical stabilization of rib fractures rib fracture colloquium clinical practice guidelines. Injury 2017;48(2):307–21.

65. Maxwell CA, Miller RS, Dietrich MS, et al. The aging of America: a comprehensive look at over 25,000 geriatric trauma admissions to United States hospitals. Am Surg 2015;81(6):630–6.

66. Tinubu J, Scalea TM. Management of fractures in a geriatric surgical patient. Surg Clin North Am 2015;95(1):115–28.

67. Simunovic N, Devereaux PJ, Sprague S, et al. Effect of early surgery after hip fracture on mortality and complications: systematic review and meta-analysis. CMAJ 2010;182(15):1609–16.

68. Leung F, Lau TW, Kwan K, et al. Does timing of surgery matter in fragility hip fractures? Osteoporos Int 2010;21(Suppl 4):S529–34.

69. Moja L, Piatti A, Pecoraro V, et al. Timing matters in hip fracture surgery: patients operated within 48 hours have better outcomes. A meta-analysis and meta-regression of over 190,000 patients. Scherer RW, ed. PLoS One 2012;7(10): e46175.

70. Zuckerman JD, Sakales SR, Fabian DR, et al. Hip fractures in geriatric patients. Results of an interdisciplinary hospital care program. Clin Orthop Relat Res 1992;274:213–25.

71. Harbrecht BG, Peitzman AB, Rivera L, et al. Contribution of age and gender to outcome of blunt splenic injury in adults: multicenter study of the Eastern Association for the Surgery of Trauma. J Trauma 2001;51(5):887–95.

72. Roth BJ, Velmahos GC, Oder DB, et al. Penetrating trauma in patients older than 55 years: a case-control study. Injury 2001;32(7):551–4.

73. Taylor MD, Tracy JK, Meyer W, et al. Trauma in the elderly: intensive care unit resource use and outcome. J Trauma Acute Care Surg 2002;53(3):407–14.

74. Demetriades D, Karaiskakis M, Velmahos G, et al. Effect on outcome of early intensive management of geriatric trauma patients. Br J Surg 2002;89(10): 1319–22.

75. Nathens AB, Rivara FP, MacKenzie EJ, et al. The impact of an intensivist-model ICU on trauma-related mortality. Ann Surg 2006;244(4):545.

76. Barr J, Pandharipande PP. The pain, agitation, and delirium care bundle: synergistic benefits of implementing the 2013 pain, agitation, and delirium guidelines in an integrated and interdisciplinary fashion. Crit Care Med 2013;41:S99–115.

77. Pandharipande PP, Girard TD, Jackson JC, et al. Long-term cognitive impairment after critical illness. N Engl J Med 2013;369(14):1306–16.

78. Brummel NE, Vasilevskis EE, Han JH, et al. Implementing delirium screening in the ICU: secrets to success. Crit Care Med 2013;41(9):2196–208.

79. Brummel NE, Jackson JC, Pandharipande PP, et al. Delirium in the ICU and subsequent long-term disability among survivors of mechanical ventilation. Crit Care Med 2014;42(2):369–77.

80. Ely EW, Shintani A, Truman B, et al. Delirium as a predictor of mortality in mechanically ventilated patients in the intensive care unit. JAMA 2004;291(14): 1753–62.

81. Inouye SK. Delirium in older persons. N Engl J Med 2006;354(11):1157–65.

82. Mangram AJ, Mitchell CD, Shifflette VK, et al. Geriatric trauma service: a one-year experience. J Trauma 2012;72(1):119–22.

83. Mangram AJ, Shifflette VK, Mitchell CD, et al. The creation of a geriatric trauma unit "g-60". Am Surg 2011;77(9):1144–6.

84. Brooks SE. Use of TQIP best practice guidelines for improved care in massive transfusion protocol (MTP) and geriatric trauma patients at a level I trauma center. American College of Surgeons Trauma Quality Improvement Program (TQIP) Annual Scientific Meeting. Nashville, 2015.

85. MacKenzie EJ, Rivara FP, Jurkovich GJ, et al. A national evaluation of the effect of trauma-center care on mortality. N Engl J Med 2006;354(4):366–78.

86. Meldon SW, Reilly M, Drew BL, et al. Trauma in the very elderly: a community-based study of outcomes at trauma and nontrauma centers. J Trauma Acute Care Surg 2002;52(1):79–84.

87. Maxwell CA, Mion LC, Mukherjee K, et al. Preinjury physical frailty and cognitive impairment among geriatric trauma patients determine postinjury functional recovery and survival. J Trauma Acute Care Surg 2016;80(2):195–203.

88. Maxwell CA, Mion LC, Mukherjee K, et al. Feasibility of screening for preinjury frailty in hospitalized injured older adults. J Trauma Acute Care Surg 2015; 78(4):844–51.

89. Rogers A, Rogers F, Bradburn E, et al. Old and undertriaged: a lethal combination. Am Surg 2012;78(6):711–5.

90. Trunkey DD, Cahn RM, Lenfesty B, et al. Management of the geriatric trauma patient at risk of death: therapy withdrawal decision making. Arch Surg 2000; 135(1):34–8.

91. Lenartowicz M, Parkovnick M, McFarlan A, et al. An evaluation of a proactive geriatric trauma consultation service. Ann Surg 2012;256(6):1098–101.

92. Cooper Z, Courtwright A, Karlage A, et al. Pitfalls in communication that lead to nonbeneficial emergency surgery in elderly patients with serious illness. Ann Surg 2014;260(6):949–57.

93. Halub ME, Sidwell RA. Cardiac risk stratification and protection. Surg Clin North Am 2015;95(2):217–35.

94. Fleisher LA, Beckman JA, Brown KA, et al. 2009 ACCF/AHA focused update on perioperative beta blockade incorporated into the ACC/AHA 2007 guidelines on perioperative cardiovascular evaluation and care for noncardiac surgery: a report of the American College of Cardiology Foundation/American Heart Association task force on practice guidelines. Circulation 2009;120(21):e169–276.

95. Cooper Z, Koritsanszky LA, Cauley CE, et al. Recommendations for best communication practices to facilitate goal-concordant care for seriously ill older patients with emergency surgical conditions. Ann Surg 2016;263(1):1–6.

96. Schwarze ML, Campbell TC, Cunningham TV, et al. You can't get what you want: innovation for end-of-life communication in the intensive care unit. Am J Respir Crit Care Med 2016;193(1):14–6.

97. Fallon WF Jr, Rader E, Zyzanski S, et al. Geriatric outcomes are improved by a geriatric trauma consultation service. J Trauma 2006;61(5):1040–6.

98. Terry S, Kaplan LJ. Ethical imperatives in staffing and managing a trauma intensive care unit. Crit Care Med 2007;35(2 Suppl):S24–8.

99. Steffens NM, Tucholka JL, Nabozny MJ, et al. Engaging patients, health care professionals, and community members to improve preoperative decision making for older adults facing high-risk surgery. JAMA Surg 2016;151(10):938–45.

100. Tapper EB, Vercler CJ, Cruze D, et al. Ethics consultation at a large urban public teaching hospital. Mayo Clin Proc 2010;85(5):433–8.

Radiology for Trauma and the General Surgeon

Patrick K. Kim, MD

KEYWORDS

- Trauma radiology • Trauma radiography • Ultrasonography • FAST
- Computed tomography • CT • Radiation effective dose

KEY POINTS

- Plain film radiography and ultrasonography (focused assessment for sonography in trauma [FAST] and extended FAST [E-FAST]) are important modalities for the initial evaluation of patients with trauma. In meta-stable or unstable patients, the combination of chest radiograph, pelvis radiograph, and FAST or E-FAST rapidly triages the torso.
- Computed tomography (CT) has become standard for imaging blunt trauma. It is unclear whether a pan-CT scan approach or selective CT scan approach is superior.
- CT is used increasingly for less stable patients because it may improve decision making about invasive procedures.
- CT angiography has become the modality of choice for imaging suspected vascular injuries of the neck and extremities.
- The impact of ionizing radiation (effective dose) of CT scans to individual patients may be infinitesimal but there may be implications at the population level. Imaging strategies in trauma should be evaluated continuously.

INTRODUCTION

Radiographic imaging is integral to the evaluation of injured patients. Conventional radiography (plain film), ultrasonography, and computed tomography (CT) are nearly universally present and immediately available in most modern facilities. In particular, ultrasonography and CT have ever-increasing roles in trauma and general surgery. Other modalities, such as conventional angiography, fluoroscopy, MRI, and nuclear medicine are important adjunct modalities. This article focuses on plain film, ultrasonography, and CT, the modalities used most often in the early phases of evaluation.

No imaging modality is perfect. Each modality has limitations, risks, and costs. The optimal use of diagnostic radiology incorporates patient physiology, mechanism of

Disclosure: No disclosures to report.
Division of Traumatology, Surgical Critical Care and Emergency Surgery, Department of Surgery, Perelman School of Medicine at the University of Pennsylvania, Penn Presbyterian Medical Center, 51 North 39th Street, Medical Office Building, 1st Floor, Philadelphia, PA 19104, USA
E-mail address: Patrick.kim@uphs.upenn.edu

Surg Clin N Am 97 (2017) 1175–1183
http://dx.doi.org/10.1016/j.suc.2017.06.014
0039-6109/17/© 2017 Elsevier Inc. All rights reserved.

surgical.theclinics.com

injury, physical examination, and an understanding of the strengths and limitations of various modalities.

PLAIN FILM

Conventional radiology (plain film) is a well-established initial modality for radiographic evaluation. Chest radiograph (CXR) and pelvis radiograph (PXR) remain recommended by Advanced Trauma Life Support as a routine in the evaluation of blunt trauma.[1] CXR is familiar, readily available, and rapid. For patients with trauma, single-view anteroposterior CXR may show a life-threatening injury requiring immediate treatment, such as pneumothorax or hemothorax, which may require tube thoracostomy. Other findings may include pulmonary contusion or aspiration, abnormal mediastinal width or contour (potentially indicating traumatic aortic injury), abnormal diaphragm contour, rib fractures, retained bullets or other objects, and extrathoracic injuries. CXR has high specificity but low sensitivity for pneumothorax, missing up to half of pneumothoraces.[2] The PXR is an appropriate initial modality in the assessment of patients with blunt trauma with hip or pelvic symptoms, abnormal hemodynamics, or unreliable examination. PXR identifies significant pelvic fractures, pelvic diastasis, hip fractures, and dislocations, all of which may require immediate treatment (eg, pelvic binder for open-book pelvic fracture, reduction of hip dislocation). In examinable patients with absent signs, symptoms, and hemodynamic issues, and if CT abdomen pelvis is planned, then PXR is low yield.[3,4]

ULTRASONOGRAPHY

Ultrasonography is rapidly becoming a favored modality in initial trauma assessment. Focused assessment for sonography in trauma (FAST) is well validated and established in the early assessment of patients with blunt abdominal trauma or penetrating precordial/transthoracic injuries.[5] As originally described, FAST comprises 4 standard views: subxiphoid pericardial, right upper quadrant, left upper quadrant, and pelvic views. The basic objective of FAST is to determine the presence or absence of hemoperitoneum. FAST has the benefits of being readily available (often performed by the surgeon or other bedside provider), noninvasive, repeatable, and without radiation. Highly operator dependent, FAST can detect intra-abdominal fluid volumes as low as 225 to 400 mL.[6] However, FAST has limited utility for diagnosing solid organ injuries, hollow visceral injuries, and retroperitoneal injuries, because these processes are potentially, but not necessarily, associated with hemoperitoneum. Furthermore, body habitus and subcutaneous or intraluminal air may decrease image quality. The role of FAST in hemodynamically stable patients with blunt trauma is minimal if CT abdomen and pelvis is indicated. If CT abdomen and pelvis is not indicated, then negative FAST, especially if repeated after an interval of time, is an appropriate component of evaluation.

The use of additional views to inspect the pleural spaces to rule out pneumothorax is known as extended FAST (E-FAST).[7] E-FAST has consistently shown excellent sensitivity and specificity in the diagnosis of pneumothorax compared with CXR.[8] In addition, E-FAST can be supplemented with dedicated views of the posterior pleural spaces to assess for hemothorax in addition to pneumothorax.

CAVITARY TRIAGE

Physiology should drive decision making regarding choice of initial imaging. Cavitary triage is the concept of rapid CXR, PXR, and FAST (or E-FAST) during or after primary and secondary survey to quickly screen for sources of life-threatening hemorrhage in hemodynamically unstable patients with blunt trauma. This rapid screen of the torso should indicate the most likely sources of hemorrhage (thoracic, abdominal, or pelvic/retroperitoneal) and guide the initial emergent treatments. In penetrating torso trauma, abdominal radiographs should be considered in addition to CXR and PXR to completely screen the torso and potentially rule out intra-abdominal trajectory. When evaluating gunshot wound injury, it is important to capture the lateral soft tissues of the torso completely. Missing a bullet may confound determination of trajectory and lead to a false sense of security.

COMPUTED TOMOGRAPHY
Computed Tomography and Unstable Patients

CT has rapidly become a standard part of the evaluation of stable patients with blunt and penetrating trauma. It is widely available, rapid, and generally accurate. In contrast with portable plain film and ultrasonography, both point-of-care modalities, CT requires sufficient patient stability for transport and time to complete the study. The traditional dictum was to never take an unstable patient to CT scan. This rule was based on many hospitals' extended distance from trauma resuscitation area to the CT scanner as well as the slow rate of CT image acquisition with earlier generations of CT scanners. These factors made active resuscitation of unstable patients logistically difficult or dangerous and potentially contributed to harm or delay in initiating a necessary procedure. However, CT scanners are increasingly located in close proximity or directly adjacent to the trauma resuscitation area and image acquisition is nearly instantaneous. Logistically, it may be possible to initiate or maintain a similar intensity of care as the trauma resuscitation area. Retrospective studies have suggested that unstable (variably defined) patients with blunt and penetrating trauma may safely undergo CT with a newer-generation CT scanner in proximity to the trauma resuscitation area.[9-12] The potential benefits of performing CT in unstable patients include differentiating patients who need operative intervention versus an interventional radiology procedure, and identifying patients who do not need an invasive procedure and can be spared an unnecessary major operation. Ultimately, the appropriateness of CT in unstable patients is patient and institution dependent.

Pan–Computed Tomography Scan Versus Selective Computed Tomography Scan

Whole-body CT scan or pan-CT scan is a term applied to a broad CT screen for blunt trauma from vertex to lesser trochanters. The alternative is selective scan of head, cervical spine, chest, abdomen, and pelvis. Proponents of pan-CT scan note that clinical judgment based on mechanism and physical examination fails to accurately predict anatomic injuries. The primary disadvantage of pan-CT scan is higher radiation dose and (presumed) associated higher radiology cost, although studies do not consistently show higher total hospital costs. Proponents of selective CT scan note that many of these additional injuries probably do not necessarily require a substantial change in plan of care. Retrospective studies have shown unexpected injuries in 20% to 38% of patients, leading to a change in management in 19% to 26% (including discharge).[13,14] A large, retrospective, multicenter study of severely injured patients with blunt trauma (injury severity score ≥16) found an association between pan-CT scan and survival.[15] Patients who underwent pan-CT scan had an absolute risk reduction of mortality between 3.1% and 5.9% compared with patients who underwent selective CT. Based on the absolute risk reductions, the number needed to treat (ie, perform CT scan) is between 17 and 32, supporting pan-CT scan for blunt trauma. (A bias toward higher anatomic injury scores may exist in patients who undergo pan-CT scan versus selective CT scan.) A large, prospective, randomized, multicenter trial of patients with blunt trauma showed no difference in mortality between pan-CT scan and selective CT scan.[16] Note that pan-CT scan was more rapid to acquire versus selective CT, the radiation exposure was statistically but not clinically different (20.9 mSv vs 20.6 mSv), and costs were not significantly different. Overall, the question of pan-CT scan versus selective CT scan remains unanswered. The final decision between pan-CT scan and selective CT scan in blunt trauma should probably incorporate physiology, mechanism, and age, favoring liberal scanning in elderly patients and more restrictive scanning in younger patients.

Blunt Cerebrovascular Injury

The diagnosis of blunt cerebrovascular injury (BCVI) is increasingly important in patients with blunt trauma as a result of increased awareness of the striking morbidity and mortality of BCVI[17] coupled with advances in CT technology that improve imaging of the carotid and vertebral arteries. At present, CT angiogram of the neck ($\geq$16 slice circa 2009, and currently much higher) is considered the standard modality for screening for BCVI. Magnetic resonance angiography is an alternative when CT angiography (CTA) is contraindicated. Screening criteria for asymptomatic patients have been recommended by trauma professional societies (**Box 1**).[18,19] Such screening criteria identify approximately 80% of patients with BCVI. The converse of this is that 20% of patients with BCVI are not identified by using established screening criteria. Given the great potential downsides of delay in diagnosis (stroke), some centers screen liberally, incorporating CTA neck vessels as a component of pan scanning.

Computed Tomography Angiography

CTA has shown effectiveness in both diagnosing and ruling out peripheral vascular injuries. A meta-analysis showed CTA sensitivity and specificity of 96% and 99%, respectively.[20] The increasing use of CTA has decreased the proportion of conventional angiography that is diagnostic and shifted the intent toward therapy.

Box 1
Western Trauma Association risk factors for blunt cerebrovascular injury in asymptomatic patients

High-energy transfer mechanism associated with:

- Displaced midface fracture (Le Fort II or III)
- Basilar skull fracture with carotid canal involvement
- CHI consistent with DAI and Glasgow Coma Scale score less than 6
- Cervical vertebral body or transverse foramen fracture, subluxation, or ligamentous injury at any level; any fracture at C1 to C3
- Near hanging with anoxia
- Clothesline-type injury or seat belt abrasion with significant swelling, pain, or altered mental status

Adapted from Biffl WL, Cothren CC, Moore EE, et al. WTA critical decisions in trauma: screening for and treatment of blunt cerebrovascular injuries. J Trauma 2009;67:1150–3; with permission.

Radiation Dose in Diagnostic Imaging

Plain film, CT, fluoroscopy, and nuclear medicine use ionizing radiation. The rational use of ionizing radiation is becoming more important with increasing use of CT. In individual patients, the risk of malignancy is infinitesimal but, over a population, the risk becomes significant.[21] The radiation energy absorbed by tissue is measured in rad or Gray (1 rad = 0.01 Gy). The biological effect of the energy is called effective dose and is measured in rem, sieverts, or millisieverts (1 rem [roentgen equivalent man] = 0.01 Sv = 10 mSv). Effective dose is the theoretic sum of all biological effects of radiation, accounting for intrinsic tissue sensitivity and mass. Conveniently, for all radiation sources (plain film, CT, and fluoroscopy), 1 rad of absorbed dose is 1 rem (10 mSv) effective dose. On average, the individual effective dose from all natural and medical radiation sources is 3.6 mSv/y. The effective doses for common CT studies are shown in **Table 1**. The effective dose for radiologic studies varies markedly, depending on many patient factors and the organ of interest. Effective dose varies inversely and strongly with age: children's tissues are more intrinsic radiosensitive and children have longer latency before detrimental effects manifest (**Fig. 1**). In contrast, elderly patients have less radiosensitivity and a shorter latency period. Based on current CT use and protocols in the United States, the estimated overall excess number of cancers attributable to CT is 1.5% to 2%.[21] The use of CT is frequently not limited to the initial evaluation but also may involve a protracted hospital course requiring many plain films and multiple CT scans.[22] The increasing use of CT scanning is an evolving public health issue.[21] For the patient-oriented Choosing Wisely campaign, sponsored by the American Board of Internal Medicine Foundation, professional societies each contributed 5 recommendations. A Choosing Wisely recommendation by the American College of Surgeons described here.

Avoid the routine use of whole-body diagnostic CT scanning in patients with minor or single-system trauma. Aggressive use of whole-body CT scanning improves early diagnosis of injury and may even positively affect survival in patients with polytrauma. However, the significance of radiation exposure, as well as costs associated with these studies, must be considered, especially in patients with low-energy mechanisms of injury and absent physical examination findings consistent with major trauma.[23]

Table 1		
Radiation effective dose (millisieverts) for commonly performed radiologic studies		
Study	**Meer et al 2012[28]**	**Sierink et al, 2016[16]**
Head CT	2	1.8
Neck or Cervical Spine CT	3	3
Chest CT	7	5.1
Abdomen CT	14	11
Extremity CT	0.1	
Trauma Total-body CT (Pan-CT Scan; Head, Cervical Spine, Chest, Abdomen)		20.9

Data from Meer AB, Basu PA, Baker LC, et al. Exposure to ionizing radiation and estimate of secondary cancers in the era of high-speed CT scanning: projections from the Medicare population. J Am Coll Radiol 2012;9(4):245–50; and Sierink JC, Treskes K, Edwards MJ, et al. Immediate total-body CT scanning versus conventional imaging and selective CT scanning in patients with severe trauma (REACT-2): a randomised controlled trial. Lancet 2016;388:673–83.

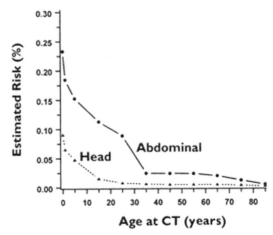

Fig. 1. Estimated lifetime attributable cancer mortality risk as a function of age at examination for a single typical CT examination of head (*broken dotted line*) and of abdomen (*broken solid line*). Note rapid increase in risk with decreasing age. (*From* Brenner D, Elliston C, Hall E, Berdon W. Estimated risks of radiation-induced fatal cancer from pediatric CT. AJR Am J Roentgenol 2001;176(2):289–96; with permission.)

In the pediatric population, the constant drive to keep the radiation dose low has given rise to the acronym ALARA (as low as reasonably achievable). This paradigm encourages critical evaluation of the number and type of studies performed as well as minimizing the effective dose for each study. In contrast, the older the patient, the less radiosensitive and the less time for detrimental effects to become manifest. Brenner and Hall[21] recommended 3 strategies to decrease CT radiation dose in the population (**Box 2**).

Pregnant patients pose a special concern. The impact of ionizing radiation is most detrimental between weeks 2 and 15 of gestation.[24] There are no high-quality observational studies on the impact of radiography on this population. The American College of Obstetrics and Gynecology (ACOG) guidelines for imaging during pregnancy and lactation are as follows[24]:

- Ultrasonography and MRI are not associated with risk and are the imaging techniques of choice for pregnant patients, but they should be used prudently and only when use is expected to answer a relevant clinical question or otherwise provide medical benefit to the patient.
- With few exceptions, radiation exposure through radiography, CT scan, or nuclear medicine imaging techniques is at a dose much lower than the exposure

---

Box 2
Strategies to minimize computed tomography radiation dose in the population

- Use automatic exposure control during CT scan
- Use alternative modalities if able
- Justify medical need for CT

Data from Brenner DJ, Hall EJ. Computed tomography–an increasing source of radiation exposure. N Engl J Med 2007;357(22):2277–84.

Table 2	
Classification of incidental findings on computed tomography	
Category 1	Requires attention before discharge
Category 2	Requires follow-up with primary doctor within 1–2 wk
Category 3	Requires no specific follow-up

From Paluska TR, Sise MJ, Sack DI, et al. Incidental CT findings in trauma patients: incidence and implications for care of the injured. J Trauma 2007;62(1):157–61; with permission.

associated with fetal harm. If these techniques are necessary in addition to ultra-sonography or MRI, or are more readily available for the diagnosis in question, they should not be withheld from a pregnant patient.

- The use of gadolinium contrast with MRI should be limited; it may be used as a contrast agent in pregnant women only if it significantly improves diagnostic performance and is expected to improve fetal or maternal outcome.
- Breastfeeding should not be interrupted after gadolinium administration.

Incidental Findings on Computed Tomography

Incidental findings are a consequence of CT imaging. Incidental findings occur in up to 45% of trauma CT scans.[25–27] A classification system for incidental findings has been proposed, stratifying by degree of significance (**Table 2**), but there is currently no common standard process for informing patients or their primary physicians. A dedicated process is necessary to ensure adherence to recommendations for category 1 and 2 incidental findings. The identification, communication, and follow-up of incidental findings is an inevitable component of trauma care.

CT technology is advancing rapidly, challenging the traditional timelines of clinical research, dissemination of knowledge, and adoption of best clinical practices. As CT image resolution and acquisition speed continue to improve, it is important to maintain the perspective of clinical relevance for optimal care of individual injured patients and the population as a whole.

SUMMARY

Diagnostic radiology plays a crucial role in the evaluation of nearly every patient with trauma. Plain film and ultrasonography can be obtained rapidly during the initial assessment. The impact of CT in decision making continues to grow as the travel distance and scan time continue to decrease. Surgeons and radiologists should collaborate to minimize unnecessary studies and radiation dose. Pregnancy should not preclude radiographic imaging in patients who are considered at risk.

REFERENCES

1. American College of Surgeons Committee on Trauma. ATLS advanced trauma life support for doctors - student course manual. 9th Edition. Chicago: American College of Surgeons; 2012. ISBN 9781880696026.
2. Ball CG, Kirkpatrick AW, Laupland KB, et al. Factors related to the failure of radiographic recognition of occult posttraumatic pneumothoraces. Am J Surg 2005; 189(5):541–6.
3. Guillamondegui OD, Pryor JP, Gracias VH, et al. Pelvic radiography in blunt trauma resuscitation: a diminishing role. J Trauma 2002;53(6):1043–7.

4. Soto JR, Zhou C, Hu D, et al. Skip and save: utility of pelvic x-rays in the initial evaluation of blunt trauma patients. Am J Surg 2015;210(6):1076–9.

5. Rozycki GS, Ballard RB, Feliciano DV, et al. Surgeon-performed ultrasound for the assessment of truncal injuries: lessons learned from 1540 patients. Ann Surg 1998;228(4):557–67.

6. Branney SW, Wolfe RE, Moore EE, et al. Quantitative sensitivity of ultrasound in detecting free intraperitoneal fluid. J Trauma 1995;39(2):375–80.

7. Kirkpatrick AW, Sirois M, Laupland KB, et al. Hand-held thoracic sonography for detecting post-traumatic pneumothoraces: the extended focused assessment with sonography for trauma (EFAST). J Trauma 2004;57(2):288–95.

8. Montoya J, Stawicki SP, Evans DC, et al. From FAST to E-FAST: an overview of the evolution of ultrasound-based traumatic injury assessment. Eur J Trauma Emerg Surg 2016;42(2):119–26.

9. Ordoñez CA, Herrera-Escobar JP, Parra MW, et al. Computed tomography in hemodynamically unstable severely injured blunt and penetrating trauma patients. J Trauma Acute Care Surg 2016;80(4):597–602.

10. Cook MR, Holcomb JB, Rahbar MH, et al. An abdominal computed tomography may be safe in selected hypotensive trauma patients with positive focused assessment with sonography in trauma examination. Am J Surg 2015;209(5): 834–40.

11. Huber-Wagner S, Biberthaler P, Haberle S, et al. Whole-body CT in haemodynamically unstable severely injured patients—a retrospective, multicentre study. PLoS One 2013;8(7):e68880.

12. Fu CY, Yang SJ, Liao CH, et al. Hypotension does not always make computed tomography scans unfeasible in the management of blunt abdominal trauma patients. Injury 2015;46(1):29–34.

13. Self ML, Blake AM, Whitley M, et al. The benefit of routine thoracic, abdominal, and pelvic computed tomography to evaluate trauma patients with closed head injuries. Am J Surg 2003;186(6):609–13.

14. Salim A, Sangthong B, Martin M, et al. Whole body imaging in blunt multisystem trauma patients without obvious signs of injury: results of a prospective study. Arch Surg 2006;141(5):468–73.

15. Huber-Wagner S, Lefering R, Qvick LM, et al, Working Group on Polytrauma of the German Trauma Society. Effect of whole-body CT during trauma resuscitation on survival: a retrospective, multicentre study. Lancet 2009;373:1455–61.

16. Sierink JC, Treskes K, Edwards MJ, et al. REACT-2 study group. Immediate total-body CT scanning versus conventional imaging and selective CT scanning in patients with severe trauma (REACT-2): a randomised controlled trial. Lancet 2016; 388:673–83.

17. Berne JD, Norwood SH, McAuley CE, et al. The high morbidity of blunt cerebrovascular injury in an unscreened population: more evidence of the need for mandatory screening protocols. J Am Coll Surg 2001;192(3):314–21.

18. Biffl WL, Cothren CC, Moore EE, et al. WTA critical decisions in trauma: screening for and treatment of blunt cerebrovascular injuries. J Trauma 2009;67:1150–3.

19. Bromberg WJ, Collier BC, Diebel LN, et al. Blunt cerebrovascular injury practice management guidelines: the Eastern Association for the Surgery of Trauma. J Trauma 2010;68(2):471–7.

20. Jens S, Kerstens MK, Legemate DA, et al. Diagnostic performance of computed tomography angiography in peripheral arterial injury due to trauma: a systematic review and meta-analysis. Eur J Vasc Endovasc Surg 2013;46(3):329–37.

21. Brenner DJ, Hall EJ. Computed tomography–an increasing source of radiation exposure. N Engl J Med 2007;357(22):2277–84.
22. Kim PK, Gracias VH, Maidment AD, et al. Cumulative radiation dose caused by radiologic studies in critically ill trauma patients. J Trauma 2004;57(3):510–4.
23. Available at: http://www.choosingwisely.org/clinician-lists/american-college-surgeons-whole-body-ct-scans/. Accessed June 8, 2017.
24. American College of Obstetricians and Gynecologists' Committee on Obstetric Practice. Committee opinion no. 656: guidelines for diagnostic imaging during pregnancy and lactation. Obstet Gynecol 2016;127(2):e75–80.
25. Paluska TR, Sise MJ, Sack DI, et al. Incidental CT findings in trauma patients: incidence and implications for care of the injured. J Trauma 2007;62(1):157–61.
26. Yeh DD, Imam AM, Truong SH, et al. Incidental findings in trauma patients: dedicated communication with the primary care physician ensures adequate follow-up. World J Surg 2013;37(9):2081–5.
27. Sierink JC, Saltzherr TP, Russchen MJ, et al. Incidental findings on total-body CT scans in trauma patients. Injury 2014;45(5):840–4.
28. Meer AB, Basu PA, Baker LC, et al. Exposure to ionizing radiation and estimate of secondary cancers in the era of high-speed CT scanning: projections from the Medicare population. J Am Coll Radiol 2012;9(4):245–50.

Trauma Education and Prevention

Richard Sidwell, MD[a,b,]*, Maher M. Matar, MD, MHA, FRCSC[c], Joseph V. Sakran, MD, MPH, MPA, FACS[d]

KEYWORDS

- Trauma education • ATLS • Injury prevention • Motor vehicle safety
- Motorcycle safety • Helmet safety

KEY POINTS

- Advanced Trauma Life Support (ATLS) is the worldwide standard for the initial management of the trauma patient, teaching a safe, common approach to this care.
- Rural Trauma Team Development Course teaches providers at small facilities how to apply the principles of ATLS in their own environment, emphasizing teamwork and communication.
- Surgical skills for trauma are taught in 3 courses, each targeting surgical trainees and attending surgeons to help them acquire and maintain the technical skills necessary for life-saving treatment.
- Motorcycle helmet laws have consistently resulted in reductions in serious injury and death owing to motorcycle crashes. Helmet law repeal has repeatedly shown increases in serious injury.

TRAUMA EDUCATION

Injury is now recognized as a disease that carries a significant public health burden. The care of the severely injured patient spans many domains—prehospital, emergency room, operating room, intensive care unit, inpatient hospitalization, and postdischarge rehabilitation. Although definitive care may occur at specialized trauma centers, the initial care after injury begins in the field and may continue at a hospital

[a] Trauma Services, The Iowa Clinic / Iowa Methodist Medical Center, 1200 Pleasant Street Des Moines, IA 50309, USA; [b] Department of Surgery, University of Iowa Carver College of Medicine, 375 Newton Road, Iowa City, IA 52242, USA; [c] Department of General surgery, The University of Ottawa Trauma and Acute Care Surgery, The Ottawa Hospital, 1053 Carling Avenue CPC, Suite 330 Ottawa, ON, K1Y 4E9, Canada; [d] Division of Acute Care Surgery and Adult Trauma Services, Department of Emergency General Surgery, Johns Hopkins Hospital, 1800 Orleans Street, Sheikh Zayed Tower/ Suite 6107B Baltimore, MD 21287, USA
* Corresponding author. Trauma Services, The Iowa Clinic / Iowa Methodist Medical Center, 1200 Pleasant Street Des Moines, IA 50309.
E-mail address: rsidwell@iowaclinic.com

Surg Clin N Am 97 (2017) 1185–1197
http://dx.doi.org/10.1016/j.suc.2017.06.010
0039-6109/17/© 2017 Elsevier Inc. All rights reserved.

surgical.theclinics.com

without trauma specialization. Because of the time critical nature of severe injury, it is important that providers across the various domains of care have training and experience in trauma management.

In the latter portion of the 20th century, and especially over the past 15 years, educational gaps and needs in trauma management have been recognized. This gap has spawned the development of multiple educational products, each targeting a specific aspect of trauma care. This article describes selected trauma educational courses, including the educational gap being filled, the target audience for each, and an assessment of effectiveness. Preference has been given to describe courses that are relevant for physicians, especially surgeons.

Advanced Trauma Life Support

Advanced Trauma Life Support (ATLS) has become the worldwide gold standard for trauma education. The story of the genesis of ATLS is well-known.[1] Dr James Styner, an orthopedic surgeon in Lincoln, Nebraska, was involved in a private plane crash on February 17, 1976. Although his wife was killed in the crash, he and his 4 children survived and first received treatment at a rural hospital. Believing that the initial care was not adequate, Dr Styner observed, "When I can provide better care in the field with limited resources than my children and I received at the primary facility, there is something wrong with the system and the system has to be changed." Modeled after Advanced Cardiac Life Support, ATLS was then born.

The pilot ATLS course was presented in Auburn, Nebraska, in 1978.[2] After this pilot program, the ATLS course was taken up by the American College of Surgeons to promulgate the course with the intent of teaching physicians an approach to the initial care of an injured person. After 37 years, ATLS has literally spanned the globe. Presently in the 9th edition, with the 10th edition set for release in 2017, more than 1 million students have been educated in more than 60 countries worldwide.[3]

ATLS is a 2- or 3-day course (most commonly 2 days) that teaches knowledge and techniques for evaluating and managing injured persons.[4] The program is presented through a combination of interactive lectures, surgical skill instruction (surgical airway, chest tube placement, focused assessment with sonography for trauma, optional diagnostic peritoneal lavage), case-based skill stations, and small group discussions. It provides a common language and approach, allowing providers—whether they frequently or infrequently treat trauma patients—to have a shared mental of the organization of the care. Specifically, the course aims to enable participants to[3]:

1. Demonstrate the concepts and principles of the primary and secondary assessment
2. Establish management priorities
3. Initiate primary and secondary management
4. Demonstrate the skills necessary to assess and manage critically injured patients

Efforts to examine the effectiveness of the ATLS education have looked at 2 areas: retention of knowledge (educational outcome) and improvement in patient outcomes (trauma mortality). Hundreds of papers have been published in this regard. The educational impact is undeniable. Participants have improvement in knowledge and organization of trauma management, practical skills, and identification of management priorities.[5] Retention in knowledge seems to decrease after 6 months, reaching a nadir at 2 years. The gained understanding of organizational skills and management priorities persists for up to 8 years.

There are many contributing components to mortality after injury, so it is difficult to precisely study the specific effect of ATLS education. A Cochrane Database review[6] attempted to examine randomized controlled trials, controlled trials, and before-and-after studies assessing the effectiveness of ATLS training. After reviewing 3109 citations, no studies existed that met these inclusion criteria. Thus, there is only a poor evidence base supporting an improvement in mortality outcome attributable to ATLS. There is also no evidence concluding that such education efforts are not valuable. It is this author's opinion that, given the near universal acceptance of ATLS, high-quality controlled trials related to ATLS education are unlikely to be conducted.

Despite the lack of high-level evidence from controlled trials, overwhelming expert opinion is that the impact of ATLS is undeniable, both in terms of provider knowledge and patient outcome. ATLS has influenced trauma education throughout the world. Past American College of Surgeons President, Dr L.D. Britt, has said, "There has been no program that has been as effective as ATLS in saving lives and decreasing morbidity of injuries. It is one of the greatest medical innovations—worldwide—in the last 75 years."[2] For more information, see https://www.facs.org/quality-programs/trauma/atls.

Trauma Evaluation and Management

The Trauma Evaluation and Management (TEAM) course in another educational offering from the American College of Surgeons Committee on Trauma. This course was originally designed as an abbreviated version of ATLS, essentially an expanded version of the ATLS lecture on "Initial Assessment and Management."[7] TEAM was meant to be used for medical student education, recognizing that undergraduate medical curricula was frequently lacking in exposure to trauma.

The TEAM program is modular in design and it introduces the evaluation and management of trauma for medical students. Instruction begins with a video demonstrating a trauma resuscitation where there are multiple errors in management. There is then a discussion, followed by a lecture on the principles of the initial assessment. A second video follows that demonstrates a properly conducted trauma evaluation. Finally, there are case scenarios for small group discussion.

The TEAM course seems to be effective in teaching the principles of trauma evaluation and management to senior medical students.[8,9] One report demonstrated that senior medical students had significant improvement in their knowledge of trauma resuscitation after the TEAM program.[9] Expectedly, the demonstrated knowledge improvement did not reach that required to pass the full ATLS course, emphasizing that TEAM cannot serve as a replacement for ATLS. However, because of the impracticality of providing ATLS for undergraduate medical students, TEAM seems to be an ideal method of teaching this group of learners.

The TEAM course has recently been reinvigorated as a potential resource for basic trauma education in developing areas of the world where the full ATLS program is not practical (personal communication). For more information, see https://www.facs.org/quality-programs/trauma/atls/team.

Rural Trauma Team Development Course

In the late 1990s, members of the ad hoc Rural Trauma Subcommittee of the American College of Surgeons recognized that there was a gap between the principles being taught to doctors in the ATLS course and the application of these concepts by a team working at smaller facilities, where resources, personnel, and experience may be limited. This began a grass roots effort to develop an educational product to address the needs of providers in rural communities. The result of this effort is the Rural Trauma Team Development Course (RTTDC).

The RTTDC is an interactive, 8-hour course that teaches a team approach to the initial care of a severely injured person. It emphasizes the early detection and treatment of critical injuries and avoidance of delay in transferring the patient to a higher level of care. Now in its fourth edition, the course is highly interactive with lectures, small group discussions, and team-based management scenarios. It includes instruction about teamwork and communication skills.[10] The course has been promulgated throughout the United States and Canada, with translations into French and Spanish. There has also been international promulgation in several locations, most recently to the Ukraine.

There are a couple of important differences between RTTDC and ATLS. First, the course is designed to presented at the local facility. Thus, the instructors come to the participants at their location, rather than the other way around. Second, the course is intentionally designed to be flexible to meet the unique needs of the providers at the local facility. Finally, participation in RTTDC is for everyone who may be a part of the initial care of the injured person at the rural facility. A typical class includes medical providers (doctors, nurse practitioners, and physician assistants), nurses, emergency medical service personnel, radiology technicians, and laboratory workers. Administrators and clerical personnel also participate.

There is emerging evidence of the effectiveness of RTTDC.[11–14] A consistent finding is that facilities where the RTTDC course has been presented have shorter times until the decision to transfer is made[11,13] and shorter total duration of stay before transfer.[12] A mortality benefit has not yet been demonstrated. Participant satisfaction has been found to be high and improvement in knowledge has been shown.[14]

An unanticipated, although possibly most important, benefit of RTTDC has been the opportunity for positive relationship building that occurs when experienced trauma providers and educators leave the trauma center to teach the course in the rural community. This opens lines of communication and fosters good relationships between facilities. As such, RTTDC is a good resource to be used by trauma centers for education and outreach. For more information, see https://www.facs.org/quality-programs/trauma/education/rttdc.

Prehospital Trauma Life Support

Just as ATLS has become the gold standard for initial physician trauma education, the Prehospital Trauma Life Support (PHTLS) course is so for prehospital providers. Because this course is intended for nonphysicians, only a limited overview is provided.

The PHTLS originated in parallel with ATLS. Because ATLS was developed as a course for physicians, PHTLS arose to meet the trauma educational needs of prehospital providers.[15] The first pilot courses were held in 1982 and 1983; the course is now in its eighth edition. It is developed and administered by the National Association of Emergency Medical Technicians with medical oversight from the American College of Surgeons Committee on Trauma.[16] New editions of the PHTLS follow each updated edition of the ATLS to maintain consistency in the educational offerings.[17] PHTLS has worldwide promulgation, now offered in more than 50 countries. Like ATLS, conventional opinion is that the educational impact is meaningful. However, also like ATLS, scientific support for improved patient outcomes is limited.[18] For more information, see http://www.naemt.org/education/PHTLS/phtls.aspx.

Advanced Trauma Operative Management

One consequence of the declining incidence of penetrating trauma in the United States and the increased nonoperative management of blunt injuries is that surgical resident trainees and practicing surgeons have fewer operative trauma cases. The

Definitive Surgical Trauma Care course is a 2-day course that has been implemented in a number of countries but has not gained a foothold in the United States. The Advanced Trauma Operative Management (ATOM) course evolved from the Definitive Surgical Trauma Care course[19] and focuses on the operative management of penetrating injury. The ATOM course is intended for senior surgical residents, trauma fellows, and fully trained surgeons (including military surgeons and those who may have infrequent exposure to patients with penetrating injury).

ATOM was established in 1998 and came under the direction of the American College of Surgeons in 2008.[20] It is an 8-hour course that begins with 6 interactive didactic sessions covering the principles of trauma laparotomy and management of abdominal and thoracic injuries.[19] The remainder of the day is spent in the surgical laboratory using a live, anesthetized 50-kg porcine model, which simulates a human operative experience. A single instructor works with a single student to create and manage multiple standardized scenarios that teach operative repair of penetrating injury to the stomach, duodenum, small intestine, kidney, ureter, bladder, pancreas, spleen, liver, inferior vena cava, and heart.

Participants in the ATOM course demonstrate improvement in knowledge and surgical confidence, both at the completion of the course[19] and at 6-month follow-up.[21] The course is offered at more than 2 dozen locations in the United States and has had international promulgation including Canada, Africa, the Middle East, and Japan.

One limitation of the traditional ATOM course is the use of 1 animal for each student, which also means that 1 instructor is required for each student. If 1 instructor could teach 2 students using 1 animal, this would increase the number of students each course could accommodate, reduce the cost per participant, and maintain sensitivity regarding efficient use of the live animal model. The 2-student to 1-instructor model has been evaluated and found to be feasible.[22] The educational experience for students seems to be maintained, and perhaps even strengthened because of the opportunity for each student to both perform and assist with each type of repair. However, this arrangement creates more difficulties with animal physiology. Presently, the 2-student ATOM teaching model is limited to selected locations. For more information, see https://www.facs.org/quality-programs/trauma/education/atom.

Advanced Surgical Skills for Exposure in Trauma

As noted, exposure to operative trauma for both surgical trainees and practicing surgeons has become more limited. This includes operations for major vascular repair. In 2005, the American College of Surgeons Committee on Trauma established a Surgical Skills Committee to develop a standardized course that could be used to train surgeons in the operative exposure of vital structures. This resulted in the Advanced Surgical Skills for Exposure in Trauma (ASSET) course.[23]

ASSET is a cadaver-based course that is completed in 1 day. Unlike most other courses, there is not a classroom component to the course. Instead, the course is conducted in the anatomy laboratory with unpreserved (fresh) human cadavers. Scenarios are presented and instructors provide a focused bedside instruction, including high-quality narrated videos, on the key aspects of the requisite operative exposure. Four students then work with 1 instructor to perform the surgical dissection on the cadaver. Using the case scenarios, students learn exposure of structures in the extremities (axillary artery, brachial artery, femoral artery, popliteal artery, and both forearm and lower leg fasciotomy), neck (carotid artery and esophagus), thorax (pulmonary hilum, subclavian artery, thoracic aorta, and heart), and abdomen and pelvis (iliac artery, aorta, left and right visceral rotation, liver, inferior vena cava, and the technique of preperitoneal pelvic packing).[23]

The target audience for the ASSET course is senior surgical residents, trauma fellows, and practicing surgeons, and the course has been shown to be valuable. Overwhelmingly, participants report gaining knowledge and learning new techniques and feel better prepared to care for injured patients.[23,24] Additionally, they nearly universally would recommend the course to colleagues.

The ASSET course is offered by more than 40 centers in the United States and Canada and has some limited additional international promulgation. One persisting challenge is the availability and cost of unpreserved (fresh) cadavers. For more information, see https://www.facs.org/quality-programs/trauma/education/asset.

Basic Endovascular Skills for Trauma

A relative newcomer to the educational courses in surgical skills for trauma, the Basic Endovascular Skills for Trauma (BEST) course recognizes that endovascular procedures are increasingly used in care of the trauma patient. Specifically, the technique of resuscitative endovascular balloon occlusion of the aorta is a life-saving maneuver than can be used to temporize noncompressible hemorrhage. The BEST course is a 4-hour course that, using a combination of lectures, simulators, and fresh cadavers, teaches participants the resuscitative endovascular balloon occlusion of the aorta procedure.[25,26]

The BEST course is new and evidence of effectiveness is just starting to emerge. One report demonstrated that participants were able to acquire the endovascular skill and that the mean time to accomplish the procedure improved with the repetitions during the course.[26] Additionally, all participants found the course to be beneficial and 85% felt ready to perform the procedure on their next call.

The BEST course is presently offered at 3 locations (the University of Maryland's RA Cowley Shock Trauma Center, the Texas Trauma Institute/University of Texas at Houston, and the University of California at Davis) and registration is open only for trauma surgeons.[25] For more information, see https://www.facs.org/quality-programs/trauma/education/best.

Simulated Trauma and Resuscitation Team Training

The RTTDC teaches that trauma management is not an individual endeavor; rather, teamwork is required. This is something that is not taught in ATLS. A newer course is the Simulated Trauma and Resuscitation Team Training (STARTT). This course recognizes that most critical errors are not a result of a knowledge deficit or technical inability; instead, they result from nontechnical skills, such as situational awareness, team leadership, and communication. Developed in Canada, STARTT brings the principles taught in Crisis Resource Management into the realm of trauma resuscitations.[27]

STARTT is an 8-hour course focused on reducing and mitigating human error in trauma resuscitations. It includes lectures that teach the principles of Crisis Resource Management.[28] The participants (physicians, nurses, and respiratory therapists) are then divided into teams who rotate through 4 standardized, high-fidelity trauma simulations. Each simulation experience lasts for 60 minutes, with 15 minutes of simulation and 45 minutes of debriefing. The course emphasizes communication and leadership skills, effective use of resources, situational awareness and problem solving, and how to enhance completion of tasks.[29,30]

The STARTT course has yet to gain a foothold of promulgation in the United States. It offers a promise, however, of filling a critical educational gap for American surgeons that is not met by the more widespread trauma educational offerings. Participant satisfaction with the course is high and it improves participant attitudes toward Crisis Resource Management training,[27] although improved patient outcomes have not yet been evaluated. The course has also demonstrated flexibility to include prehospital providers and simulation of a mass casualty event.[29] For more information, see http://www.traumacanada.org/page-1811219.

Summary

Over the past 4 decades, and especially in the last 15 years, multiple high-quality trauma educational products have been developed. These courses provide a standardized approach to the instruction of how to care for the injured person through development of knowledge, technical skills, and teamwork. Each has been developed to address an educational gap and most began as a grass roots effort after recognition of the need. The courses have been met with positive perception from participants and are widely seen as promoting improvements in patient outcomes. Although they are all found to be educationally effective, demonstrating significant improvements in patient outcome has been elusive. There are still aspects of care of the injured patient where structured and standardized education has not been developed; hospital care (after the initial assessment), rehabilitation from injury, and trauma system development are among these. It is the opinion of this author that, as injury is increasingly recognized as a public health burden, there will continue to be development of educational products to assist teaching the various components of the comprehensive care of trauma patients. For more information regarding all of these educational offerings, see **Table 1**.

INJURY PREVENTION
Public Health

The junior surgical resident on the trauma service is presenting patients at morning report: Mr A Doe, a 25-year-old man status post motor vehicle accident with a

Table 1 Trauma education websites	
Course	**For More Information**
Advance Trauma Life Support (ATLS)	https://www.facs.org/quality-programs/trauma/atls
Trauma Evaluation and Management (TEAM)	https://www.facs.org/quality-programs/trauma/atls/team
Rural Trauma Team Development Course (RTTDC)	https://www.facs.org/quality-programs/trauma/education/rttdc
Prehospital Trauma Life Support (PHTLS)	http://www.naemt.org/education/PHTLS/phtls.aspx
Advanced Trauma Operative Management (ATOM)	https://www.facs.org/quality-programs/trauma/education/atom
Advanced Surgical Skills for Exposure in Trauma (ASSET)	https://www.facs.org/quality-programs/trauma/education/asset
Basic Endovascular Skills for Trauma (BEST)	https://www.facs.org/quality-programs/trauma/education/best
Simulated Trauma and Resuscitation Team Training (STARTT)	http://www.traumacanada.org/page-1811219

traumatic brain injury, Mrs B Doe, a 65-year-old woman had an "accident" at home falling down the stairs with multiple rib fractures, and Mr. C Doe, a 38-year-old man had an accident at work having his arm traumatically amputated by an auger.

An accident is "an unfortunate incident that happens unexpectedly and unintentionally, typically resulting in damage or injury," or "An event that happens by chance or that is, without apparent or deliberate cause." These are some of the definition that Google provides for the definition of accident. Synonyms include the words mishap, mischance, and misfortune. This implies that the event was unavoidable, leading us to believe that nothing can be done to prevent this outcome. When viewed as an accident, the motor vehicle collision, the fall, and the event at work simply become reportable statistics. If we examine these events from a public health perspective, we then change the statistical into a preventable outcome. The Centers for Disease Control and Prevention define public health as "the science of protecting and improving the health of families and communities through promotion of healthy lifestyles, research for disease and injury prevention and detection and control of infectious diseases."[31] Using the public health perspective opens an entirely new opportunity dimension to a given event, with opportunity for research, implementation of policies, and room for public awareness and education.

Trauma

Trauma continues to be the leading cause of death in individuals 1 to 46 years of age, and is the third leading cause of death overall across all age groups, claiming the lives of up to 200,000 individuals annually. In the United States, it accounts for 41 million emergency department visits annually, and results in 2.3 million hospital admission. It leads to 30% of the total life-years lost annually, ahead of both cancer and heart disease, which account for 16% and 12%, respectively. Given the uniqueness of this disease process in that all age groups are implicated, the life-years lost to trauma are equal to those lost owing to cancer, heart disease, and human immunodeficiency virus infection combined. It also costs up to $671 billion annually in health care costs and losses to productivity owing to disability.[32] Worldwide, 973 million people were injured by trauma requiring some health care, and 4.8 million of those succumb to their injuries, making this a global issue.

It is not until we delve deeper into these statistics that we truly understand what these numbers mean. On the global front, injury leads to 247.6 million disability-adjusted life-years annually, with 210.8 million and 36.8 million of those coming from years loss to life and years of live with disability, respectively.[33] Deeper dissection into the data reveals that the largest contributors to this phenomenon are unintentional injuries such as falls, drownings, and poisonings; transport-related injuries; and intentional injuries such as self-harm and interpersonal violence.[33] This information empowers public health experts by highlighting potential areas for further research and intervention.

Injury Prevention Initiatives

Some of the earliest work in injury prevention comes from Dr William Haddon in the 1970s. He proposed a matrix to assess events that led to injury by dividing them into separate factors that may have contributed to the incident including human factors, vehicle and equipment factors, and environmental factors. He further examines the crash in 3 phases: the precrash, the crash, and the postcrash phases, that have led to the incident at hand[34] (**Table 2**). By examining each event in this manner, we can identify modifiable factors at different phases of the unwanted event, be it a crash, fall, abuse, or fire. The Haddon Matrix is actively used by public health researchers to help identify points of potential intervention.

Table 2
Basic matrix for classification of road loss factors in each of the 3 phases of interactions that lead to the end result in energy-damaged people and property

Phases	Factors		
	Human	Vehicle and Equipment	Environment
Precrash			
Crash			
Postcrash			
Results→			

Adapted from Haddon W Jr. A logical framework for categorizing highway safety phenomena and activity. J Trauma 1972;12:206; with permission.

Injury prevention strategies can be either passive or active. A passive intervention is one that does not require the user to make conscious modifications to their behavior to protect them from the event, and are most effective. Interventions such as this include safety caps on medication bottles, leading to the reduction in poisoning in children. An active intervention is labeling on the medication bottle with warning that inform the user of safeguarding the medication from children. These interventions are seen as less effective.[35]

Motor Vehicle and Traffic Safety

Although the number of people driving motorized vehicles has dramatically increased since the mid 1920s leading to the total number of miles traveled annually to be 10 times higher, the death rate has declined from 18 per 100 million vehicle miles traveled in 1925, to 1.7 per 100 million vehicle miles traveled in annually in the United States in 1997.[36] The road to these dramatic changes was paved years ago.

In 1966, the dramatic increase in the number of fatalities owing to motor vehicle crashes, accounting for up to 41% of all unintentional injuries in the United States, caught the attention of congress. Public Works Chairman, George Fallon, with strong support from then-President Lyndon B. Johnson, shepherded the Highway Safety Act in an attempt to empower and force each state to implement a highway safety program. The legislation addressed driver education, traffic control, accident prevention, and emergency services. Given the importance of the matter, the legislation had strong bipartisan support in the House of Representatives, which led to its passing into law on September 9, 1966.[37] This later gave birth to the National Highway Safety Bureau, which is today known as the National Highway Traffic Safety Administration. Under the leadership of Dr Haddon, the National Highway Safety Bureau led the taskforce that would pioneer and revolutionize automotive safety, as a whole.

Automobiles

Using the Haddon matrix, the team studied crashes identifying areas to be addressed, with the goal of minimizing injury and death. This included changes to vehicles' safety features, such as the implementation of head rests and shatter-resistant windshields. Increased lighting on roadways and reflectors on the roads, and breakaway signs and utility poles, along with the implementation of strict seatbelt laws and speed limits are the injury prevention initiatives that have led to thousands of lives being saved.[36]

Fifty years later, although the numbers are better, motor vehicle crashes remain the number 1 cause of death for those aged 5 to 24 and the number 2 cause of death for toddlers and adults 25 years and older. The most recent insult to injury is the increased use of electronic devices while driving, referred to as distracted driving. Since the advent of text messaging in 1992, and later the evolution and popularization of so-called smartphones, the use of cell phones while driving has become problematic.[38] It is reported that 22% of all motor vehicle crashes can be directly attributed to driving while manipulating a mobile device. Simulation studies have shown that manipulating a cell phone while driving is equated to driving under the influence of alcohol, leading to delayed braking time, a 140% increase in missed lane changes, and a 6-fold increase in crashes. Currently, 54% of adults reported talking on the phone while driving, and 50% admitted to texting while driving.[38] Based on a review by members of the Injury Control Prevention Committee of the Eastern Association for the Surgery of Trauma, they recommended that all drivers should not text, and that all young drivers should not use cell phones or any messaging system while driving.[38] At this time in the United States, laws against cell phone use while driving are not standardized across all states, an opportunity for intervention.

Motorcycles

Motorcycles are referred to as "a hazardous means of transportation, with death rates per 100 million person-miles of travel reaching more than 35 times that of cars."[35] In the United States, motorcycles account for less than 1% of the vehicle miles traveled, yet claim the lives of up to 14% of those killed on roads.[39] Injuries to the head after motorcycle collision is one of the main causes of morbidity and mortality in this patient population.[40] A Cochrane review examining the literature surround the effectiveness of helmets in protecting patients involved in motorcycle collisions demonstrated that wearing a helmet reduced head injuries by 69% and death by 42%.[40] Implementing mandatory helmet laws has consistently led to an increase in helmet use, and has led to decrease in the incidence of head injuries by 34% and 22% in California and Nebraska, respectively. The risk of death was also reduced by 12% and 26%, respectively.[35] A study that reviewed the effects of repealing helmet laws in Arkansas showed that patients not wearing helmets had significantly higher Abbreviated Injury Scale head injury scores, longer durations of stay in the intensive care unit and hospital in general, and posed an increased economic burden on the system owing to nonreimbursement.[41] This shows the positive impact that such injury prevention programs can have on a population, and the negative impact of repealing such measures as well.

Bicycles

Bicycling is an excellent source of exercise, and a great mode of transportation; it also leads to 1.2 million emergency department visits—500,000 injuries and 900 fatalities—with a total productivity loss of approximately $10 billion annually.[42] Children 5 to 14 years of age are the most affected by his mechanism of injury. One of the main issues with bike safety involves the use of helmets, or the lack thereof. Helmet use has proven to be effective in minimizing serious injuries as a consequence of a crash while on a bicycle. One study demonstrated that the use of helmets decreased the risk of head injury and traumatic brain injury by 85% and 88%, respectively.[43] Legislative action and educational interventions have led to increased helmet use in this population by up to more than 50%, leading to a reduction in head injury in users.[44]

Other Interventions

Injury prevention is not only focused on traffic-related events. It is a needs-based process. Using data from institutes such as the Centers for Disease Control and Prevention, one can identify the needs of a given community and address the issues related to that specific community as they arise. A systematic literature review and metaanalysis published in the *Journal of Adolescent Health* demonstrated that injury prevention initiatives successfully decreased sports-related incidence of injuries in adolescents.[45] The use of training plus education and the use of safety equipment was the culprit in reducing the number of unwanted incidences.[45]

Community-based injury prevention programs are not all the same. In a review of the effectiveness of 16 injury prevention programs, the author found programs that had statistically significant improvements in outcomes, and those that had no impact. One of the factors cited that helped to improve the successful implementation of a program was community cohesion, which could be effected by cultural homogeneity. The lack of the latter can lead to a loss of cohesion, and failure of the program implementation. Before the implementation of a program, knowledge of the community's cultural needs and diversity will help to address this factor. Another cited factor was the structure of the program, and how long it was implemented. Time is needed within a community to allow for successful adoption of new behaviors, and thus needs to be factored into the program. Last, certain projects may benefit more from passive interventions versus active interventions, depending on the intervention at hand.[46]

Summary

This is an ever-evolving field of health care that must adapt to the ongoing changes in the environment. In the 1970s, cell phone use in automobiles was not a contributor to unintentional collisions; rather, the lack of safe roadways and cars without proper safety mechanisms in place to protect its occupants was paramount. With the implementation of newer technologies in vehicles, some cars are now capable of identifying pedestrians in its path, alerting the driver of the potential collision, or applying the brakes automatically. There has also been the development of self-deploying helmets that inflate before impact, protecting the bicycle rider from serious head injuries. The number of tools at our disposal to help minimize morbidity and mortality are increasing. This is only possible through ongoing research and development, and continuously monitoring trends and statistics that we can truly have a positive impact on the overall well-being of our population. This is possible through the eyes of public health.

REFERENCES

1. Styner JK. The birth of ATLS. Surgeon 2006;4:163–5.
2. Hoyt DB. Looking forward. Bull Am Coll Surg 2013;98(4):7–8.
3. Advanced Trauma Life Support, student course. 9th edition. American College of Surgeons; 2012.
4. American College of Surgeons. Advanced Trauma Life Support. Available at: https://www.facs.org/quality-programs/trauma/atls/about. Accessed April 10, 2017.
5. Abu-Zidan FM. Advanced Trauma Life Support training: how useful is it? World J Crit Care Med 2016;5(1):12–6.
6. Jayarman S, Sethi D, Chinnock P, et al. Advanced Trauma Life Support training for hospital staff (review). Cochrane Database Syst Rev 2014;(8):CD004173.
7. American College of Surgeons. Trauma evaluation and management. Available at: https://www.facs.org/quality-programs/trauma/atls/team. Accessed April 10, 2017.
8. Ali J, Danne P, McColl G. Assessment of the Trauma Evaluation and Management (TEAM) Module in Australia. Injury 2004;35:753–8.

9. Ali J, Adam R, Williams JI, et al. Teaching effectiveness of the Trauma Evaluation and Management module for senior medical students. J Trauma 2002;52:847–51.

10. Rural Trauma Team Development Course. 4th edition. Chicago: American College of Surgeons.; 2016.

11. Kappel DA, Rossi DC, Polack EP, et al. Does the Rural Trauma Team Development Course shorten the interval from trauma patient arrival to decision to transfer? J Trauma 2011;70:315–9.

12. Dennis BM, Vella MA, Gunter OL, et al. Rural Trauma Team Development Course decreases time to transfer for trauma patients. J Trauma 2016;81:632–7.

13. Malekpour M, Neuhaus N, Martin D, et al. Changes in rural trauma prehospital times following the Rural Trauma Team Development Course training. Am J Surg 2017;213(2):399–404.

14. Zhu TH, Hollister L, Scheumann C, et al. Effectiveness of the Rural Trauma Team Development Course for educating nurses and other health care providers at rural hospitals. J Trauma Nurs 2016;23(1):13–22.

15. McSwain N. Judgment based on knowledge: a history of Prehospital Trauma Life Support, 1970-2013. J Trauma 2013;75:1–7.

16. National Association of Emergency Medical Technicians. What is PHTLS. Available at: http://www.naemt.org/education/PHTLS/whatisPHTLS.aspx. Accessed April 10, 2017.

17. Chapleau W. Prehospital Trauma Life Support: a history of 25 Years of PHTLS on the release of its 6th edition. EMS News Network 2006;42–3.

18. Blomberg H, Svennblad B, Michaelsson K, et al. Prehospital Trauma Life Support training of ambulance caregivers and the outcomes of traffic-injury victims in Sweden. J Am Coll Surg 2013;217(6):1010–9.

19. Jacobs L, Burns KJ, Kaban JM, et al. Development and evaluation of the Advanced Trauma Operative Management course. J Trauma 2003;55(3):471–9.

20. American College of Surgeons. Advanced Trauma Operative Management. Available at: https://www.facs.org/quality-programs/trauma/education/atom. Accessed April 10, 2017.

21. Jacobs LM, Burns KJ, Luk SS. Followup survey of participants attending the Advanced Trauma Operative Management (ATOM) course. J Trauma 2005; 58(6):1140–3.

22. Ali J. The Advanced Trauma Operative Management course—a two student to one faculty model. J Surg Res 2013;184:551–5.

23. Bowyer MW, Kuhls DA, Haskin D, et al. Advanced Surgical Skills for Exposure in Trauma (ASSET): the first 25 courses. J Surg Res 2013;183:553–8.

24. Kuhls DA, Risucci DA, Bowyer MW, et al. Advances surgical skills for exposure in trauma: a new surgical skills cadaver course for surgery residents and fellows. J Trauma 2013;74(2):664–70.

25. American College of Surgeons. Basic Endovascular Skills for Trauma. Available at: https://www.facs.org/quality-programs/trauma/education/best. Accessed April 10, 2017.

26. Brenner M, Hoehn M, Pasley J, et al. Basic Endovascular Skills for Trauma course: bridging the gap between endovascular techniques and the acute care surgeon. J Trauma 2014;77(2):286–91.

27. Ziesmann MT, Widder S, Park J, et al. S.T.A.R.T.T.: development of a national, multidisciplinary trauma crisis resource management curriculum—results from the pilot course. J Trauma 2013;75(5):753–8.

28. Gillman LM, Brindley P, Paton-Gay JD, et al. Simulated Trauma and Resuscitation Team Training course - evolution of a multidisciplinary trauma crisis resource management simulation course. Am J Surg 2016;212:188–93.

29. Gillman LM, Martin D, Engels PT, et al. S.T.A.R.T.T. plus: addition of prehospital personnel to a national multidisciplinary crisis resource management trauma team training course. Can J Surg 2016;59(1):9–11.

30. Trauma Association of Canada. S.T.A.R.T.T. (Simulated Trauma and Resuscitation Team Training). Available at: http://www.traumacanada.org/page-1811219. Accessed April 10, 2017.

31. What is Public Health? Centers for Disease Control and Prevention Foundation. Available at: http://www.cdcfoundation.org/print/content/what-public-health. Accessed January 22, 2017.

32. Trauma Statistics. National Trauma Institute. Available at: http://www. nationaltraumainstitute.org/home/trauma_statistics.html. Accessed January 15, 2017.

33. Haagsma JA, Graetz N, Bolliger I, et al. The global burden of injury: incidence, mortality, disability-adjusted life years and time trends from the Global Burden of Disease study 2013. Inj Prev 2016;22(1):3–18.

34. Haddon W Jr. A logical framework for categorizing highway safety phenomena and activity. J Trauma 1972;12:193–207.

35. Rivara F, Grossman D, Cummings P. Injury prevention. N Engl J Med 1997;337: 543–8.

36. Achievements in Public Health, 1900-1999 Motor-Vehicle Safety: A 20th Century Public Health Achievement. 1999. Available at: https://www.cdc.gov/mmwr/ preview/mmwrhtml/mm4818a1.htm.

37. The Highway Safety Act of 1966. History, Art & Archives: United States House of Representatives. Available at: http://history.house.gov/Historical-Highlights/1951-2000/The-Highway-Safety-Act-of-1966/. Accessed January 23, 2017.

38. Llerena LE, Aronow KV, Macleod J, et al. An evidence-based review. J Trauma Acute Care Surg 2015;78(1):147–52.

39. Naumann R, Shults R. Helmet use among motorcyclists who died in crashes and economic cost savings associated with state motorcycle helmet laws — United States, 2008–2010. 2012. Available at: https://www.cdc.gov/mmwr/preview/ mmwrhtml/mm6123a1.htm. Accessed January 15, 2017.

40. Liu BC, Ivers R, Norton R, et al. Helmets for preventing injury in motorcycle riders. Cochrane Database Syst Rev 2008;(1):CD004333.

41. Bledsoe GH, Schexnayder SM, Carey MJ, et al. The negative impact of the repeal of the Arkansas motorcycle helmet law. J Trauma 2002;53(6):1077–8.

42. Centers for Disease Control and Prevention. Bicycle safety. 2016. Available at: https://www.cdc.gov/motorvehiclesafety/bicycle/. Accessed January 15, 2017.

43. Thompson R, Rivara F, Thompson D. A case-control study of the effectiveness of bicycle safety helmets. N Engl J Med 1989;320:1361–7.

44. Rivara FP, Thompson D, Thompson R. The Seattle children's bicycle helmet campaign: changes in helmet use and head injury admissions. Pediatrics 1994;93:567–9.

45. Salam RA, Arshad A, Das JK, et al. Interventions to prevent unintentional injuries among adolescents: a systematic review and meta-analysis. J Adolesc Health 2016;59(4 Suppl):S76–87.

46. Nilsen P. What makes community based injury prevention work? In search of evidence of effectiveness. Inj Prev 2004;10(5):268–74.

UNITED STATES POSTAL SERVICE® Statement of Ownership, Management, and Circulation
(All Periodicals Publications Except Requester Publications)

1. Publication Title	2. Publication Number	3. Filing Date
SURGICAL CLINICS OF NORTH AMERICA	529 – 800	9/18/2017

4. Issue Frequency	5. Number of Issues Published Annually	6. Annual Subscription Price
FEB, APR, JUN, AUG, OCT, DEC	6	$386.00

7. Complete Mailing Address of Known Office of Publication *(Not printer) (Street, city, county, state, and ZIP+4®)*

ELSEVIER INC.
230 Park Avenue, Suite 800
New York, NY 10169

Contact Person
STEPHEN R. BUSHING
Telephone *(Include area code)*
215-239-3688

8. Complete Mailing Address of Headquarters or General Business Office of Publisher *(Not printer)*

ELSEVIER INC.
230 Park Avenue, Suite 800
New York, NY 10169

9. Full Names and Complete Mailing Addresses of Publisher, Editor, and Managing Editor *(Do not leave blank)*

Publisher *(Name and complete mailing address)*

ADRIANNE BRIGIDO, ELSEVIER INC.
1600 JOHN F KENNEDY BLVD. SUITE 1800
PHILADELPHIA, PA 19103-2899

Editor *(Name and complete mailing address)*

JOHN VASSALLO, ELSEVIER INC.
1600 JOHN F KENNEDY BLVD. SUITE 1800
PHILADELPHIA, PA 19103-2899

Managing Editor *(Name and complete mailing address)*

PATRICK MANLEY, ELSEVIER INC.
1600 JOHN F KENNEDY BLVD. SUITE 1800
PHILADELPHIA, PA 19103-2899

10. Owner *(Do not leave blank. If the publication is owned by a corporation, give the name and address of the corporation immediately followed by the names and addresses of all stockholders owning or holding 1 percent or more of the total amount of stock. If not owned by a corporation, give the names and addresses of the individual owners. If owned by a partnership or other unincorporated firm, give its name and address as well as those of each individual owner. If the publication is published by a nonprofit organization, give its name and address.)*

Full Name	Complete Mailing Address
WHOLLY OWNED SUBSIDIARY OF REED/ELSEVIER, US HOLDINGS	1600 JOHN F KENNEDY BLVD. SUITE 1800 PHILADELPHIA, PA 19103-2899

11. Known Bondholders, Mortgagees, and Other Security Holders Owning or Holding 1 Percent or More of Total Amount of Bonds, Mortgages, or Other Securities. If none, check box ► ☐ None

Full Name	Complete Mailing Address
N/A	

12. Tax Status *(For completion by nonprofit organizations authorized to mail at nonprofit rates) (Check one)*
The purpose, function, and nonprofit status of this organization and the exempt status for federal income tax purposes:
☒ Has Not Changed During Preceding 12 Months
☐ Has Changed During Preceding 12 Months *(Publisher must submit explanation of change with this statement)*

13. Publication Title	14. Issue Date for Circulation Data Below
SURGICAL CLINICS OF NORTH AMERICA	JUNE 2017

15. Extent and Nature of Circulation			Average No. Copies Each Issue During Preceding 12 Months	No. Copies of Single Issue Published Nearest to Filing Date
a. Total Number of Copies *(Net press run)*			928	610
b. Paid Circulation *(By Mail and Outside the Mail)*	(1)	Mailed Outside-County Paid Subscriptions Stated on PS Form 3541 *(Include paid distribution above nominal rate, advertiser's proof copies, and exchange copies)*	333	289
	(2)	Mailed In-County Paid Subscriptions Stated on PS Form 3541 *(Include paid distribution above nominal rate, advertiser's proof copies, and exchange copies)*	0	0
	(3)	Paid Distribution Outside the Mails Including Sales Through Dealers and Carriers, Street Vendors, Counter Sales, and Other Paid Distribution Outside USPS®	338	276
	(4)	Paid Distribution by Other Classes of Mail Through the USPS *(e.g., First-Class Mail®)*	0	0
c. Total Paid Distribution *(Sum of 15b (1), (2), (3), and (4))* ►			671	565
d. Free or Nominal Rate Distribution *(By Mail and Outside the Mail)*	(1)	Free or Nominal Rate Outside-County Copies included on PS Form 3541	58	45
	(2)	Free or Nominal Rate In-County Copies Included on PS Form 3541	0	0
	(3)	Free or Nominal Rate Copies Mailed at Other Classes Through the USPS *(e.g., First-Class Mail)*	0	0
	(4)	Free or Nominal Rate Distribution Outside the Mail *(Carriers or other means)*	0	0
e. Total Free or Nominal Rate Distribution *(Sum of 15d (1), (2), (3) and (4))* ►			58	45
f. Total Distribution *(Sum of 15c and 15e)* ►			729	610
g. Copies not Distributed *(See Instructions to Publishers #4 (page 63))* ►			199	0
h. Total *(Sum of 15f and g)* ►			928	610
i. Percent Paid *(15c divided by 15f times 100)* ►			92.04%	92.62%

* If you are claiming electronic copies, go to line 16 on page 3. If you are not claiming electronic copies, skip to line 17 on page 3.

16. Electronic Copy Circulation	Average No. Copies Each Issue During Preceding 12 Months	No. Copies of Single Issue Published Nearest to Filing Date
a. Paid Electronic Copies ►	0	0
b. Total Paid Print Copies (Line 15c) + Paid Electronic Copies (Line 16a) ►	671	565
c. Total Print Distribution (Line 15f) + Paid Electronic Copies (Line 16a) ►	729	610
d. Percent Paid (Both Print & Electronic Copies) (16b divided by 16c × 100) ►	92.04%	92.62%

☒ I certify that 50% of all my distributed copies (electronic and print) are paid above a nominal price.

17. Publication of Statement of Ownership

☒ If the publication is a general publication, publication of this statement is required. Will be printed
in the __OCTOBER 2017__ issue of this publication.   ☐ Publication not required.

18. Signature and Title of Editor, Publisher, Business Manager, or Owner	Date
Stephen R. Bushing	9/18/2017

STEPHEN R. BUSHING - INVENTORY DISTRIBUTION CONTROL MANAGER

I certify that all information furnished on this form is true and complete. I understand that anyone who furnishes false or misleading information on this form or who omits material or information requested on the form may be subject to criminal sanctions (including fines and imprisonment) and/or civil sanctions (including civil penalties).

PS Form **3526**, July 2014 *(Page 3 of 4)*   PRIVACY NOTICE: See our privacy policy on www.usps.com.

PS Form **3526**, July 2014 *(Page 1 of 4 (see instructions page 4))*   PSN: 7530-01-000-9931   PRIVACY NOTICE: See our privacy policy on www.usps.com.

Printed and bound by CPI Group (UK) Ltd, Croydon, CR0 4YY

03/10/2024

01040397-0009